Nursing Management of Women's Health

Debra Holloway
Editor

Nursing Management of Women's Health

A Guide for Nurse Specialists and Practitioners

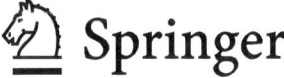 Springer

Editor
Debra Holloway
Guy's Hospital
Guy's and St Thomas NHS Foundation Trust
London
UK

ISBN 978-3-030-16114-9   ISBN 978-3-030-16115-6   (eBook)
https://doi.org/10.1007/978-3-030-16115-6

This Springer imprint is published by the registered company Springer Nature Switzerland AG
The registered company address is: Gewerbestrasse 11, 6330 Cham, Switzerland

Preface

The role of the specialist nurse within gynaecology has developed and grown over time; there are no training courses that cover all aspects of this diverse role.

This book written by specialist nurses for specialist nurses or those aspiring to be specialist nurses covers the fundamentals needed by nurses within each of the unique and specialist parts of women's health.

The nurses who have written the chapters are working as clinical nurse specialists, advanced nurse practitioners or nurse consultants within gynaecology and women's health and have a wealth of experience between them.

Each chapter covers history taking, diagnostics, management and treatment and referral if needed.

The chapters are laid out so that they can be used by specialist and those with an interest in women's health and indeed sib specialist nurses who may come across women from another subsection of women's health who may need to update on current practices. They also point out references and resources that are useful and tips on courses that are needed for nursing staff such as scanning or hysteroscopy.

London, UK   Debra Holloway

Contents

The Role of the Specialist Nurse Within Gynaecology

Debra Holloway

As in many specialities, the role of the specialist nurse within gynaecology and women's health has developed in an ad hoc way. Like all fields of nursing, there are many different roles, such as clinical nurse specialist (CNS), nurse practitioner (NP), advanced nurse practitioner (ANP) and nurse consultant (NC), with little guidance on or regulation of the educational background and qualifications that these nurses require.

Recent work by the Royal College of Nursing (RCN) [1] has looked at credentialing these roles but there is still no part of the Nursing and Midwifery Council register for advanced practice and it does not look like this is going to be forthcoming in the next few years. The RCN credentialing system assesses the background and the legitimacy of the nurse to practice at an advanced level, looking at experience, qualifications and competence. Nurses need to look at advanced practice, and ask is this a level of practice or a task [2]. With changes to the pre-registration criteria, non-medical prescribing may change and become one of the skills of a qualified nurse in normal practice. The problems with clarity related not only to nurses, but also to other health care professionals and patients who may be unsure of the scope of practice and the limits or remits of the role. In addition, the roles may be grouped by bands of pay and some may have a specific skill attached to the title, such as colposcopist or hysteroscopist. If the practitioner is working to a job description devised by the employer, then they are within their remit. Thus, for example, non-medical prescribing should be within the person specification and role description. It should then be expected that there would be an organisational policy regarding non-medical prescribers that would lay out the ongoing CDP requirements needed to maintain skills and competencies within that role.

D. Holloway (✉)
Guys and St Thomas NHS Foundation Trust, London, UK
e-mail: Debra.Holloway@gstt.nhs.uk

© Springer Nature Switzerland AG 2019
D. Holloway (ed.), *Nursing Management of Women's Health*,
https://doi.org/10.1007/978-3-030-16115-6_1

Other countries, such as USA, Canada and Australia, have defined and grouped roles and these have been written into law. [3]

Many will ask, is there any difference in the roles and is there any difference from a medic doing the same job?

Advanced nursing practice stems from a nurse's development of themselves and will always be underpinned by nursing education and thinking, so a nurse may approach a hysteroscopy in a different way from a medical doctor. Advanced nursing practice is about having the right professional in the right place at the right time to ensure that the patient has the correct care needed, and is not necessarily about having a doctor in the clinic. All advanced practice roles must meet the four pillars of advanced practice (Table 1.1), which are:

- Leadership and management.
- Education.
- Research.
- Advanced clinical practice [4].

The key points on working at an advanced level are:

- Advanced knowledge and clinical skills.
- Accountable practitioners normally working at the boundaries of the profession.
- Innovation.
- Skilled at assessing and managing risks.
- Freedom and authority to act and take responsibility for these decisions and actions taken.
- Very experienced and highly educated experts.
- Holistic assessment and addressing of medical and nursing and all the needs of the patient.
- Look at the whole person through fusions of different models from health promotion, caring, counselling, assessment, diagnosis, referral, treatments and discharge.
- The solution to work force challenges [1].

Some ANP roles have educational courses behind them such as hysteroscopy (Master's module at Bradford University), colposcopy (educational module undertaken by anyone who trains in colposcopy via the British Society for Colposcopy and Cervical Pathology) and scanning (PgDip). Some may have combined many different courses at Master's level to gain the competencies needed, where no one educational course meets all the needs of the role.

The areas in which nurses have advanced and developed their practice are widespread in gynaecology and in each different educational courses have been developed and adapted. There is currently no one course or one educational way of covering all areas of advanced practice in gynaecology. The various areas in which nurses are working within gynaecology and women's health are:

Table 1.1 Four pillars of advanced practice

Leadership and management	Identify change Innovate Manage change Service development Build and develop cases for change Negotiate and influence skills Significant network Development of team/s
Education	Understand the principles of teaching and learning and the different styles Support others to develop both knowledge and skills Promote and foster a culture and environment of learning Teach clients/patients Give information to patients in appropriate language and develop materials to support this Teach Mentor Coach
Research	Use research in clinical and educational practice Have critical appraisal skills Be involved in research Be involved in or lead audits Be involved in or lead service redesign Apply research findings to practice Develop guidelines and protocols that are evidence-based. Undertake or be involved in research Write publications Give presentations/lectures/talks
Advanced clinical practice	Undertaken high-level-decision making Have clinical judgement skills Be able to problem solve Apply critical thinking Reflect Manage patients with complex needs or in complex systems Carry out assessment Make diagnosis Make referrals Treat Discharge Be autonomous Non-medical prescription Carry out therapeutic interventions Have high levels of communication skills Be able to use public and service users in designing care

- Pre-assessment
- Colposcopy
- Hysteroscopy
- Scanning
- Fertility
- Urogynaecology

- Early pregnancy
- Endometriosis
- Contraception and sexual health
- Menopause
- Gynaecological cancer
- Termination of pregnancy
- General gynaecology
- Adolescent and paediatric gynaecology
- Theatre and post-op

The following chapters refer to this wide range of specialities and the role that nurses can play in them.

The expanded practice in nursing comes from the changing needs of the population, the lack of other health care staff and practitioners. In all areas, nurses who are able and willing to expand their scope of practice and push at the boundaries of care are needed. Some are consultation-based with physical skills, or psychological, or a combination, whereas others take on roles that have previously been undertaken by other professionals. On the whole, nurses have looked at the competencies needed and then undertaken learning at work or have found courses that underpin the education needed. Although there can be a lack of guidance, the RCN has produced some documents to guide nurses who are in those roles or working towards them, and these should be looked at in connection with the credentialed process [5–8]. In addition, there is debate around CNS and ANP. The roles do differ; thus, there can be further debate around generic and speciality ANP.

The roles that have the most research behind them are those of the CNS in gynaecology oncology, whereas in some of the newer roles there is no research that is nationally evaluated at all. There is one commissioned role currently available via specialist commissioning in the UK [9] and that is at an endometriosis centre that has a given status by the British Society for Gynaecological Endoscopy that requires that the jobholder to be a CNS.

Whatever the career path, there are many sources of help and inspiration in practice, from identifying the gaps to developing the skills and knowledge required, devising new roles and networking with others.

There are many factors that can have an impact on the expansion and development of the roles. These include:

- Clarity around the role
- Credentialing
- Availability of education for expanded roles in finance and provider terms
- Individuals ideas about the role
- Support from peers and other professionals, patients and organisations
- Overall costs and salary

To ensure that the roles are sustainable and to ensure success, the planning costs and benefits need to be clearly shown, and nurses have traditionally been very poor at this and the economics of health care [10]. Nurses need to ensure that all encounters with patients are logged and monitored and their work audited to show the impact of their role to the organisation. For example, the CNS in gynaecological oncology initiates telephone contact and subsequent discussion with a GP, which has meant that a patient did not have to attend hospital or indeed become an inpatient.

Whatever the area or the title there are some clear components and skills the nurse should have:

- Holistic and through assessment—taking a structured history to ensure that they have the information needed to make a provisional diagnosis or to direct which tests and investigations are likely to be needed. This would encompass interview techniques, open and closed questioning, and active listening. Paramount is good communication and the ability to discuss and question sensitive areas such as sexual history, contraception and pregnancy including pregnancy loss.
- Ordering appropriate tests and investigations such as bloods, scans, magnetic resonance imaging, dual-energy X-ray absorptiometry.
- Physical examinations—speculum, bi-manual and abdominal, depend on the area of work. The RCN [11] has guidance for training on this as it is not widely covered within the advanced assessment skills modules within an ANP Master's.
- Advanced skills—hysteroscopy, hysteroscopic polyp removal, intrauterine system insertions, implant insertions, colposcopy, urodynamics, scans, cystoscopy, endometrial biopsy, urodynamics, ring pessary care and conservative management follow-up in many the women, all of whom have their own related course and competency documents to be completed and audits of practice that need to be maintained, along with the appropriate continuing professional development to ensure ongoing competencies.

Specialist nurses can work in any part of women's health and have normally developed in response to patient's needs, organisational changes, NICE guidance and a desire to retain experienced nurses within the clinical setting.

As the following chapters show, nurses within gynaecology are able to utilise skills of advanced practice and those of a CNS to enhance care and ensure that a woman is seen by the right practitioner with the right skills at the right time to obtain high-quality care that is tailormade for that woman.

References

1. Advanced level of nursing practice: introduction. RCN—June 2018. Publication code 006894. Accessed 10 Aug 2018
2. Bryant-Lukosius D, DiCenso A (2004) A framework for the introduction and evaluation of advanced practice nursing roles. J Adv Nurs 48(5): 530–540
3. Leary A, Maclain K, Trevatt P, Radford M, Punshon G (2017) Variations in job titles within the nursing workforce. J Clin Nursing 26(23–24):4945–4950
4. https://www.hee.nhs.uk/sites/default/files/documents/Multi-professional%20framework%20for%20advanced%20clinical%20practice%20in%20England.pdf. Accessed 10 Aug 2018

5. RCN credentialing. https://www.rcn.org.uk/professional-development/publications/pub-006897
6. RCN CNS endometriosis. https://www.rcn.org.uk/professional-development/publications/pub-004776
7. RCN CNS menopause. https://www.rcn.org.uk/professional-development/publications/pub-005701
8. RCN CNS early pregnancy. https://www.rcn.org.uk/professional-development/publications/pub-006394
9. https://www.england.nhs.uk/commissioning/wp-content/uploads/sites/12/2014/04/e10-comp-gynae-endom-0414.pdf
10. Fulton J (2013) Making outcomes of clinical nurse specialist practice visible. Clin Nurse Spec 27(1):5–6
11. Genital examination in women. RCN. https://www.rcn.org.uk/professional-development/publications/pub-005480

Suggested Reading

England: 'Advanced level nursing: a position statement'. www.dh.gov.uk/en/Publicationsandstatistics/Publications/PublicationsPolicyAndGuidance/DH_121739
https://www.rcn.org.uk/professional-development/advanced-practice-standards
Scotland: 'Advanced nursing practice toolkit' in Scotland. www.advancedpractice.scot.nhs.uk.
The Association of Advanced Nursing Practice Educators—Educational networking for advanced nursing practice in the UK. www.aape.org.uk
Wales: 'Framework for advanced nursing, midwifery and allied health professional practice in Wales'. www.wales.nhs.uk/sitesplus/documents/829/NLIAH%20advanced%20Practice%20Framework.pdf

2

Anne Teasdale, Katharine Gale, and Debra Holloway

2.1 Heavy Menstrual Bleeding

Heavy menstrual bleeding (HMB) is one of the most common reasons for gynaeco-logical consultations in both primary and secondary care. About 1 in 20 women aged between 30 and 49 years [1] consult their GP each year because of heavy periods or menstrual problems, with menstrual disorders comprising 12% of all referrals to gynaecology services. Many women tolerate problematic heavy bleed-ing for years as they think that this is normal, having spoken to family members who have experienced the same, or because they are too embarrassed to speak to anyone about it, so they manage the best that they can. When some women eventually do seek help they can be feeling fairly desperate.

Over the past 30 years, this subject has been the focus of much research, improv-ing our clinical knowledge and also our understanding of the psychological effects. This research has led to the development of guidelines and clinical pathways that allow clinicians to offer a more consistent and evidence-based approach to manag-ing the condition.

The National Institute for Health Care and Excellence (NICE) guideline on HMB, published in 2007 (updated in 2018) [2], defined HMB as excessive men-strual blood loss that interferes with the woman's physical, emotional, social and material quality of life, and that can occur alone or in combination with other symptoms [1].

A. Teasdale · D. Holloway (✉)
Guys and St Thomas NHS Foundation Trust, London, UK
e-mail: Debra.Holloway@gstt.nhs.uk

K. Gale
North Bristol NHs Trust, Bristol, UK

© Springer Nature Switzerland AG 2019
D. Holloway (ed.), *Nursing Management of Women's Health*,
https://doi.org/10.1007/978-3-030-16115-6_2

Any intervention should aim to improve quality of life rather than focusing on blood loss, as women have differing ideas of what normal bleeding is [2]. Treatment and care should take into account women's needs and preferences. Good communication is essential, supported by evidence-based information, to allow women to make informed decisions about their care [2].

2.1.1 Signs and Symptoms

Heavy menstrual bleeding is an abnormally heavy and prolonged menstrual period occurring at regular intervals and preventing normal activities such as working and socialising. HMB may cause one or all of the following:

- Flooding through to clothes or bedding.
- Frequent changes of sanitary protection.
- Double sanitary protection—tampons and towels.
- Passing blood clots—larger than a 50 pence piece.

Frequent, unpredictable and painful periods are also common reasons for presentation, as they also interfere with daily life.

Additionally, long-term HMB may lead to anaemia, low ferritin and iron levels, which can lead to fatigue, tiredness and a further impact on quality of life.

2.1.2 Causes of HMB

- In younger women, heavy periods are most often due to a temporary hormonal imbalance, which eventually corrects itself.
- In many of women with heavy periods between the ages of 25 and 40 years no underlying cause is found.
- In the years close to menopause, heavy periods are also usually a sign of hormonal imbalance; however, the possibility of underlying disease does increase with age.
- Table 2.1 below summarises the causes of HMB [1–3], which are then examined in more detail.

1. *Fibroids*: Fibroids are benign tumours of uterine smooth muscle, termed leiomyomas. They are relatively common, particularly in women of Afro-Caribbean origin [3]. The actual prevalence of uterine fibroids is unknown and most likely underestimated, as 50% of women are asymptomatic and the identification may be an incidental finding on an ultrasound scan, following a hysterectomy or post-mortem. The estimated lifetime chance of women having fibroids is likely to be around 60%.
   These are covered in more detail in a later section.
2. *Endometrial polyps*: Polyps are outgrowths of the endometrium [4], as shown in Fig. 2.1. They may be pedunculated or sessile, single or multiple and vary in size

Table 2.1 Causes of HMB [1–3]

None
Fibroids
Anovulatory cycles—such as PCOS (see a later section)
Endometrial polyps
Tamoxifen
Adenomyosis
Endometrial hyperplasia
Hormone dysfunction—PCOS, extremes of reproductive life
IUCD—can increase blood loss during periods by 45–50%
Medications such as warfarin
Thyroid disorders
Blood clotting disorders—Von Willebrand disease, thrombocytopaenia
Infections and endometritis
Other chronic conditions such as renal and liver disease
Dysfunctional uterine bleeding—when all other causes have been excluded

PCOS polycystic ovary syndrome, *IUCD* intrauterine contraceptive device

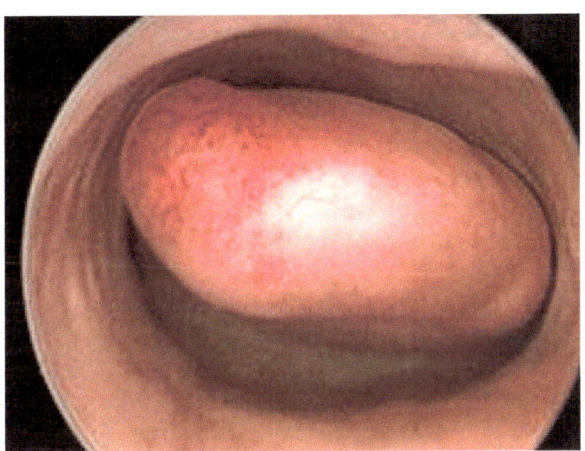

Fig. 2.1 Endometrial polyp

(0.5–4 cm). The prevalence of endometrial polyps in women presenting with pre- or post-menopausal bleeding is around 25%. It is unlikely that the increased endometrial surface area caused by the presence of polyps causes excessive menstrual loss. However, different expressions of sex steroid receptors in the endometrium overlying polyps may result in light, unscheduled bleeding (spotting) and vaginal discharge, or heavier bleeding if hyperplastic or malignant. However, many women report an improvement in their symptoms of heavy bleeding once the endometrial polyps have been removed. Endometrial polyps can be diagnosed using ultrasound; however, accuracy is limited, and hysteroscopy is the gold standard, offering the opportunity for removal of the polyp, or at least biopsy, at the same time. The risk of polyps harbouring serious endometrial disease is increased after the menopause and with the use of tamoxifen, with approximately 1% being malignant.

3. *Tamoxifen*: An effective and widely used therapy for women with breast cancer because it reduces the recurrence rates and prolongs disease-free survival. It is a non-steroidal, partial oestrogen agonist; it exhibits anti-oestrogenic activity in the breast, but has a stimulatory effect on the endometrium. This hormonal activity results in a higher incidence of heavy bleeding, post-menopausal bleeding and endometrial pathological conditions such as endometrial polyps, hyperplasia and cancer.

   Endometrial evaluation is indicated for a woman on tamoxifen with abnormal bleeding, primarily to exclude serious endometrial disease but also to detect and treat endometrial polyps, which are more common with tamoxifen (30–80%). Some gynaecologists advocate endometrial screening in asymptomatic women on tamoxifen.

4. *Adenomyosis*: Adenomyosis [3] occurs when the tissue that normally lines the uterus (endometrial tissue) grows into the muscular wall of the uterus, the myometrium. The displaced tissue continues to act normally—thickening, breaking down and bleeding—during each menstrual cycle. An enlarged uterus and painful, heavy periods can result. More recently, diagnosis has been made using ultrasound based on previously noted histology post-hysterectomy. The exact cause of adenomyosis is not known.

5. *Endometrial hyperplasia*: Hyperplasia refers to an increase in cell numbers [5]. In the case of endometrial hyperplasia this results in a thickened lining of the uterus which, in turn, can result in heavy bleeding.

Risk factors for developing endometrial hyperplasia relate mainly to unopposed oestrogen exposure:

- Increased body mass index (BMI) with excessive peripheral conversion of androgens in adipose tissue to oestrogen.
- Anovulation associated with polycystic ovarian syndrome (PCOS) or the peri-menopause.
- Oestrogen-secreting ovarian tumours.
- Drug-induced endometrial stimulation, e.g. the use of tamoxifen or unopposed oestrogen HRT.

Diagnosis is histological and requires an endometrial biopsy, preferably taken during a hysteroscopy [5], which allows a full assessment of the uterine cavity. The importance of endometrial hyperplasia relates not only to the symptoms of bleeding it can cause, but also to its oncogenic potential. The Royal College of Obstetricians and Gynaecologists (RCOG) Green Top Guideline (2016) [5] categorises endometrial hyperplasia into two groups, with or without atypia, and the management is very much influenced by the presence of atypia. Malignant progression has been reported to occur in 30% of cases of hyperplasia with atypia if left untreated. A proportion of hyperplasia regresses without treatment; however, treatment is advised. Hyperplasia without atypia is treated with progestogen therapy. The Mirena intrauterine system (IUS) is the recommended option; however, if this is not acceptable, oral progestogens are a second choice. The RCOG recommends endometrial surveillance with endometrial biopsy at a minimum of 6-monthly intervals. At least two consecutive 6-monthly negative biopsies should be obtained before the woman is discharged [5].

For women with atypical hyperplasia, hysterectomy is recommended unless fertility is an issue, in which case progestogen therapy is advised.

In addition to this, the importance of reversing risk factors and long-term monitoring, as outlined in the guidelines, is often within the scope of the specialist nurses e.g. weight management.

2.1.3 History-Taking

The clinical history of women presenting with HMB helps to identify the likelihood of pelvic pathological conditions including endometrial or cervical polyps and uterine fibroids or endocrine dysfunction such as PCOS. Whether further investigations and referral to secondary care are required needs to be determined [2]. Women with fibroids often report a palpable pelvic mass, or a sensation of abdominal pressure causing urinary or bowel symptoms.

In addition to a full general medical history, a clinical history specific to bleeding should include [1, 2]:

- Number of pregnancies and desire for future pregnancies.
- Current contraception.
- How long has the problematic bleeding existed? Is it a recent change or have the periods always been heavy?
- The nature of the bleeding—how many days a period lasts, how often the period comes, what type of sanitary protection is used and how often it is changed, whether blood clots are passed or flooding is experienced.
- Cervical smear history.
- History of STI.
- Related symptoms, such as persistent intermenstrual bleeding (IMB), post-coital bleeding (PCB), pelvic pain and/or pressure symptoms, that might suggest uterine cavity abnormality, histological abnormality, adenomyosis or fibroids.
- Other factors that may affect treatment options, such as comorbidities or previous treatment for HMB.
- Are there any signs of a clotting problem, e.g. problematic bleeding after dental treatment or nose bleeds or bleeding after childbirth or operations?
- Impact on quality of life.
- Tiredness and breathlessness or other signs of anaemia.

2.1.4   Physical Examination and Blood Tests

If the woman has a history of heavy bleeding with other related symptoms, such as pain or IMB, a physical examination, including speculum, bi-manual and abdominal, should be performed. This establishes the size of the uterus and gives an indication of the presence of fibroids [2].

A full blood count should be performed on all women with HMB; testing for coagulation disorders should only be considered for women who have had HMB since their periods started, and for those with a personal or family history suggesting a coagulation disorder [2]. Whilst initiating investigations, it is worth discussing medical treatment options that can be started whilst awaiting the results of any tests.

2.1.5   Investigations to Discover the Cause of HMB

If a woman presents with HMB and her history suggests a low risk of pathological condition or abnormality, pharmacological treatment could be considered without further investigation. A 3-month trial of pharmacological treatment followed by a review and further investigation if unsuccessful would be appropriate management [2]. However, if there are any other symptoms, such as pain, IMB or PCB, further investigations are indicated.

The NICE guideline [2] suggests taking into account the woman's history and examination when deciding whether to offer hysteroscopy or ultrasound as the first-line investigation. However, both have their advantages and limitations; therefore, if both investigations are available a more comprehensive clinical picture will be ascertained. More often than not, the resources available are the deciding factor, and most units have easier access to ultrasound rather than hysteroscopy.

Hysteroscopy allows the assessment of the uterine cavity through direct vision, using a small telescope. The development of miniature hysteroscopes (diameter 3.5 mm or less) have enabled the procedure to be safely performed in the outpatient setting, often without significant discomfort [6]. Hysteroscopy is the most reliable investigation for identifying intrauterine pathological conditions such as submucosal fibroids or endometrial polyps.

Outpatient hysteroscopy should be offered to women with HMB if their history suggests submucosal fibroids, polyps or endometrial pathology. They may have symptoms such as persistent IMB or they may have risk factors for endometrial pathological conditions such as obesity, PCOS, tamoxifen therapy or unsuccessful medical management. An endometrial biopsy can be taken during a hysteroscopy. NICE does not recommend taking a "blind" biopsy on women with HMB, as any pathological condition is likely to be missed [2].

A transvaginal ultrasound should be offered to women with HMB if any of the following apply [2]:

• The uterus is palpable abdominally, suggesting large fibroids.
• History or examination suggests a pelvic mass.

- Examination is inconclusive or difficult, for example, when women are obese.
- Suspicion of adenomyosis (bulky uterus and dysmenorrhoea).

If a uterine pathological condition is suspected, then medical management of HMB should be considered whilst awaiting a hysteroscopy or ultrasound scan, potentially avoiding a delay in managing the patient's symptoms. It is important to remember that failed medical management of HMB would increase the likelihood of pelvic pathological conditions, uterine fibroids or endometrial hyperplasia or carcinoma.

2.1.6   Other Investigations

Cervical screening should be up to date and swabs for infections should be taken dependent on history and if there are any reports of discharge. Bloods should be taken for FBC [2] and/or iron and ferritin levels and depending on the history, including TSH and investigations for bleeding disorders. In addition, irregular bleeding may suggest PCOS; therefore, a hormone profile may need to be taken.

2.1.7   Increased Risk of Endometrial Pathological Conditions

- Persistent intermenstrual or.
- Persistent irregular bleeding.
- Infrequent heavy bleeding.
- Infrequent heavy bleeding with obesity and or PCOS.
- Women taking tamoxifen.
- Women for whom treatment for HMB has been unsuccessful.

2.1.8   Management of HMB

When considering treatment options with women consideration should be given to [2]:

- The woman's preferences
- Any comorbidities
- The presence or absence of fibroids (including size, number and location), polyps, endometrial pathological conditions or adenomyosis
- Other symptoms such as pressure and pain

  Discussions should also cover

- The benefits and risks of various options
- Suitable treatments if the patient is trying to conceive
- Whether she wants to retain her fertility and/or her uterus

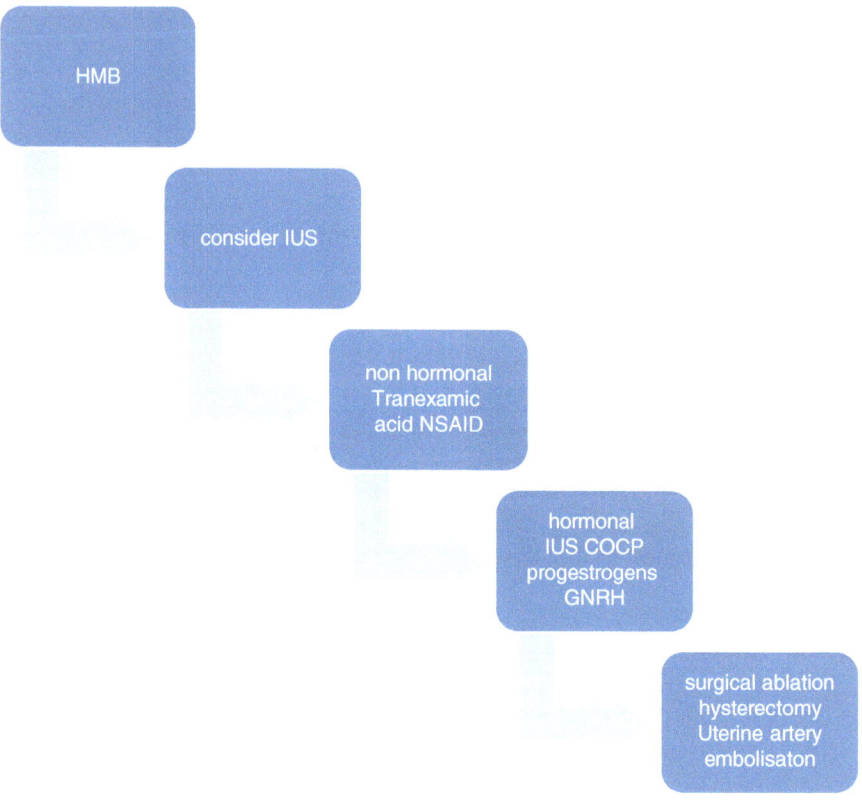

Fig. 2.2 Recommended treatment options in line with the NICE guideline on HMB [2]

Figure 2.2 below shows a summary of the treatments that can be used. Pharmacological options are generally encouraged before surgery as they can often have a successful outcome and involve less risk. Pharmacological options include:

- *Mirena IUS—levonorgestrel-releasing intrauterine system (LNG-IUS)*. Releases a small amount of synthetic progesterone called levonorgestrel. The effect is to prevent proliferation of the endometrium. Periods normally become either very light or stop altogether within 3–6 months of insertion; however, irregular spotting can also occur during this time. Period pain is often reduced. The IUS reduces bleeding by 71–90% and is seen to be an effective, safe and cost-effective treatment for HMB (ensure that the system being used is licensed for the treatment of HMB).

  It is important to ensure the woman understands that 1 in 20 devices are expelled, particularly during the first year, with heavy menstrual loss. Nurses can teach women how to self-check for the threads and if they are unsure or unable to feel them then encourage a check-up at 6 weeks with the practice nurse. If the threads are not visible on examination, an ultrasound scan should be arranged to check the device's location.

- *Tranexamic acid—anti-fibrinolytic agent.* Can reduce the heaviness of the bleeding by 40–50% in most cases. However, the number of days of bleeding is not reduced, nor is period pain. Tranexamic acid works by reducing the breakdown of blood clots in the uterus. It is associated with gastrointestinal symptoms and may not suitable for women with a history of thromboembolic disease. A trial of 3 months is recommended [2, 7].
- *NSAIDS—non-steroidal anti-inflammatory drugs, including mefenamic acid.* Can reduce the amount of blood loss by about a third. They work by reducing the high level of prostaglandin in the uterus lining, which seems to contribute to heavy periods and period pain. They do not reduce the number of days bleeding. Common side effects are gastrointestinal and therefore not suitable for women with stomach ulcers and can increase symptoms in women with asthma.
- *COCP—combined oral contraception pill.* Reduces bleeding by about a third in most women. Often reduces period pain too. Can be taken in addition to NSAIDS if required.
- *Long-acting progestogen contraceptives—*The injection and the implant tend to reduce heavy periods. Up to half of women using these methods have no periods after a year. These are not used just as a treatment for heavy periods; however, if contraception is an issue for a woman with heavy periods these could be suitable options (for both of the above, please see the Chap. 13 on contraception for more guidance on the criteria for prescribing).
- *Oral progestogens—synthetic progestogen.* It is not commonly used to treat heavy periods because of the many common side effects; however, it is sometimes considered if other treatments have not worked. It should be taken on days 5–26 of the cycle to have the best effect.
- *GnRH analogues—gonadotrophin-releasing hormone.* Down-regulation of GnRH receptors, thereby reducing the release of follicle-stimulating hormone (FSH) and luteinising hormone (LH), which in turn leads to inhibition of androgen and oestrogen production leading to a medically induced menopause. Long-term use can cause a risk to bone density; therefore, add-back therapy such as HRT should be provided.

For those women with no identified pathological condition, fibroids less than 3 cm in diameter that are not causing distortion of the uterine cavity, or suspected or diagnosed adenomyosis, the LNG-IUS should be considered as the first-line treatment. If a woman declines or it is not suitable, other pharmacological treatments can be considered. Medical management options are:

- LNG-IUS
- Non-hormonal
  - Tranexamic acid
  - NSAIDS (non-steroidal anti-inflammatory drugs)

- Hormonal
  - Combined hormonal contraception
  - Progestogen-only contraception (pills, injection, implant)
  - Cyclical oral progestogens
  - GnRH analogue

Surgical options are:

- Endometrial ablation
- Hysterectomy

Endometrial ablation (by a second-generation technique) is the destruction of the endometrial lining by heat. Patient suitability for the ablative procedure needs careful consideration. Women need to be sure that they have completed their family before opting for this procedure. The best outcomes are seen in women with a small regular uterine cavity of less than 10 cm. The most likely outcome will be normal or lighter periods rather than a complete absence of periods. Women should be aware that common side effects include pelvic cramping and vaginal discharge.

For those women with larger fibroids, management will be very dependent upon their wish to maintain their fertility or their reluctance to lose their uterus. The LNG-IUS is an option only if the uterine cavity is not distorted by fibroids; otherwise, the same pharmacological options are suitable.

2.1.9   Management of Fibroids

If the patient is asymptomatic, then treatment is unnecessary, which is the case in 50% of women [8]. When considering treatment options, the woman's expectations and the following factors should be taken into account: the location and size of the fibroids, any comorbidities, the age of patient and her desire to retain her fertility and her uterus, the severity of her symptoms and the impact on their quality of life. Nurses can provide information about all possible treatment options. They can support the women to make the right decision for them based on the risks and benefits of each treatment option and whether she is trying to conceive or wanting to having children in the future. The nurse should make every attempt to understand what matters most to each individual woman and support her personal priorities and choices.

The actual cause of fibroids is unknown, but they [9].

- Are more common in nulliparous women
- Common in Afro-Caribbean women
- More common in women with a family history of fibroids
- More common in older women
- May have a genetic link
- May be related to diet and vitamin D

- Have an increased risk in patients with PCOS
- Have an increased risk in women with obesity
- Have an increased risk in patients with co-morbidities such as diabetes and hypertension

Fibroids can be located within the uterine cavity (intracavity), within the myometrium but extending significantly into the uterine cavity (submucosal), centrally within the myometrium (intramural), at the outer border of the myometrium (subserosal), or attached to the uterus by a pedicle (pedunculated). Figure 2.3 below shows the different positions of fibroids. Fibroids can also arise separately from the uterus, especially in the broad ligament, presumably from embryonal remnants.

A clear diagram in Fig. 2.4 shows where these are positioned.

They vary in size and site and this often determines their presentation; however, there can be huge differences between one person and the next. Some women with large fibroids can be asymptomatic and women with small fibroids can be very symptomatic [8]. A third of women with uterine fibroids report HMB that is having

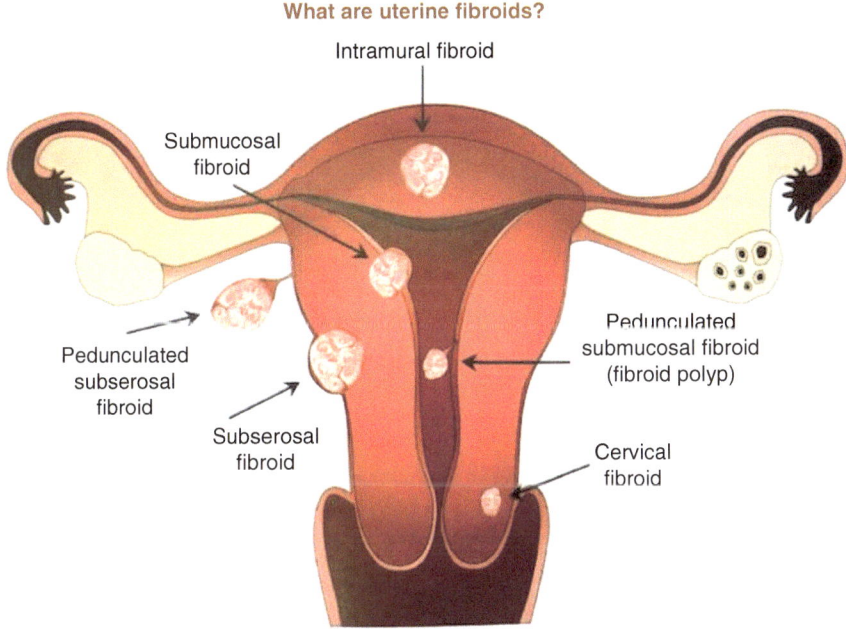

Fig. 2.3 Types of fibroids: 1. Subserosal fibroids project outwards from the uterus and are maybe pedunculated. They are more likely to become large, causing pressure symptoms and pelvic pain. 2. Intramural fibroids are the most common and grow within the wall of the myometrium of the uterus. 3. Submucosal (5%) are the least common growing between the myometrium and the endometrium and therefore may affect fertility. They may be pedunculated or partially within the myometrium. Type 0 is entirely within the cavity and type 1 is 50% within the cavity and type 2 is less than 50% in the cavity

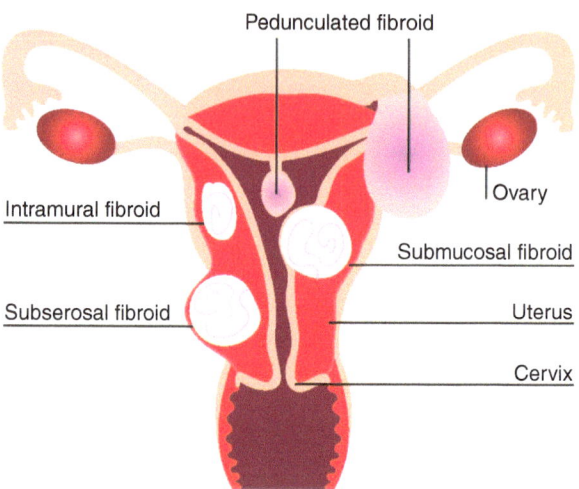

Fig. 2.4 Position of fibroids

Pedunculated fibroid

Intramural fibroid

Subserosal fibroid

Ovary

Submucosal fibroid

Uterus

Cervix

a negative impact on their home, work and social life and frequently leads to anaemia.

In addition to bleeding issues, women with fibroids also report:

- HMB
- PCB
- IMB
- Pain
- Pressure
- Bloating
- Difficulty opening bowels
- Difficulty passing urine
- Painful sex
- Links with miscarriages
- Links with infertility

2.1.10 Investigations

In addition to the investigations for heavy bleeding as above, women with fibroids need an examination and a pelvic scan, which may be both transvaginal and abdominal, dependent on the size of the fibroids. This needs to detail the size, position, location of the fibroids and any impact on the uterine cavity. Women with large fibroids also need a renal scan to look at her kidneys for signs of hydronephrosis.

If these lack clarity, then she may go on to have a hysteroscopy to assess the cavity, MRI and tubal patency testing dependent on the presentation and the desired outcomes [10].

Submucosal and intramural fibroids tend to be more associated with heavy bleeding. Submucosal fibroids are covered with endometrium and their presence gives rise to an increased surface area from which to bleed. The presence of intramural fibroids can also increase the general size of the uterus, resulting in more bleeding. There is evidence to suggest that blood flow might be greater in the presence of fibroids because of the inability of the blood vessels supplying the endometrium overlying the fibroid to undergo the usual progestogenic changes.

2.1.10.1 Treatments

Figure 2.5 shows a summary from NICE for the management of fibroids dependent on size

- *Hysteroscopic resection*: HMB is caused by submucosal fibroids in around 15% of women. If submucosal fibroids are identified, then hysteroscopic removal

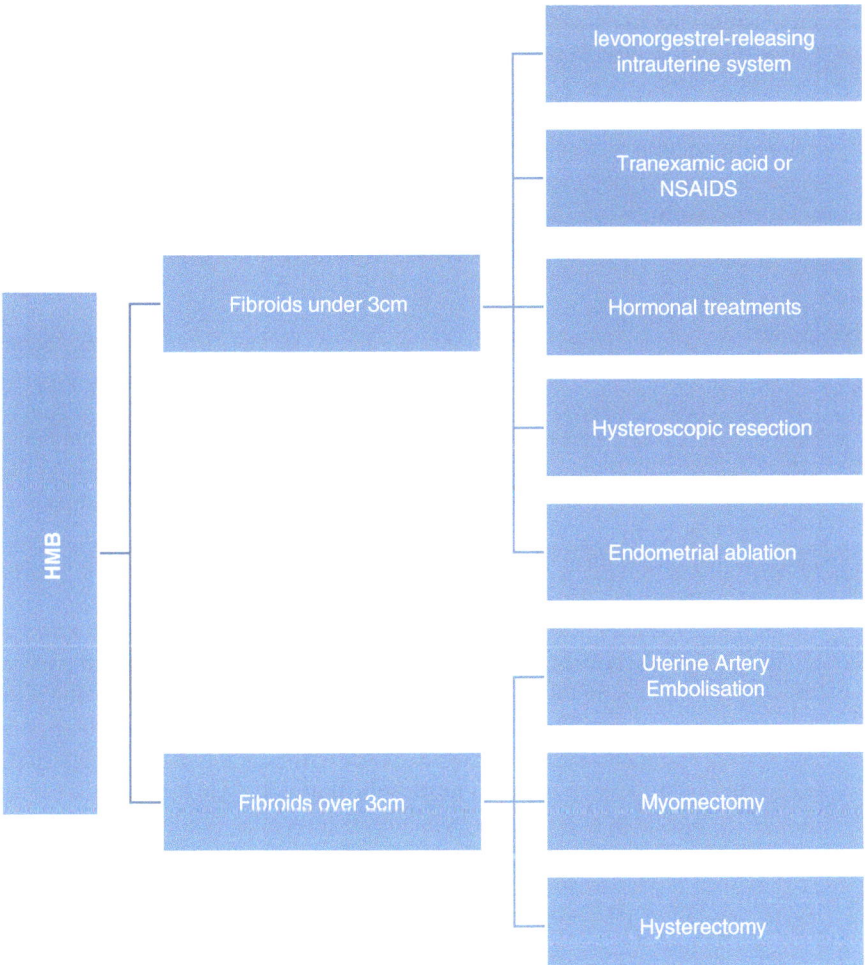

Fig. 2.5 Management of HMB

should be considered [2] especially for women wishing to conceive. This procedure can be performed in the outpatient setting using a hysteroscopic device, called a morcellator, for small fibroids, where the hysteroscopy is inserted into the uterus and the fibroids are cut into small pieces that are removed through the suction tube. It can also be carried out under a general anaesthetic by transcervical resection of fibroid. There is a 70–80% improvement in HMB and women report that they do not require ongoing medical treatment following the procedure.

For those women with larger fibroids, management is very dependent upon their wish to maintain fertility or reluctance to lose their uterus. The LNG-IUS is an option only if the uterine cavity is not distorted by fibroids; otherwise, the same pharmacological options are suitable.

- *Uterine artery embolisation*: This is indicated for symptomatic fibroids and is an effective alternative to surgical myomectomy [2, 7]. It is an image-guided procedure carried out by interventional radiologists under local anaesthetic and sedation to block the blood supply to the fibroids. A small catheter is fed through the femoral artery in the groin until it reaches the uterine artery when small particles are injected to cause a blockage and infarct the fibroid tissue. The average permanent reduction in size of fibroids is up to 70% and therefore similar to the semi-permanent reduction associated with GnRH agonists. It is usually only carried out in women who have completed their family; however, with informed consent, some women who wish to conceive opt for UAE over myomectomy. An improvement in symptoms in 83–84% of women at 6 and 12 months has been shown. Women require an overnight stay in hospital to ensure optimal pain relief and they should be aware of the potential rare but serious complications, including allergic reaction, infection, bleeding from the incision in the groin, and perforation of the uterine artery.

- *Magnetic resonance-guided focused ultrasound (MRgFUS)*: Although not generally available within the national health service, MRgFUS is a non-surgical procedure that is performed by a interventional radiologist using MRI and ultrasound to identify the fibroids and then apply ultrasound-generated energy to heat up the fibroids to destroy them. This procedure is suitable for women with fibroids between 7 and 10 cm, but no more than six fibroids in total.

- *Pre-surgery treatment*: Before surgery, medical treatment may be given to women as a pre-treatment to reduce the size of the fibroid and reduce the bleeding and risk of anaemia. GnRH downregulates the pituitary, which reduces the follicle-stimulating and luteinising-hormone, which in turn reduces the oestrogen levels. The reduction in oestrogen causes a drop in the blood supply to the uterus and reduces the size of the fibroids by up to 50% [11]. The GnRH injection is administered every 28 days for up to 6 months, but is associated with symptoms similar to those seen around the menopause. Side effects include, hot flushes with night sweats, loss of libido and vaginal dryness, and changes in mood.

- *Selective progesterone receptor modulators*: This is an oral tablet that may be used in the same way as GnRH for women pre-surgery. The tablet is taken once a day for 3 months. It also reduces heavy bleeding and the size of the fibroid with results lasting for up to 6 months. It is also indicated for women with moderate to severe HMB who are not suitable for surgery. It should only be prescribed after careful diagnosis. Liver function tests are undertaken before starting treatment and cannot be used in conjunction with any hormonal contraception. The schedule is shown in Fig. 2.6. It is taken with a treatment break, but the 3-month course can be repeated and restarted during the week of their second menstruation. Progesterone receptor modulator-associated endometrial changes can be seen on the recommended annual ultrasound, which should be arranged during their treatment break after their first menstruation. If the thickening persists for 3 months, then an endometrial biopsy should be taken. Side effects include usually welcomed amenorrhoea, breast tenderness, headaches, changes in mood and tiredness [12]. There have been some concerns around the safety of progesterone receptor modulators with liver interactions; thus, the new guidance does suggest a liver function test, before initiation of the medication, while on the medication for the first few courses, and then after this [13].

- *Myomectomy*: This is a surgical procedure to remove the fibroids, performed either via laparoscopy (key hole) or laparotomy (open abdominal surgery) [14]. It is particularly useful for fibroids that are intramural, subserosal or pedunculated. Only women with one or two fibroids that are no larger than 7 cm are usually suitable for laparoscopic myomectomy, which is associated with a shorter length of stay. It is suitable for women who are keen to retain their fertility, but that may not always be an option depending on the size, number and location of fibroids. Women should be informed of the small risk of an emergency hysterectomy at the time of surgery owing to excessive bleeding if larger fibroids cause it

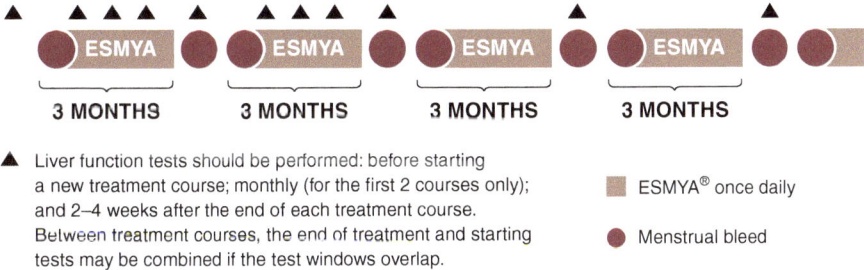

ESMYA® DOSING AND LIVER MONITORING SCHEDULE

The diagram below shows at what point you should:

- start each ESMYA® course in your menstrual cycle

- have liver tests during treatment

▲ Liver function tests should be performed: before starting a new treatment course; monthly (for the first 2 courses only); and 2–4 weeks after the end of each treatment course. Between treatment courses, the end of treatment and starting tests may be combined if the test windows overlap.

■ ESMYA® once daily

● Menstrual bleed

Fig. 2.6 Care of women on ESMYA

to be a technically difficult procedure. For women with large fibroids, the effectiveness of the procedure may be limited. Therefore, women who are approaching the menopause or who have completed their family, then hysterectomy may be a reasonable consideration.

- *Hysterectomy*: This is the only treatment that ensures amenorrhoea and removes the possibility of pregnancy. It is a common surgical procedure involving the removal of the uterus plus or minus the ovaries and cervix via either laparoscopy or laparotomy. Women should be informed that even if their ovaries are preserved, there is a possible risk of loss of ovarian function, and of its consequences.

Nurses should ensure that women have an opportunity for a detailed discussion before opting for a hysterectomy and they need to be made aware of the implications of surgery before they make their decision.

The pre-hysterectomy discussion should include:

- Sexual feelings
- Impact on fertility
- Bladder function
- Need for further treatment
- Treatment complications
- Her expectations
- Alternative surgery
- Use of HRT if ovaries are removed
- Psychological impact

In the updated NICE guidelines on HMB [2], there is acknowledgement that although hysterectomy is an possible option for women following the failure of first-line treatments, a small number of women voice a preference for hysterectomy without willing to try other potential treatment options. Endometrial ablation may be a less invasive procedure, but hysterectomy is usually associated with great patient satisfaction.

It is not without risks and the overall risk of serious complications from an abdominal hysterectomy is quoted at 4 in every 100 women. Women should be made aware of the increased risk of serious complications, which include haemorrhage and perforation of other abdominal organs when uterine fibroids are present.

For benign conditions, the ovaries are usually retained during a hysterectomy; however, women should be informed about the risk of potential loss of ovarian function and the associated earlier onset of symptoms (see Chap. 10). Nurses should discuss with women the options for management of the menopausal symptoms in advance of surgery.

2.1.11 Intermenstrual and Post-coital Bleeding

Intermenstrual bleeding (IMB) refers to vaginal bleeding (other than post-coital) at any time during the menstrual cycle other than during normal menstruation.

Post-coital bleeding (PCB) is non-menstrual bleeding that occurs immediately after sexual intercourse [15]. Breakthrough bleeding is irregular bleeding associated with hormonal contraception.

Unscheduled bleeding causes anxiety and concern because it can be a presenting symptoms for gynaecological cancer, particularly cervical and endometrial, and although rare in young women, it should be investigated.

2.1.12 Causes of Post-coital Bleeding

- Infection
- Cervical ectropion—especially in women taking the combined hormonal contraceptive pill
- Cervical or endometrial polyps or submucosal fibroids
- Vaginal cancer
- Cervical cancer
- Trauma

No specific cause is found in approximately 50% of cases.

2.1.13 Causes of Intermenstrual Bleeding

- Pregnancy-related, including ectopic pregnancy and gestational trophoblastic disease
- Physiological
  - 1–2% of women experience spotting around ovulation
  - Hormonal fluctuation during the peri-menopause
- Cervical causes
  - Infection, e.g. chlamydia
  - Cervical polyps
  - Cervical ectropion
- Uterine causes
  - Fibroids
  - Endometrial polyps
  - Adenomyosis
  - Endometritis

2.1.14 Iatrogenic Causes

- Tamoxifen.
- Missed oral contraceptive pills.
- Following cervical smear or treatment to the cervix.

- Drugs altering clotting parameters—e.g. anticoagulants, selective serotonin reuptake inhibitors (SSRIs), corticosteroids.
- Alternative remedies when taken with hormonal contraceptives—e.g. ginseng, gingko, soy supplements and St John's wort.

2.1.15 History-Taking

Menstrual history

- Regularity and cycle length
- Duration of abnormal bleeding—how long has this problem persisted
- Timing of bleeding in the menstrual cycle
- Associated symptoms—pain, fever, vaginal discharge, dyspareunia
- Any factors that make the bleeding worse—exercise, intercourse

  Obstetric history

- Previous pregnancies and deliveries, including time since last delivery/miscarriage/termination
- Current breast-feeding

  Gynaecological history

- Current use of contraception
- Cervical smear history, including the most recent result and any previous abnormalities
- Previous gynaecological investigations or surgery
- Previous infections

  Sexual history

- Risk factors for sexually transmitted infections (STIs), past history and treatment for STIs.

  Medical history, including family or personal history of bleeding disorders, and current medication.

2.1.16 Examination

First, establish that the bleeding is from the vagina, not the rectum or in the bladder. An abdominal examination should be performed noting the presence or absence of pelvic masses. A PV examination should be performed (speculum and bimanual) looking for obvious pathological conditions. Note whether any contact bleeding occurs, friability of tissue, cervical "excitation" or tenderness, and the presence of ulceration, polyps or discharge. Common findings include:

- Cervical ectropion—appears as a red area around the external os due to extension of the endocervical columnar epithelium over the ectocervix.
- Cervical polyp—a growth of tissue arising from the endocervix and usually protruding through the external os. They are normally attached by a thin stalk and can be avulsed and sent to histology. Occasionally, endometrial polyps can be seen extruding through the cervix.
- Cervicitis—the cervix appears red, congested and sometimes oedematous. There may be discharge and the cervix is usually tender to the touch.

2.1.17 Investigation

The possibility of pregnancy and an STI should first be excluded as the cause if bleeding [16]. A pregnancy test and STI screen should be performed, in addition to a cervical screening if it is due. If the bleeding is heavy, then a full blood count (FBC) could be considered and a hormone profile if PCOS is suspected (see later section) [15].

A transvaginal ultrasound scan can be performed to look for any structural abnormality, including endometrial polyps and fibroids. Evidence of endometrial thickening should prompt referral for outpatient hysteroscopy and endometrial biopsy, particularly in women over the age of 40 [6].

For women with persistent PCB, colposcopy is recommended because of its higher sensitivity (see Chap. 3).

2.1.18 Management

Management is dependent on the cause of the bleeding.

2.1.19 Infection

- Appropriate antibiotics depending on the organism involved.
- Contact tracing if STI (see Chap. 13).

2.1.20 Hormonal

Women should be advised that unscheduled bleeding in the first 3 months after starting a new hormonal contraceptive method is common, and this can be up to 6 months with the IUS or progestogen implant [17].

- COCP users.
  - The same pill should be trialled for at least 3 months as the bleeding may settle.
  - If the bleeding does not settle, a different pill with a maximum dose of 35 mcg of oestrogen can be tried.
  - A different COCP may be tried, or a different dose or type of progestogen.

- Progestogen-only contraceptive pill users.
  - A different pill may be tried.
  - An NSAID, such as mefenamic acid, may shorten the duration of the bleeding episode.
- Progestogen implants, depot and IUS users.
  - A first-line COCP may be considered for up to 3 months continuously or in the usual cyclical regime, in addition to the progestogen method.
  - An NSAID can be used to shorten the duration of the bleeding.

2.1.21 Cervical Ectropion

- May resolve spontaneously if the COCP is stopped, or following pregnancy.
- Can be cauterised with silver nitrate.
- If silver nitrate is not effective, other treatment options include thermal cautery and diathermy, or cryosurgery (after a normal colposcopy and biopsy).

Cervical polyps should be avulsed and sent for histology.

2.1.22 Endometrial Polyps

If endometrial polyps are a possibility, further investigation with outpatient hysteroscopy is appropriate. This is the gold standard investigation for suspected uterine pathological conditions and it allows removal of the polyps at the same time. Endometrial polyps should be removed owing to the small risk of abnormality.

If there is a suspicion of symptomatic fibroids, women should be referred to secondary care for further management.

Of note, there is a high rate of spontaneous resolution of IMB and PCB in menstruating women, particularly during the peri-menopausal years.

2.2   Post-menopausal Bleeding

There are many causes of PMB and therefore many different treatments depending on the cause. It can be entirely normal and there may be no cause found; as long as the woman has been investigated, then she can be reassured. Of paramount importance in the woman's mind and that of the health care professional is to exclude cancer, as PMB is a common sign of cancer, although only about 10% of women with PMB have cancer.

Any women with post-menopausal bleeding should be referred to secondary care. The nurse specialist can still be responsible for their care pathway using ultrasound, diagnostic and operative hysteroscopy, and then discharging women if suspected cancer is ruled out.

2.2.1 Definition and Prevalence

Post-menopausal bleeding is a common complaint that represents about 5% of referrals [18].

The number of episodes and amount can vary. Most women have either no cause or a benign cause, but about 10% of women have endometrial cancer [19]. Endometrial cancer accounts for 1 in 18 of every female cancers and is increasing [20].

It is defined as:

- Unscheduled bleeding that occurs a year after the last natural menstrual period [19].
- Any breakthrough bleeding on cyclical hormone replacement therapy (HRT).
- Breakthrough bleeding after 6 months on continuous combined therapy (CCT) after amenorrhea has been established.

2.2.2 Presentation

- No symptoms—found as an incidental finding with imaging for other conditions
- PMB
- Abnormal bleeding
- Vaginal discharge

  More advanced disease may present with:

- Pelvic/back pain
- Pelvic lump
- Pain on intercourse
- Weight loss
- Other presentations of endometrial cancer are abnormal cells on routine cervical screening or persistent vaginal discharge.

The NICE guidance identifies women presenting with PMB as suspected cancer and dictates the need for fast track referral and specific treatment times for these patients [21]. Figure 2.7 below shows a summary for the care of women with PMB.

The main care that women require consists of:

- Pelvic examination with cervical screening and infection screen if needed
- Pelvic or abdominal ultrasound
- Hysteroscopy and endometrial biopsy

2.2.3 Causes of Bleeding

There are many causes of PMB:

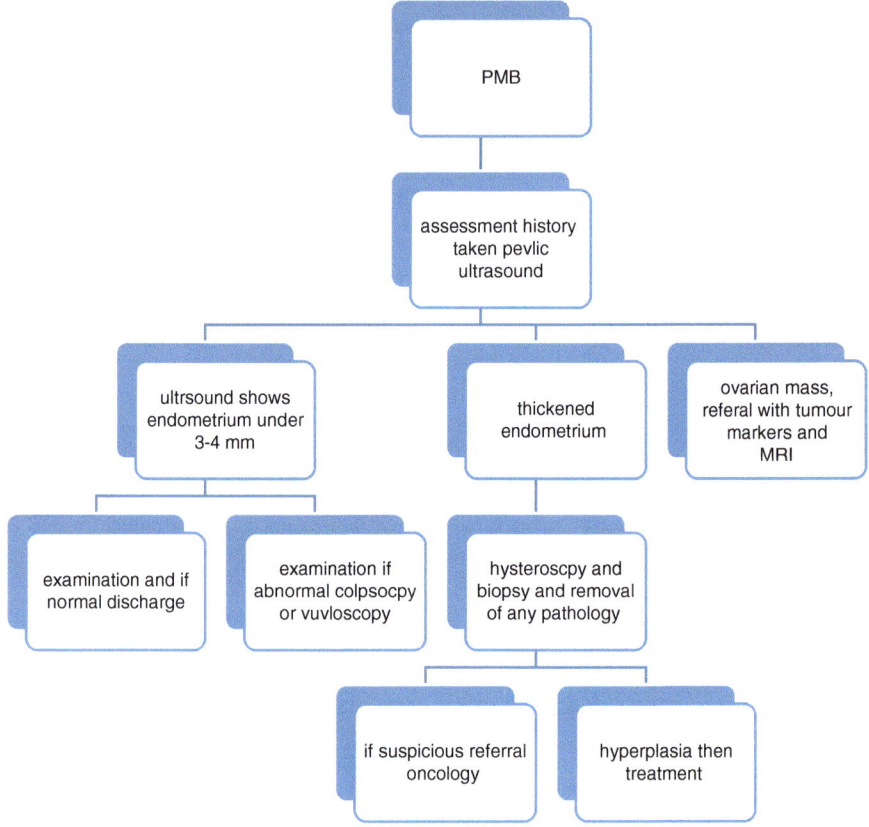

Fig. 2.7 Care of women with PMB

- Once investigated with a scan and then possibly hysteroscopy and biopsy, there may be no cause found. This in itself can be reassuring.
- Atrophic vaginitis—see Chap. 10.
- Cervical polyps.
- Endometrial polyps.
- Submucosal fibroids.
- Bleeding from the bladder.
- Endometrial hyperplasia [5].
- Endometrial cancer—the most common female cancer with a rising incidence. The average age at presentation is during the menopause and post-menopause, but a small percentage are diagnosed before the menopause. The reason for the rise in incidence are multiple and include fewer hysterectomies, as women undergo conservative treatments for HMB, increase in obesity and increased use of tamoxifen. A woman with a BMI of 42 has a tenfold increase in endometrial cancer compared with that of a woman with a normal BMI [22]. There are many different types of endometrial cancer (adenocarcinomas, endometrioid type, papillary serous and clear cell endometrial carcinomas) most commonly endo-

Table 2.2 Risk factors for endometrial cancer

• Over 50 years of age
• Use of unopposed oestrogen
• Obesity, as the circulating oestrogen can impact on the endometrium
• Nulliparity
• Late menopause—due to prolonged stimulation with oestrogen
• Diabetes
• Previous endometrial hyperplasia
• Tamoxifen use, which increases the risk by two- to threefold [23]
• History of polycystic ovaries with a history of long-term non-ovulation, thus increasing endometrial stimulation by oestrogen
• History of HNPCC or lynch syndrome with a lifetime risk of up to 60% [24]
• Hypertension
• Women with a high BMI over 30 have a three times higher risk [25]

metrioid adenocarcinoma, which is often against a background of endometrial hyperplasia. Table 2.2 below shows the risk factors for endometrial cancer.
• Cervical cancer—most of the cervical cancers are squamous cell cancers (80–90%) with the rest being adenocarcinomas. Cervical cancer does not typically present as PMB, but can present as PCB after the menopause. On examination, there may be a tumour of the cervix or it may appear normal. If an abnormality is suspected, then a colposcopy and biopsy should be undertaken.
• Vaginal and vulva cancers and pre-cancerous changes such as VIN and VAIN can also cause bleeding. Any suspicion in this regard will require a vaginoscopy or vulvoscopy and a biopsy.
• *Oestrogen-secreting tumours. These are rare and are normally found with a mass on examination.* They are normally found on the ovary and the oestrogen that is secreted from these can then stimulate the endometrium. If these are suspected, then ultrasound and tumour markers are needed followed by MRI. The treatment would normally be surgery under the care of a gynaecologist–oncologist.

2.2.4 Tamoxifen

Women using tamoxifen can have bleeding, which increases the risk, in addition to benign pathological conditions such as polyps [25]. The effects of tamoxifen on the endometrium are often difficult to fully assess on ultrasound as the picture of the myometrial and endometrial junction makes the endometrium appear thicker with cystic spaces, which does not correlate with the endometrium on hysteroscopy and direct biopsy.

2.2.5 HRT

A common reason for PMB can be HRT (see Chap. 10). This can lead to a discontinuation of HRT and a fear amongst health professionals that it will lead to cancer, but in fact the incidence of endometrial cancer is lower on the CCT HRT than on no therapy or sequential therapy. Bleeding on HRT has the same causes as women who are not on HRT, and thus can be due to polyps and fibroids or it can be related to the HRT itself, such as too much oestrogen or too little progestogen, the wrong type of HRT (such as CCT when they are not post-menopausal).

Other causes can be:

- Poor absorption.
- Compliance.
- Drug interactions.
- Underlying cycle.
- Women on CCT may have atrophy and inactive endometrium due to the use of continuous progesterone. However, there can still be breakthrough bleeding, which is not fully understood.

2.2.6   Conclusion

There can be many different causes of bleeding within the post-menopause and treatments differ from medication and reassurance to complex surgery.

When looking at bleeding it is important to try and classify the cause of the bleeding to try and tailor the treatments. There are some classification systems to help with this. PALM-COEIN (polyp, adenomyosis, leiomyoma, malignancy and hyperplasia, coagulopathy, ovulatory dysfunction, endometrial, iatrogenic and not yet classified) is one of these and as a chapter summary is included in Table 2.3 below [26].

2.3   Polycystic Ovarian Syndrome

Polycystic ovarian syndrome affects 6–8% of women of reproductive age and up to 10% of women worldwide, normally beginning during puberty [27]. It is the most common endocrine disorder [28], with its true prevalence not known.

The syndrome accounts for 80% of cases of hyperandrogenism in women and is a leading cause of infertility [27].

Table 2.3 PALM-COEIN classifications of bleeding [26]

Polyp	Coagulation disorders
Adenomyosis	Ovarian dysfunction
Leiomyomas	Endometrial
Malignancy and hyperplasia	Iatrogenic
	Not yet classified

PALM-COEIN polyp, adenomyosis, leiomyoma, malignancy and hyperplasia, coagulopathy, ovulatory dysfunction, endometrial, iatrogenic and not yet classified

Polycystic ovarian syndrome is a heterogenous multifactorial endocrine disorder with two of the following three criteria [27]:

- Oligo (infrequent bleeding) and/or anovulation (menstrual cycle disturbance).
- Hyperandrogenism (increase in testosterone), which causes increased facial hair, acne.
- Polycystic ovaries that are seen on ultrasound.

The aetiology of PCOS is still unknown; it is a complex disorder that affects multiple systems and the point of origin is still not clear. There is currently no way to prevent PCOS; however, there is a role for lifestyle interventions to prevent long-term complications, but little research into this area has been undertaken [27].

The key to the secondary prevention of long-term conditions is lifestyle and weight loss, which can be seen to increase ovulation in women and prevent the development of diabetes [27].

It has been suggested that there might be defects within the hypothalamic–pituitary axis that lead to an increase in LH or defects in the ovaries, leading to overproduction of androgens or links with insulin resistance. However, it appears to be an inherited disorder with multiple genes involved and multiple organs with a poorly understood pathophysiology. It involves the ovary, adrenal, hypothalamus, pituitary and insulin-sensitive tissues and to compound the complexity, there are subtypes of women with different issues and presentations [27].

Resistance to insulin can lead to compensation by the pancreas, and this promotes ovarian and to some extent adrenal androgen productions. The high insulin also inhibits the hepatic production of sex hormone binding globulin (SHBG), which then compounds the issue, as there is more circulating free androgens. Within the ovary, the higher and continuous exposure to LH also promotes the production of ovarian androgens. The LH, being high, stimulates increased pulses of GnRH, which in turn lead to poor and incomplete follicular development [27].

There are many theories about the cause and its effect on women and this is developing rapidly as the long-term consequences of PCOS are likely to have an impact on women's fertility, reproduction, self-esteem and cardiovascular health into the future [29]. Specialist nurses can undertake the management of women with PCOS in the short and long term and when accessing fertility services.

As the presentation and symptoms can be different for different women there is no formal classification system; however, some have been proposed [27]:

- Mild (16% of women).
- Ovulatory PCOS (16%) with varying symptoms and unknown long-term health risks.
- Hyper-androgenesis and chronic anovulation (7%) with potential health risks.
- Severe PCOS (61%), with irregular periods, PCOS on imaging, elevated androgen, increased insulin concentrations and potential long-term risks.

Women are likely to present with symptoms, or an inability to conceive or concern because of a family history.

2.3.1 Symptoms

As with all conditions, women suspect that they have PCOS based on the symptoms that they have; these can vary from woman to woman, but polycystic ovaries on ultrasound without any symptoms does not constitute PCOS.

- Obesity and weight gain—45% of women with PCOS are obese—central obesity with increased waist hip ratio.
- Menstrual disturbances/lack of ovulation—manifests as amenorrhoea, oligo-menorrhoea (in 70%), abnormal menstrual cycles (in 30%).
- Hirsutism in 60–70%. The presence of thick pigmented hairs on the upper lip, chin, chest, back, arms, peri-umbilical area, thighs and buttocks.
- Acne in 15–25% that lasts beyond adolescence. However, this is a non-specific feature.
- Male pattern balding in 5–10%; in PCOS, this loss is at the vertex or crown.
- All the hyperandrogenism symptoms are exacerbated by obesity.
- Infertility due to anovulation.
- It can be difficult to diagnosis in a younger woman around menarche, when the cycles may well be anovulatory while menstruation starts. In younger women, it is suggested that all three of the Rotterdam criteria are present, as the irregular periods last for at least 2 years after menarche [27].

2.3.2 Diagnosis

The basis of a diagnosis and the guide for future investigations lies with a good history being taken. In addition to a general gynaecology history, the specific points are listed below:

- Age at menarche and cycles after this.
- Reproductive history including contraception used, number of pregnancies and the outcomes (including miscarriages and terminations).
- Family history of PCOS.
- Past menstrual cycles, present cycles, amenorrhoea and/or episodes of menorrhagia or any irregular cycles or IMB.
- Androgenic symptoms of acne, hirsutism, rapid onset virilisation, alopecia, and ask about any treatments used for hair removal or acne treatment.
- Family history of CAD, obesity, diabetes, hyperandrogenism and premature baldness in male relatives.
- Medication history as anti-epileptics can cause hirsutism.
- Lifestyle questions.

There are a few basics that must be undertaken in the examination.

- Measurement of height, weight, BMI, waist and hip circumference.
- Assessment of acne, facial, chest and abdominal hair.
- Blood pressure.
- Breast examination.
- Abdominal striae.
- Familial balding, deepening of voice, broadening of shoulders, decrease in breast size.
- Pelvic bimanual examination, clitoral examination, loss of vaginal rugae is compatible with virilisation (rare) [27].

2.3.3 Diagnostic Criteria

There has been debate over the different diagnostic criteria used with PCOS, the most common is the Rotterdam [29] system that states that two out of the three must be present for diagnosis: hyperandrogenism, oligo- or anovulation and PCOS on imaging. In 2006, the Androgen Excess Society proposed that all three of the following should be present: hyperandrogenism, ovarian dysfunction (infrequent or no periods and PCOS on imaging) and exclusion of other disorders. However, the advice from the RCOG [29] is to use the Rotterdam criteria.

2.3.4 Investigations

- Transvaginal ultrasound is normally the first-line investigation if a woman is sexually active. One polycystic ovary is sufficient to provide a diagnosis of an increase in ovarian volume to more than 10 ml and more than twelve 2- to 9-mm ovarian follicles seen in the ovary [27].
- Polycystic ovaries are seen in 75% of women with PCOS, but also in 25% of women who do not have PCOS.
- Scanning is also used to assess the endometrium and triage women with a thickened endometrium, who would then need further investigation, such as endometrial biopsy and hysteroscopy; however, routine scanning for this is not recommended.

2.3.5 Blood Tests

- Androgens—the decreased SHBG means that there will be a rise in free testosterone in the total testosterone measured, which should be <5 nmol/l. If >5 nmol/l, there is no evidence to measure dehydroepiandrosterone sulphate (DHEA-S); however, androstenedione may also be checked if other androgens are normal and then referral to endocrinologist to exclude adrenal causes [27, 30].

- LH and FSH measurement—day 1–3 of the cycle. LH is elevated and the ratio of LH to FSH is >2:1 (this is normally the only condition that gives an increase in LH over FSH).
- Check FSH and LH to rule out other causes of no periods such as POI or hypothalamic amenorrhoea.
- Thyroid function tests, 17-hydroxyprogesterone and prolactin only if there is amenorrhoea, to exclude disorders that may mimic PCOS symptoms (thyroid dysfunction, hyperprolactinaemia and adrenal hyperplasia).
- Oestradiol is elevated, but there is no indication to measure.
- Oral glucose tolerance test and fasting lipids. Women with PCOS who are overweight and those who are not but have other risk factors should undergo a 2-h oral glucose tolerance test. Women with impaired fasting glucose and/or impaired glucose tolerance test should have an oral glucose test annually [29].

Table 2.4 below shows the test results.

Table 2.4 Test results

Test	Results
Total and serum testosterone The levels can be difficult to measure in women In women with PCOS, 70% have elevated free testosterone, 40% elevated total testosterone and 25% elevated DHEA-S Caution in obese women as SHBG levels are low = increased free and normal total testosterone. Aim to measure in follicular stage	Elevated Do not measure other androgens unless the testosterone level is over 5
DHEA-S	Raised and in 10% of patients, it may be the only androgen raised
Serum 17 hydroxyprogesterone	To exclude adrenal hyperplasia
Prolactin To exclude pituitary problems in women with no ovulation. However, it can be raised in some women with PCOS up to 1300 ng/ml without the need for additional investigations	
TSH	To check that the menstrual dysfunction is not connected thyroid dysfunction
Glucose tolerance test As per local guidelines to check for diabetics Abnormal results are seen in 40% of women with PCOS Women with normal GTT should be screened every 2 years for changes and those with impaired GTT should be screened every 2 years for diabetes A fasting insulin test can be undertaken if needed	
Fasting lipids Abnormal lipids are often seen in women with PCOS and a fasting lipid screen is recommended in women with PCOS	Increased total cholesterol and LDL with low HDL

PCOS polycystic ovary syndrome, *DHEA-S* dehydroepiandrosterone sulphate, *SHBG* sex hormone binding globulin, *TSH* thyroid-stimulating hormone, *GTT* glucose tolerance test, *LDL* low-density lipoprotein, *HDL* high-density lipoprotein

2.3.6 Causes

There is evidence for inheritance. CYP21 and CYP11A genes have been implicated in studies [27]. If a woman has PCOS, her sister has a 20–40% chance of having it as well, and this risk is increased further if they are twins [27].

Current research suggests that PCOS might be a condition that is formed when the women is a foetus in relation to raised anti-Müllerian hormone (AMH), allowing more testosterone to pass to the foetus [31]. The rise in AMH is due to the multiple follicles; with this rise, it keeps the LH high, which supresses ovulation and increases testosterone. In non-PCOS, AMH decreases during pregnancy, but it has been found to remain high and it can inhibit aromatase, which increases testosterone as it is not converted to oestrogen.

However, various aspects of the syndrome may be differentially inherited. Polycystic ovaries have a smooth thickened vascular capsule with hyperplasia of thickened stromal cells surrounding the arrested follicles and microscopic examination shows thickened luteinised theca cells.

2.3.7 Differential Diagnosis

- Thyroid dysfunction
- Hyperprolactinaemia
- Cushing's syndrome
- Androgen-secreting cancers
- Insulin resistance
- Androgen or anabolic drug use
- Hypogonadotropic hypogonadism
- Premature ovarian insufficiency [27]

2.3.8 Treatments

The treatments for PCOS are varied and depend on the presenting complaint and the needs of each individual women, which are usually dependent on fertility wishes. In general, all women should be advised about lifestyle and weight loss.

Treatments can be for: fertility, hirsutism or periods.

Psychologically, excess hair can have a negative impact on women's self-esteem [27–29]. The treatments for this are normally mechanical or hair removal with the topical eflornithine cream helping in some women. If the symptoms of excess androgens are mild, then the COCP can be used [27–29].

The COCP inhibits hormone production of FSH and LH via the feedback system. This in turn increases the production of SHBG, which decreases free testosterone and improves symptoms. Combined pills with androgen progestogens (levonorgestrel and norethisterone) should be avoided in favour of desogestrel or drospirenone. Drospirenone is a spironolactone analogue with anti-androgen properties [27]. However, the newer pills have a higher risk of venous thromboembolism

(VTE); therefore, this needs to be balanced with the women's risks for taking the COCP such as weight, smoking, CVD risks and blood pressure (see Chap. 13) [32].

2.3.9 Hyperandrogenism

If there is more significant hirsutism, then anti-androgens can be used, with assessment at 3 months and if no effect consideration should be given to an androgen secreting tumour. Examples of anti-androgens are spironolactone, cyproterone and finasteride. They should not be taken in pregnancy and used for at least 6 months and sometimes the effectiveness on hair growth is not seen until 12 months of treatment, whereas the effect on acne is much quicker [28]. Some women may need a combination of therapy such as COCP and anti-androgens, and metformin may be added to a COCP as well.

Excess hair should be treated by mechanical means and a combination of hormones such as Dianette, or topically with eflornithine cream. Acne responds to some contraceptive pills, but if it is persistent, then a referral to a dermatologist is required [28].

The use of metformin in women who are not planning to conceive has been covered by NICE [33]. They have concluded that there is not enough evidence to suggest it over and above regimes for hirsutism or acne. There was also no current evidence for the benefits of preventing diabetes and CVD and it also has side effects that may affect compliance with treatment.

2.3.10 Diet and Lifestyle

Obesity increases women's symptoms and worsens the endocrine profile; therefore, women should be encouraged and supported in losing weight. With weight loss, periods may return, meaning a decrease in symptoms, and even achievement of pregnancy [30]. Along with changes in diet, an increase in physical activity is essential. In addition, women may need behavioural therapies to help with lifestyle changes.

- Women with BMI >30 should be encouraged to lose weight and discuss lifestyle issues.
- Weight loss is a desirable outcome in obese women and improves the endocrine profile and likelihood of ovulation.
- Start with decreasing the intake of carbohydrate and fat in every meal and moderately increase protein.
- Low glycaemic index diets may be preferable to diets with a high glycaemic index.
- Moderate physical activity should be encouraged.
- Anti-obesity drugs—orlistat has been studied and is being used in primary care, with small studies in PCOS.
- Metformin may improve insulin resistance and aid weight loss, its role in PCOS and in combination with orlistat is still being evaluated [33].

2.3.11 Menstrual Irregularity

Women with menstrual dysfunction need to ensure that they have adequate progestogen cover for the endometrium to prevent irregular bleeding, hyperplasia and in some cases cancer. This can be achieved by treatments to promote ovulation or they can be given progestogen, such as in contraception, progesterone or the IUS. Weight loss, as always, helps too.

- The easiest way to achieve this is with COCP if there are no current fertility wishes and the woman has no contra-indications to the COCP [32]. The COCP enables regular endometrial shedding, improves the androgen profile and regulates the cycle.
- Cyclical progestogens to induce withdrawal bleeds every 3 months in amenorrhoeic women.
- Levonorgestrel intra-uterine system. The IUS provides endometrial protection in women in anovualtion, controls bleeding and provides contraception.

2.3.12 Infertility

Weight loss can restore ovulation, and this can be as little as 5–7% in overweight women resulting in restoration of ovulation in up to 80% of women [27]. For more information on fertility see Chap. 6.

If this is unsuccessful, then metformin may be added, as this can restore ovulation, but it may take up to 9 months to see the full effects. Data from studies are lacking and this method may not work in all women with PCOS.

Metformin has been shown to increase the conception rate but not the live birth rate. The side effects of metformin are anorexia, nausea, flatulence and diarrhoea [27].

If these do not help, then the drug clomiphene given over 5 days increases gonadotrophin production, promoting the development of follicles, and should be used but only up to six cycles. Women undergoing clomiphene ovulation induction have a 40% chance of conceiving and should be informed about the risk of multiple pregnancy. Nurse specialists have an important role to play in seeing women during ovulation induction and supporting them through fertility treatment [34].

If unsuccessful, women then move on to fertility treatments. Caution must be observed as women with PCOS are more at risk of ovarian hyperstimulation syndrome (OHSS) with fertility treatments [27].

In women who do not respond to treatments, IVF or laparoscopic ovarian diathermy (LOD) may be used. This can increase ovulation, but carries risks such as those associated with laparoscopy, including adhesions. There is a suggested pregnancy rate of 60%, there is no risk of OHSS and a low risk of post-operative adhesions, the effect of LOD is not long-lasting; therefore, it is followed by ovarian stimulation.

2.3.13 Long-TERM Complications

All women with a diagnosis of PCOS should be counselled about the long-term implications and health risks of the condition [27–30].

1. Infertility.
2. Risk of gestational diabetes, and women should be referred to a specialist team if this is detected.
3. Women should be screened for diabetes with a glucose tolerance test (GTT). 10% of obese women with PCOS have type II diabetes by the age of 40 and 35% of obese women have impaired GTT by the age of 40. Insulin resistance with abdominal obesity accounts for a higher prevalence of non-insulin-dependent diabetes mellitus.
4. Women should be aware that there is a risk of sleep apnoea.
5. Increased risk of non-alcoholic fatty liver [35].
6. Risks of CVD—all women should be assessed for risk factors such as obesity, lack of exercise, smoking, family history of diabetes, dyslipidaemia, hypertension and impaired GTT at the initial diagnosis. Abnormal findings should be treated. Women with PCOS are more likely to develop subclinical atherosclerosis of carotid vessels and have a higher risk of myocardial infarction compared with age-matched controls, metabolic disturbances associated with insulin resistance are known to increase cardiovascular risk. Prevalence of treated hypertension is three times higher in women with PCOS. The standard cardiovascular risk calculators have not been validated in women with PCOS [29].
7. Depression, poor self-esteem and anxiety are common, and women should be screened and referred to appropriate counsellors if needed. Psychosocial complications – quality of life is decreased and anxiety and depression increased owing to multiple factors; thus, there is a huge role for the specialist nurse within this area of long-term monitoring and care. Nurses can support women and facilitate onward referrals to other support groups if needed.
8. Risks of cancer—women with scanty or no periods have a risk of endometrial hyperplasia because of the stimulation of the endometrium with oestrogen. As before, it is best to protect the endometrium with an IUS or with oral progesterone stipulating a withdrawal bleed every 3 months. If women have not had endometrial protection, then an ultrasound scan is needed and endometrial biopsy for detection of endometrial hyperplasia owing to the increased risk of endometrial cancer.

   There is no increased risk of breast or cervical cancer. PCOS in combination with ovarian cancer has been poorly studied, but inducing multiple ovulations in chronic anovulation may confer a slightly elevated risk.

2.3.14 Long-Term Management

1. Lifestyle changes, which include diet, weight loss, exercise.

2. Many women and health care professionals ask about the use of metformin in women with PCOS and yet there is no evidence that this has a long-term impact on the outcome of women who are not wanting to conceive [33].
3. Some women may need to be referred for bariatric surgery [27–29].

2.3.14.1 Long Term

Once started on any medication its effectiveness and women's tolerance should be monitored at 3 months and then 6-monthly after that. This may change as the needs of the woman change from symptom management to fertility. All women should be encouraged to increase their physical activity and have a healthy diet; it is often useful to refer them to a dietitian for helpful advice and support. Women should be advised that it is a long-term condition and once under control, symptoms can reoccur if weight is increased or treatments stopped.

2.4 The Future

There are many different treatment options being researched as we become more aware of the complex nature of PCOS and the impact that studies, however small, can have on future health.

Aromatase inhibitors [27]—these reduce the conversion of androgens to oestrogens, which has an impact on the feedback system and allows FSH to increase to stimulate ovarian activity and ovulation. Some studies have shown that the results are similar to those associated with clomiphene for women who wish to conceive and they provide an option for women resistant to clomiphene. Aromatase inhibitors may even become the first-line treatment for women.

Statins—given with the COCP statins reduce androgen levels [27]. This can lead to improved lipids, a decrease in hair and decreased testosterone. Although studies are small, this may be an emerging area that would help many women.

Weight loss medicines—they are beneficial in reducing weight.

Bariatric surgery—small studies have found this beneficial and improved symptoms and chances of conception.

Women can be managed by a specialist nurse in women's health with PCOS in both a community and a hospital setting. Much of the support needed is around lifestyle. Some women will need to be referred on and these are women with a raised testosterone (to exclude other causes), infertility, rapid onset of hirsutism and those who endometrial hyperplasia is suspected.

2.5 Premenstrual Syndrome

2.5.1 Definition

Premenstrual syndrome (PMS) is defined as a condition that manifests with distressing physical, behavioural and psychological symptoms, in the absence of organic or underlying psychiatric disease [36].

The syndrome is always cyclical, regularly recurs during the luteal phase of each cycle and disappears by the end of menstruation [37]. As with many conditions, the degree and type of symptoms can vary significantly. Many women have mild symptoms that do not cause them much trouble; however, at the other end of the spectrum there are women whose symptoms are so severe that they have an impact on everyday life and can cause the breakdown of relationships and normal activities. This severe form of PMS is called premenstrual dysphoric disorder by the American Psychotic Association [37].

Symptoms of PMS are distinguished from normal physiological premenstrual symptoms because they cause significant impairment of daily activity. Additional terms used are premenstrual disorders (PMDs), which cover all sub-groups of PMS.

Within the spectrum of PMS, the following categories are defined [38]:

- Mild PMS—symptoms do not interfere with personal/social and professional life.
- Moderate PMS—interferes with life, but able to function, though sub-optimally.
- Severe—unable to interact.
- Premenstrual exaggeration or exacerbation or an underlying disorder—where conditions flare up premenstrually with incomplete relief of symptoms when menstruation ends. Examples of this can be diabetes, depression, asthma, migraines and epilepsy.
- Premenstrual dysphoric disorder. This condition is recognised in the USA, with some strict criteria for diagnosis of five out of 11 categories, one of which must be mood, but this diagnosis can be restrictive and miss out other women with severe symptoms. It defines severe PMS, which occurs in 3% of the at-risk population.
- Non-ovulatory PMDs is a new classification within the updated RCOG guidelines [38]. The symptoms occur without ovulation and the mechanism is not understood.
- Progesterone-induced PMDs—caused by exogenous progestogens such as the COCP or HRT, where the symptoms like those they had with PMS return. They are not cyclical and are more common in women who are progestogen-sensitive.
- PMDs without menstruation—for women with an ovarian cycle, but no bleeding owing to surgery or IUS.

2.5.2   Causes and Prevalence

There is no consensus on the precise aetiology of PMS [36–38]. However, it revolves around cyclical ovarian activity and the effect of the levels of oestrogen and progesterone on neurotransmitters serotonin and gamma-aminobutyric (GABA) appears to be the key factor [37]. PMS is not seen in pregnancy, before puberty or after the menopause, which supports the notion of ovarian cycle involvement. However, changes in oestrogen levels postnatally and post-menopause can give rise to similar depressive symptoms, often in women who had experienced PMS before [36]. The two current theories are:

1. Some women are sensitive to progestogens, as when measured in women with PMS and without the blood levels of both oestradiol and progesterone being the same.
2. Implicated in PMS are the neurotransmitters serotonin and GABA. Serotonin receptors are responsive to oestrogen and progestogen and SSRIs which can known to reduce PMS symptoms. GABA levels are modulated by the metabolite of progestogen and in women with PMS, these metabolite levels are reduced [37].

The prevalence of clinical PMS is as high as 40% [38] but severe PMS is thought to affect 5–8% of the at-risk population [38]. However, this is probably under-reported. Women who are on hormonal contraception and who have normal weight and regular exercise appear to have a lower prevalence. There is some ongoing work looking at genetic disposition to PMS, but nothing conclusive as yet.

Establishing the diagnosis is essential. Symptoms should be recorded prospectively over two to three cycles using a symptom diary/menstrual chart and not made on recall of retrospective events. This should be in a chart of a diary specially designed to record symptoms [38].

2.5.3 Assessment and Diagnosis

History and prospective symptom charting are the basis for establishing a diagnosis, in addition to general history, which includes gynaecological and obstetric, as PMS can be common in women who have had postnatal depression. There should be discussion and questions on lifestyle such as diet, exercise, smoking and alcohol and drug habits. If there is a doubt a symptom diary has been used, then a 3-month trial of GnRH can be used to establish a definitive diagnosis [38].

2.5.4 Symptoms

There is a vast array of symptoms that can vary, but generally are psychological such as mood swings, anxiety, depression, and physical such as bloating and breast pain (Table 2.5). With PMS it is the timing and the cyclical nature of the symptoms. There is no limit or weighting applied to any of the symptoms to aid in diagnosis [37].

No blood tests or physical examinations are needed to diagnose PMS; however, if there is any doubt over the diagnosis, then differential diagnoses can be thyroid disorder; thus, TSH is needed, peri-menopause (FSH and LH are needed) depression (depression screening tools) [36].

Table 2.5 Typical symptoms of PMS

Psychological symptoms	Physical symptoms	Behavioural changes
Irritability	Headache	Reduced cognitive ability
Mood swings	Bloating	Increased risk of accidents
Depression	Breast tenderness	Poor concentration
Aggression	Swelling of the limbs or fingers	
Irrational thoughts	Weight gain	
Tiredness/fatigue	Clumsiness	
Reduced cognitive function	Backache	
Sleep disorders	Hot flushes before period (20%)	
Food cravings	Palpitations (20%)	
Forgetfulness and difficulty concentrating	Gastrointestinal upset	

2.5.5 Treatment and Management

Once diagnosed, explained and explored there are some simple measures that can be discussed:

- Reduction in stress, although there is no evidence base that can be helpful in reducing the reaction to the symptoms [37].
- Changes to diet, such as reducing carbohydrates and alcohol and caffeine, can help in the premenstrual phase, as can exercise; however, in moderate to severe cases in addition to this, treatment will need to be started [37]. This may include referral for psychological or psychiatric therapy and for CBT [37, 38].
- The treatment of women with PMS needs to be an integrated holistic approach with a multidisciplinary team (MDT) composed of GP, gynaecologist, mental health practitioner and a dietitian.

Table 2.6 shows lifestyle advice.

The use of complementary and alternative medicines and therapies.

The evidence is often limited or conflicting; however, women do benefit from an integrated holistic approach and the following are some complementary and alternative medicines (CAMs) that women may try [37, 38].

- Vitamin B6—mixed results, but caution should be taken with a large dosage because of peripheral neuropathy.
- Magnesium—there is some evidence that this may help PMS.
- Calcium and vitamin D—some studies have suggested that women might be at a higher risk of PMS if they have lower calcium and that a high intake of vitamin D and calcium may help to prevent the symptoms, but more data are needed.

Table 2.6 Lifestyle advice

Avoidance of smoking
Avoidance of alcohol
Avoidance of caffeine
Vitamin B6
Balanced diet, which includes magnesium-rich food, potassium-rich food and drinking plenty of water
Exercise and relaxation strategies; recent studies have shown an unbeneficial effect of exercise on PMS [39]
Diet of small, frequent meals with complex carbohydrates to ensure steady blood sugar, and reduce the tendency to overeat

- There are limited data to support the use of soy isoflavones and red clover in women with PMS and menstrual migraines.
- Agnus castus is the best research CAM and does help some women with PMS; as with all CAMs, larger randomised controlled trials (RCTs) are needed and the dosage needs to be standardised.
- St John's wort also helps in mild to moderate cases of PMS, but caution is needed because of its multiple drug interactions. It helps behavioural symptoms, but there is a high drop-out rate because of the side effects.
- Evening primrose oil is often suggested for PMS because of its content of gamma-linolenic acid.
- Reflexology—small studies showing some benefit.
- Ginkgo biloba—some benefit.
- Acupuncture—some benefit.

2.5.6 Medical Treatments

The medical treatments of PMS are split into two groups: one is the suppression of ovulation and the other targets SSRIs. Many of the treatments are off-licence, but do have evidence behind them.

- Suppression of ovulation [36–38].
    - Normally with the COCP.
        This suppresses ovulation; however, when given in the cyclical contraceptive way and used with some of the progestogens such as LNG, then the symptoms may remain. Therefore, in women with PMS it should be given continuously and with different progestogens (drospirenone, products Yasmin and Yaz); however, prescribers need to be aware of the increased risk of VTE with these preparations [32].
    - Transdermal oestrogen—transdermal oestradiol patches can be used at 100 mcg (off-license with no long-term safety data on breast and endometrial safety); therefore, an individual risk and benefits assessment is needed. Women need to use additional contraception as suppression of ovulation can

in theory not be guaranteed. In addition, to protect the endometrium, progestogen needs to be used and this can enhance the PMS-like symptoms; thus, the lowest dose possible needs to be used such as the IUS or vaginal pessaries or micronised progesterone. The progestogen is to prevent endometrial hyperplasia so this needs to be a minimum of 10–12 cyclical progestogens or IUS. On these regimes, there should be a low threshold for investigating unscheduled bleeding. Women should be counselled that even the low levels from the IUS can give PMS-like symptoms and bleeding initially.
- A treatment that is effective for PMS is danazol, but because of its masculinising side effects, the risks are not thought to outweigh the benefits; therefore, it is not normally administered, but can be used at 200 mg twice daily during the luteal phase with additional contraception.
- Gonadotrophin-releasing hormone (GnRH) analogues. These have been used for a long time in many different conditions to suppress ovulation, and they should be reserved for women with severe PMS after different treatments have been tried because of side effects and long-term effects. They can be used alone for 6 months and to prevent menopausal symptoms and bone density loss. HRT in the form of tibolone or continuous combined HRT should be used. In addition to the add-back HRT, bone density scans should be undertaken yearly and the treatment stopped if the density falls significantly. GnRH analogues can also be taken for a couple of months to assess symptoms and to aid diagnosis before surgery.
- Progestogen therapy has not been shown to be beneficial and although progestogen-only contraception such as injections (Depo), implants and Cerazette do suppress ovulation, they may replace the cyclical symptoms with long-term low-level symptoms. As with the other progestogen-only contraception, there is no evidence for treating PMS with the IUS, except as part of endometrial protection.

- Surgical suppression of ovulation.
    Women with severe symptoms that are resistant to treatment but do respond to GnRH analogues may benefit from a total abdominal hysterectomy (TAH) and a bilateral oophorectomy. This is obviously not without risk and should be used as a last resort. Women need adequate counselling that they will need to use HRT, which may include testosterone, and that the ovaries need to be removed in addition to the uterus.

- Selective serotonin reuptake inhibitors [36–38].
    As serotonin is thought to be a cause of PMS, SSRIs have been used in the treatment. RCTs show their benefits over placebo. SSRIs should be considered one of the first-line treatments in severe PMS [38]. The treatment should be with a specialist and the evidence suggests that using them for the second half of the cycle might be just as effective as using them continuously. This cyclical use reassures the user that these are not habit-forming; however, if used on a continu-

ous basis, then they will need to be withdrawn gradually. As with this medication for any indication, the women need to be warned of side effects such as nausea, insomnia, somnolence, fatigue and reduction of libido. This can be minimised by use during the luteal phase. This treatment should be discontinued before and during pregnancy. Examples are fluoxetine (20–60 mg daily), sertraline (50–100 mg daily) and citalopram (20–30 mg daily).

- Diuretics.
  Spironolactone (100 mg) has been shown to help with mood and physical symptoms, especially weight gain [38].
- Cognitive behavioural therapy.
  Cognitive behavioural therapy (CBT) [38] can be used with SSRIs or by itself and should be made available to women with PMS symptoms. CBT is associated with better maintenance of the symptoms in the long term.

Women with severe PMS should be managed by an MDT, which should consist of GP, gynaecologist, mental health care professional and dietitian. However, very few specialist centres exist in the UK.

2.5.7 Surgical Treatment

In women who have severe PMS, hysterectomy and bilateral salpingo-oophorectomy (BSO) has been shown to be of benefit, if medical and other treatments have failed. However, it should normally be carried out after a trial of GnRH and add-back to check that HRT is tolerated in younger women, as after the TAH and BSO she will need to use oestrogen and possibly testosterone if under the age of 45 (See Chap. 10). Women often ask for the ovaries to be removed and this should not be undertaken without the uterus; HRT would then need to involve progestogen, which can bring back PMS-like symptoms [38].

Table 2.7 shows a summary of treatments for PMS.

Table 2.7 Summary of treatments (adapted from the RCOG Green Top Guideline)	
	First line:
	Exercise, CBT, vitamin B6
	Combined pills—new generation
	Continuous or luteal phase—SSRIs (citalopram 10 mg)
	Second line:
	Estradiol patches (100 mg) and progestogen
	Higher-dose SSRI (citalopram 20–40 mg
	Third line:
	GnRH analogues and add-back
	Fourth line:
	Surgical treatment and HRT

References

1. BMJ Best Practice (2018) Assessment of menorrhagia. BMJ Publishing
2. NICE Clinical Guideline (2018) Heavy menstrual bleeding. Lumsden MA, Rees M (2014) Menstrual problems, 2nd edn. RCOG, London. https://www.nice.org.uk/guidance/ng88
3. Alexandra I et al (2016) Women's health care in advanced practice nursing. Chapter 28: Peri menstrual and pelvic symptoms and syndromes. Springer, New York
4. AAGL practice report (2012) Practice guidelines for the diagnosis and management of endometrial polyps. J Minim Invasive Gynecol 19(1):3–9
5. https://www.rcog.org.uk/globalassets/documents/guidelines/green-top-guidelines/gtg_67_endometrial_hyperplasia.pdf. 2016
6. Royal College of Obstetricians and Gynaecologists/BSGE (2011) Best practice in outpatient hysteroscopy (Green Top Guideline No. 59). https://www.rcog.org.uk/en/guidelines-research-services/guidelines/gtg59/. Accessed 7 Jul 2018
7. Bryant Smith A, Lethaby A, Farquhar C, Hikey M (2018) Antifibrinolytics for heavy menstrual bleeding. Cochrane Database Syst Rev 4: CD000249
8. Buttram VC, Reiter RC (1981) Uterine leiomyomata: etiology, symptomatology and management. Fertil Steril 36:433–445
9. Holloway D (2017). https://www.guidelinesfornurses.co.uk/womens-health/practical-tips-for-the-diagnosis-and-management-of-fibroids/453725.article
10. BMJ Best Practice (2018) Fibroids. BMJ, London
11. Lumsden MA, West CP, Thomas E, Coutts J, Hillier H, Thomas N, Baird DT (1994) Treatment with the gonadotrophin releasing hormone-agonist goserelin before hysterectomy for uterine fibroids. BJOG 101:438–442
12. Chabbert-Buffet N, Kolanska K et al (2018) Selective progesterone receptor modulators: current applications and perspectives. Climacteric 21(4):375–379. https://doi.org/10.1080/13697 137.2017.1386650
13. https://www.rcog.org.uk/en/guidelines-research-services/guidelines/esmya-ulipristal-acetate%2D%2D-mhra-safety-alert/
14. Lumsden MA (2010) Modern management of fibroids. Obstet Gynaecol Reprod Med 20(3):82–86
15. BMJ Best Practice (2018) Assessment of vaginal bleeding. BMJ
16. Sweet MG, Schmidt-Dalton TA, Weiss PM et al (2012) Evaluation and management of abnormal uterine bleeding in premenopausal women. Am Fam Physician 185(1):35–43
17. Management of Unscheduled Bleeding in Women Using Hormonal Contraception; Faculty of Sexual and Reproductive Healthcare (2009). https://www.rcog.org.uk/globalassets/documents/guidelines/unscheduledbleeding23092009.pdf
18. Guruwadayarhalli B, Jones SE, Srinivasan V (2007) Hysteroscopy in the diagnosis of postmenopausal bleeding. Menopause Int 13(3):132–134
19. Scottish Intercollegiate Guidelines Network (2002) Investigation of post-menopausal bleeding: a national clinical guideline. SIGN publication no 61. SIGN, Edinburgh
20. Bray F, Dos S, Silva I, Moller H, Weiderpass E (2005) Endometrial cancer incidence trends in Europe: underlying determinants and prospects for prevention. Cancer Epidemiol Biomark Prev 14(5):1132–1142
21. National Institute of Clinical Excellence (2017) https://www.nice.org.uk/guidance/ng12
22. Mackintosh M, Crosbie E (2012) Obesity driven endometrial cancer: is weight loss the answer? BJOG 120:791–794
23. Kalampokas T, Sofoudis C, Anastasopoulos C et al (2013) Effects of tamoxifen on postmenopausal endometrium. Eur J Gynaecol Oncol 34(4):325–328
24. Manchanda R, Menon U, Michaelson-Cohen R, Beller U, Jacobs I (2009) Hereditary non-polyposis colorectal cancer or Lynch syndrome: the gynaecological perspective. Curr Opin Obstet Gynecol 21(1):31–38

25. Humphrey MM, Apte SM (2009) The use of minimally invasive surgery for endometrial cancer. Cancer Control 16(1):30–37
26. https://www.figo.org/sites/default/files/uploads/IJGO/papers/AUB%20Classification.pdf
27. BMJ Best Practice (2018) Polycystic ovary syndrome. BMJ
28. Connolly A (2018) Polycystic ovary syndrome requires long term holistic care. Guidelines in practice
29. RCOG Green Top Guidelines (2014) Long term consequences of polycystic ovary syndrome. RCOG Green Top Guideline number 33
30. ESHRE. https://www.monash.edu/medicine/sphpm/mchri/pcos/guideline
31. Brooke T, Mimouni NEH, Barbotin A et al (2018) Elevated prenatal anti-Müllerian hormone reprograms the fetus and induces polycystic ovary syndrome in adulthood. Nat Med 24:834–846
32. https://www.fsrh.org/ukmec/
33. https://www.nice.org.uk/advice/esuom6/chapter/key-points-from-the-evidence
34. Morris EJ (2001) The role of infertility nurses in ovulation induction programmes. Hum Fertil 4(1):14–17
35. Kumarendran B, O'Reilly M, Manolopoulos K et al (2018) Polycystic ovary syndrome, androgen excess, and the risk of nonalcoholic fatty liver disease in women: a longitudinal study based on a United Kingdom primary care database. PLoS 15(3):e1002542
36. BMJ Best Practice (2017) Premenstrual syndrome and dysphoric disorder. BMJ
37. Panay N. NAPS guidelines on premenstrual syndrome. https://www.pms.org.uk/assets/files/guidelinesfinal60210.pdf
38. Green LJ, O'Brien P, Panay N, Craig M, on behalf of RCOG (2017) Management of premenstrual syndrome. RCOG Green Top Guideline 48
39. Dehnvi M, Jafarnejad F, Sadeghu Goghary S (2018) The effect of 8 weeks of aerobic exercise on the severity of physical symptoms of premenstrual syndrome: a clinical trial study. BMC Womens Health 18(1):80

Colposcopy and Cervical Problems

3

Jennie Deeks

Women experiencing symptoms suggesting a cervical problem should initially visit their GP or practice nurse for a primary consultation.

Although this chapter discusses colposcopy and cervical problems, not all cervical problems will require referral to a colposcopy clinic.

3.1 The Cervix

Often referred to as the neck of the womb, the cervix is the lower part of the uterus (womb) which extends into the upper vagina. See Fig. 3.1.

3.2 Human Papillomavirus (HPV)

The HPV family of viruses contains more than 100 types; some types of HPV cause benign skin warts, or papillomas, which gave this group of viruses its name. Approximately 40 HPV types affect the genital area. They can be subdivided into those that are low risk for cervical cancer (such as HPV-6 and HPV-11, which are responsible for causing genital warts) and those which are high risk for cervical cancer.

HPV is the most common sexually transmitted infection; however cervical cancer is initiated by high-risk types of HPV; the two high-risk HPV types that most commonly cause cervical cancer are HPV-16 and HPV-18, which together are responsible for approximately 70% of cervical cancer [1].

HPV is so common that it can almost be considered a normal consequence of having sex. Estimates suggest that between 50% and 79% of all women who have

J. Deeks (✉)
Quality Matron United Lincolnshire Hospitals NHS Trust, Lincolnshire, UK

Basildon and Thurrock University Hospitals NHSFT, Basildon, UK

© Springer Nature Switzerland AG 2019
D. Holloway (ed.), *Nursing Management of Women's Health*,
https://doi.org/10.1007/978-3-030-16115-6_3

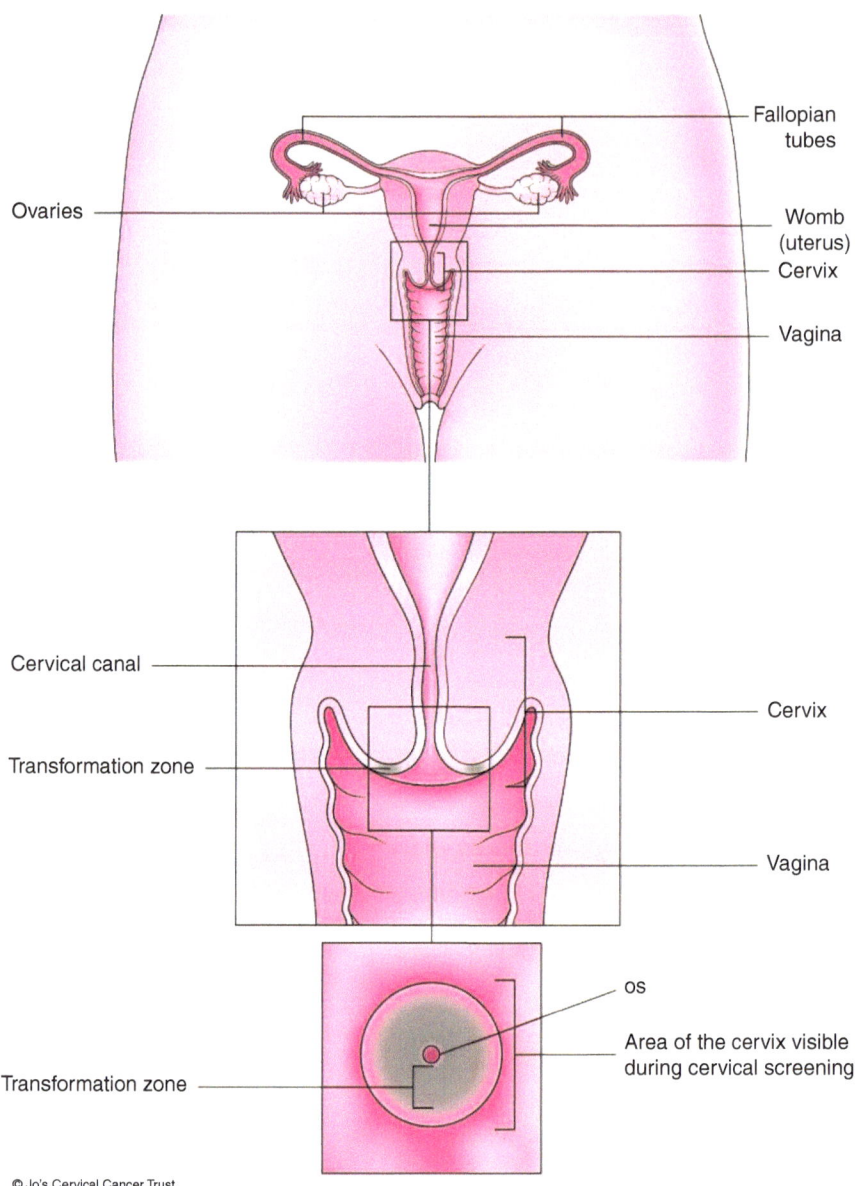

Fallopian tubes

Ovaries

Womb (uterus)

Cervix

Vagina

Cervical canal

Cervix

Transformation zone

Vagina

os

Area of the cervix visible during cervical screening

Transformation zone

Fig. 3.1 Position of the cervix. Figure is taken from Jo's Cervical Cancer Trust (2018)

had sexual intercourse have a lifetime risk of becoming infected with one or more of the sexually transmitted HPV types. Often the infection is transient, and it is only when it becomes persistent, and in a small minority of women, that this may lead to cervical intraepithelial neoplasia, better known as CIN—the abnormal growth of precancerous cells in the cervix. Figure 3.2 shows HPV under a microscope and a view on the cervix at colposcopy.

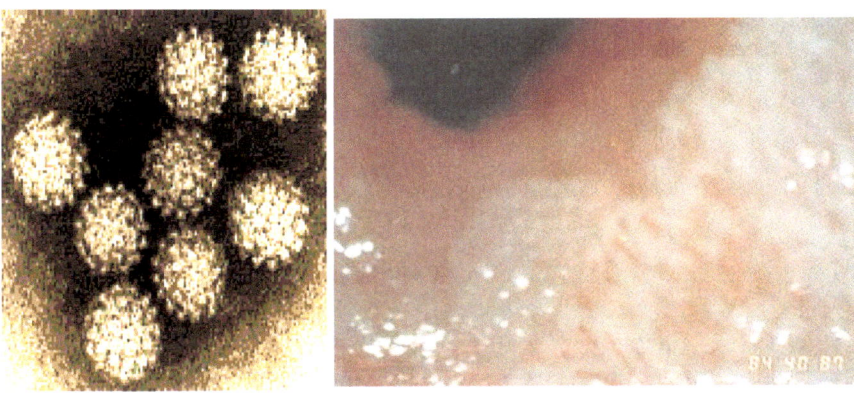

Fig. 3.2 HPV under microscope and colposcope

In summary:

- HPV infection is almost a normal consequence of sex.
- In most women, HPV will cause no long-term harm and will be eradicated by the immune system.
- Genital warts do not cause cervical cancer.
- There are no externally visible physical signs of high-risk HPV; you can only tell you have it by undergoing specific tests.
- Regular cervical screening (smear tests) can pick up the changes which could progress to cancer.
- The HPV vaccination programme was introduced in September 2008 for girls aged 12–13 years in year 8 of school. Whilst effective, it doesn't eradicate HPV risk completely.

3.3   Colposcopy

3.3.1   Colposcopy and Cervical Screening Within the UK

All eligible women, in the UK, have a right to access a National Cervical Screening Programme (NCSP) and to have a cervical screening test taken by an appropriately trained, competent and skilled sample taker. Since the introduction of the NHS' computerised call and recall system for cervical screening, the majority of cervical samples are now undertaken in the primary care setting. However, some patients who have had previous abnormal history, or are known to be difficult to sample, may be referred to a colposcopy clinic for a colposcopist to perform their cervical screening. Figure 3.3 shows the colposcope used in colposcopy appointment.

Cervical colposcopy is part of the NHS cervical screening service. Screening tests are undertaken to monitor the health of an individual and are designed to detect diseases, precursors or factors which predispose asymptomatic people to disease [2].

Fig. 3.3 Colposcope

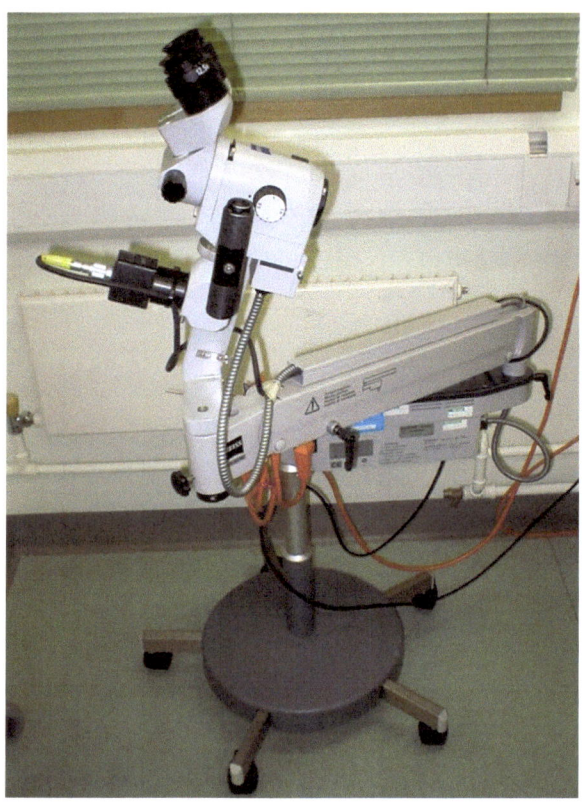

The UK National Screening Committee (UK NSC) defines screening as:

'...a public health service in which members of a defined population, who do not necessarily perceive they are at risk of, or are already affected by a disease or its complications, are asked a question or offered a test, to identify those individuals who are more likely to be helped than harmed by further tests or treatment to reduce the risk of a disease or its complications' [3].

Cervical screening is unique, as it allows signs of changes to be identified at an early stage when treatment—which can be carried out on an outpatient basis—effectively prevents the vast majority of cases progressing to cervical cancer. Poor technique in cervical screening, however, may result in a failure to detect precancerous abnormalities hence sample takers within the NHSCSP must be appropriately trained and updated to reduce the chance of a woman undergoing poor quality screening (see Sec. 3.4.4). Screening intervals vary as a woman gets older, and intervals will change in response to an abnormality being detected. A decision to cease screening will depend on the patient's screening history. Any decisions regarding changes to a screening routine will be made by the responsible clinician.

Approximately 6% of women will have an abnormal cervical screening result, and these are reported as low-grade squamous intraepithelial lesions (LSIL) or high-grade squamous intraepithelial lesions (HSIL) [3]. If a screening result shows a low-grade result in the absence of HPV DNA, the this will mean a return to routine 3 or 5 yearly recall. Low-grade abnormalities with HPV DNA present, and high-grade abnormal results, these women are referred to their local colposcopy clinic for assessment and/or treatment.

If treatment is required, women will require one further screening test 6 months after treatment, known as 'test of cure'. If this result is normal, they will be returned to routine 3 or 5 yearly recall. If an abnormality is identified, the woman will be seen again in the colposcopy clinic.

The investigation and actual diagnosis of an abnormal test result can only be confirmed following histological assessment of a cervical tissue biopsy, usually undertaken at a colposcopy clinic. Histological precancerous abnormalities (CIN) if detected can be treated or monitored in colposcopy clinic. CIN or cervical intraepithelial neoplasia literally means the presence or formation of new, abnormal cell growth within the layer of cells forming the surface or lining of the cervix. CIN can be either low grade (CIN 1) or high grade (CIN 2 or 3). In some cases the abnormality will be classed as cervical glandular intraepithelial neoplasia (CGIN). These abnormalities affect the inner part of the cervix (endocervix) whereas CIN affects the outer part of the cervix (ectocervix).

CIN is primarily detected through the National Cervical Screening Programme (NCSP), and depending on the grade, this will dictate the treatment or management plan. All low-grade cytology results are automatically referred for HPV testing; if this is negative, the woman is at negligible risk and will be returned to normal call/recall. If the HPV test is positive, colposcopy referral is required. Current guidelines recommend that all ladies who are referred to a colposcopy clinic with a low-grade, HPV-positive cytology result associated with atypical transformation zone should have directed punch biopsies of the cervix at their first visit where possible. If there is no atypical transformation zone present, a colposcopic biopsy is not indicated. The screening programme is consistently evolving as is the development of HPV knowledge, and there will be moves in the future to have HPV as the primary test, followed by cytological screening if necessary.

3.4 Treatment of CIN

3.4.1 Local Destruction/Cryotherapy

Women with low-grade cytology results can be managed conservatively as CIN 1 can regress. In some cases treatment may be the preferred course of action, and for these low-grade abnormalities, cryotherapy is acceptable. Any kind of destructive therapy must not be performed unless there has been a previous directed biopsy result alternatively through application of nitrous oxide through a probe indicating that the woman definitely has low-grade disease. This can be undertaken by a cold coagulator as seen in Fig. 3.4. The British Society for Colposcopy and Cervical pathology (BSCCP) recommends that prior to performing any such treatment, colposcopists must review cytology, histology and colposcopy results, to avoid likelihood of something more sinister being present and undiagnosed.

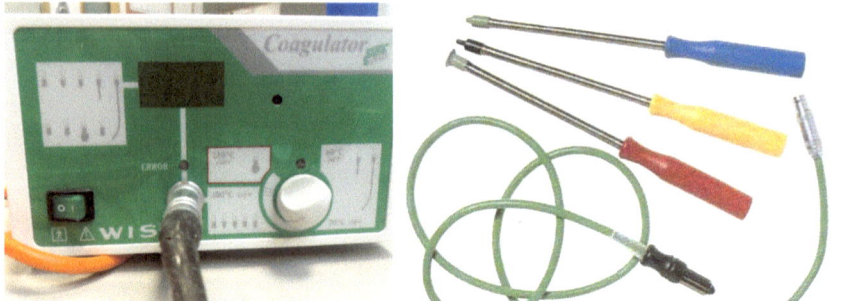

Fig. 3.4 Cold coagulator and probes

3.4.2 Excisional Treatment

In the case of high-grade cytology or a biopsy result indicating CIN 2 or above, excisional treatment is recommended. A common form of excisional treatment is the large loop excision of the transformation zone (LLETZ). This can usually be performed very easily in an outpatient colposcopy clinic, with minor discomfort to the woman. The advantage of LLETZ treatment over ablative techniques is the ability to confirm diagnosis histologically by sending the piece of removed cervix for testing. Ablative techniques cannot offer this level of reassurance.

3.4.3 Post Treatment

Following treatment for CIN, most women will have an uneventful recovery; however some women may experience symptoms. Mild period style pain is expected but will normally pass within a few hours. Paracetamol or ibuprofen should be adequate relief for this. Cryotherapy can cause excessive watery discharge, whereas women who have had LLETZ may experience some bleeding and brown discharge. These symptoms are expected as part of the normal healing processes. Infection is relatively unlikely as all colposcopy equipment is sterile or single use; it is often dependent on how compliant the woman has been with her post-procedure guidance. Offensive discharge, excessive bleeding and low abdominal pain can all be indicators that an infection is developing.

There is a minimally higher risk of premature birth in pregnancies following a cervical LLETZ. This is a rare complication but will be more likely in cases where multiple treatments or excessively large treatments are required. The risks associated with treatment should be discussed with women but will generally be outweighed by the benefits the treatment offers.

3.4.4 Cytology Training for Nurses

Public Health England (PHE) has a set of resources available to those working within the NHSCSP, and these include e-learning packages and videos; however there are only five NHS CSP-approved cervical cytology training centres in the UK, four in England and one in Scotland. More detailed information can be accessed from the PHE website.

3.4.5 Colposcopy Training for Nurses

The joint BSCCP/RCOG training programme is currently the only recognised colposcopy training and certification programme for colposcopists who wish to practise within the NHSCSP [4].

Colposcopy training currently involves colposcopic assessments initially under supervision and, additionally, completion of an electronic logbook of cases. Trainees must also attend histopathological and cytopathological sessions. Once the trainee is ready, they will undergo an OSCE (Objective Structured Clinical Examination).

As with any skill, practice must be maintained and, in the case of colposcopy, must be evidenced in order for a colposcopist to retain their accreditation. Colposcopists practising within the NHSCSP must see at least 50 new referrals per year arising from the NHS screening programme and attend an update at least once in a 3 yearly period. Performance is also monitored on an ongoing basis by the lead colposcopist and hospital-based programme coordinator within each colposcopy clinic.

3.5 What Is the Relationship Between HPV and Cervical Cancer?

Women who test positive for a high-risk HPV may not necessarily go on to develop cervical cancer. It's not certain why in some women, persistent HPV infection causes more serious problems than in others. A positive test does, however, indicate that a woman is at greater risk than one who tests negative. In most women, the immune system successfully deals with any initial HPV infection. This happens before the HPV can completely incorporate itself into the cell DNA and disrupt cell reproduction, leading to CIN. Regular cervical screening (smear tests) can pick up the changes which could progress to cancer [5]. Confirmation of the presence of high-risk HPVs can only be achieved using biomolecular HPV testing.

There are co-factors which can increase the risk of cervical cancer. These include smoking and having more than four full-term pregnancies. Some studies have also suggested that experiencing first intercourse at an early age, having multiple sexual partners or having intercourse with a male partner who has had multiple sexual partners can contribute to a woman's risk; also immune suppression has been identified as a co-factor [6].

Around 30 HPV types are transmitted through sexual contact, including the high-risk HPVs implicated in cervical cancer. An increase in the incidence of genital HPV infection occurs when individuals begin to engage in sexual activity. The great majority of genital HPV infections never cause any overt symptoms and are spontaneously cleared by the immune system in a matter of months. It's not known whether the immune system clears the HPV virus from the body or whether the virus remains but causes little harm.

Genital HPV infection is very common, and all sexually active women are at risk.

Transmission of HPV infection occurs through skin-to-skin contact; in the case of genital HPVs, this transition takes place as a result of sexual activities. Some low-risk HPV types, such as genital warts, have however been found where an individual has not had a sexual experience.

Studies into vaccine efficacy are finding HPV vaccines are well tolerated whilst being effective against high-risk HPV [7]. Whilst 99% effective [8], acknowledges the current vaccines do not offer protection against all types of HPV that can cause cervical cancer; however there is evidence of some cross protection.

3.6 Cervical Cancer

Cervical cancer is a largely preventable disease, but worldwide it is one of the leading causes of cancer death in women, with most deaths occurring in low- to middle-income countries [1]. The primary cause of cervical precancer and cancer is persistent or chronic infection with one or more of the 'high-risk' (or oncogenic) types of human papillomavirus (HPV). In most women and men who become infected with HPV, these infections will resolve spontaneously; however for a minority, this may lead to precancerous changes to the cervix, which, if not treated, may progress to cancer 10–20 years later. Understanding and identification of HPV are important public health concerns and form part of the national screening programme [9].

Healthcare practitioners must support informed sensitive care for women, enabling them to take full advantage of the UK cervical screening programme from vaccination to cervical treatment.

3.6.1 Types of Cervical Cancer

There are two main types of cervical cancer:

• Squamous cell carcinoma (SCC)
• Adenocarcinoma

SCC is the most common and accounts for approximately 90–95% of all cervical cancers.

The precursor lesions for SCC are identified as dyskaryosis (cell change) through cervical screening (smear tests) and identified histologically through colposcopy and biopsy as cervical intraepithelial neoplasia (CIN)—the abnormal growth of precancerous cells in the cervix.

There are three distinct CIN classifications or grades for categorising abnormal (precancerous) cell growth: CIN 1, CIN 2 and CIN 3.

These generally correspond to the smear results of mild (CIN 1), moderate (CIN 2) or severe dyskaryosis (CIN 3), respectively.

In most women it takes many years to progress from a normal cervix to CIN 3.

However, it should be noted that not all women with CIN 3, even if left untreated, will go on to develop cancer [10].

The challenge is in identifying those women who have the potential to progress to cancer and those who do not. As a result, all women with CIN are treated as if they have the potential to develop cervical cancer.

Adenocarcinoma is far more difficult to detect at a precancerous stage. Cervical cytology is unreliable at picking up the glandular changes that indicate that an adenocarcinoma could develop.

As well as cervical problems detected as part of the NHSCSP, women may have cause to seek advice from medical or nursing staff regarding concerns about their cervical health during their screening interval. There are various reasons why women could be experiencing symptoms; the remainder of this chapter intends to demystify some of these conditions.

3.6.2   Cervical Trauma

Anyone involved in caring for women should be aware that domestic violence is not uncommon and cervical symptoms may be due to trauma. Any woman with new and/or unexplained cervical symptoms should have a physical examination. This can not only rule out evident pathology but assess for injury and inflammation/ infection. Genital examination can reveal external abnormalities such as *Candida albicans*, lichen sclerosis or vulval lesions; additionally during the internal examination, abnormal vaginal discharge or signs of infection may be seen.

Should a woman disclose domestic violence during a consultation, clinicians should be prepared to give her information regarding local or national support services; the Department of Health website has a number of useful resources. In all cases identified, the healthcare professional should consider the need to discuss safeguarding intervention with their patient.

3.6.3   Cervical Ectropion

Also known as cervical erosion, this is a very common cervical condition in women of menstrual age. There are two types of cells on the cervix, the tougher shiny appearance 'ectocervical' cells which usually cover the outside of the cervix and the rougher looking 'endocervical' cells which are usually found within the endocervical canal. A cervical ectropion is where some endocervical tissue has protruded to the outside of the cervix. Figure 3.5 shows how this looks during the colposcopy examination.

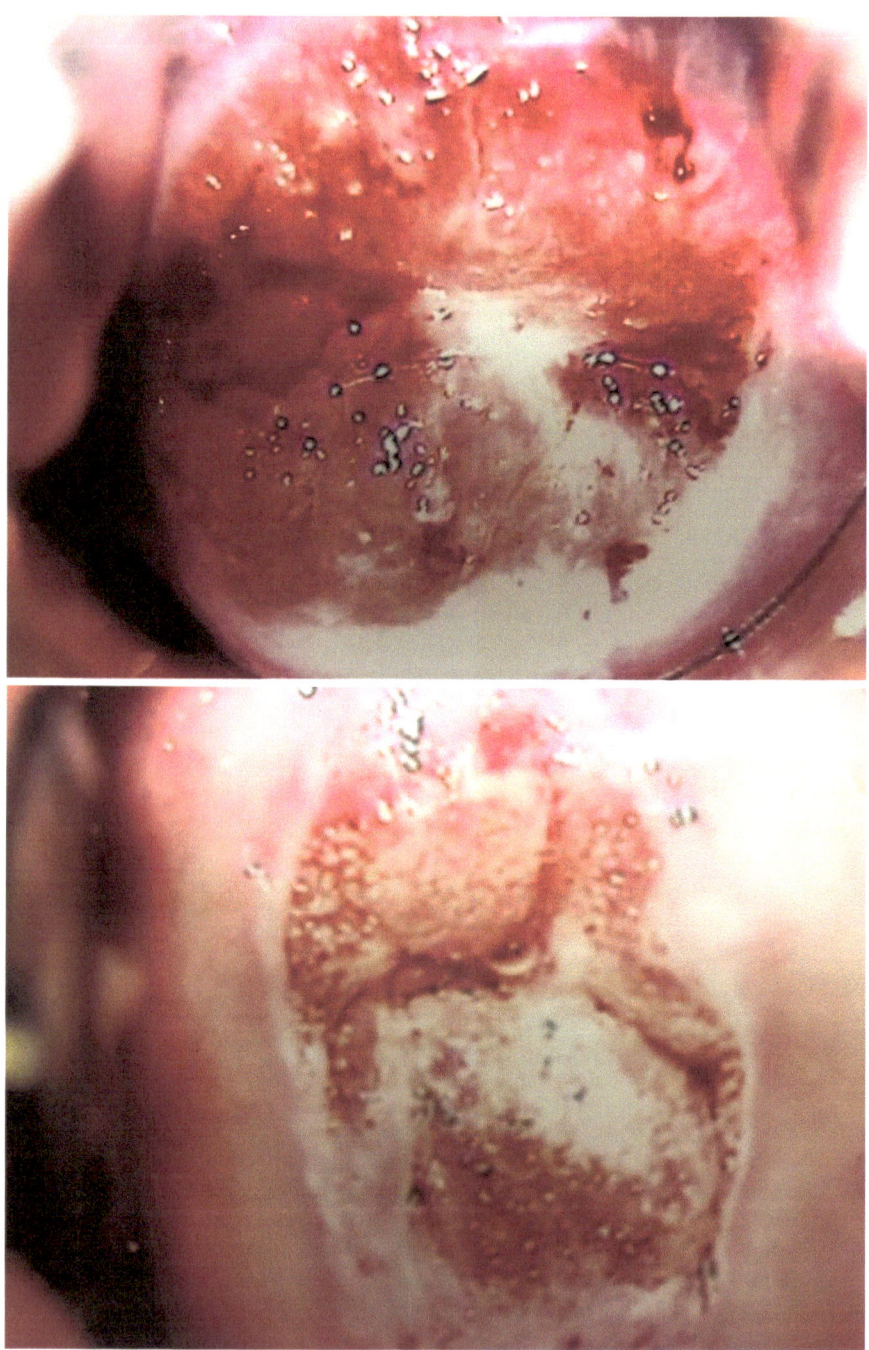

Fig. 3.5 Cervical ectropion via colposcope

Both types of tissue are healthy tissue, but the displacement of endocervical tissue to the ectocervix can cause unwelcome symptoms these are generally related to oestrogen such as in COCP and in pregnancy.

As the endocervical cells are not used to the vaginal environment, they will generate discharge to protect themselves. In some cases this discharge can become very heavy, which some women will find difficult to manage. Endocervical cells are also not designed to withstand the effects of vaginal penetration and will bleed when subjected to even a gentle touch. This may cause distress to women as they will often suffer with post-coital bleeding (bleeding after sex) and intra-menstrual bleeding (bleeding between periods). Women may often report a constant period, as they are experiencing daily bleeding; however the colour and flow may differ during their actual menstruation. This can also induce contact bleeding when taking cytology screening samples. Contact bleeding during cervical screening is not an adequate reason to refer a woman into colposcopy if there are no further symptoms. If contact bleeding is persistent and cervical cytology is negative, gynaecological referral is recommended. If adequate cytology cannot be obtained on three consecutive occasions, then a colposcopy referral is necessary to facilitate adequate sampling and ensure the cervix is visually assessed in the absence of cytology data.

A cervical ectropion is not life-threatening, but women can find the effects limiting. It can dictate what they are comfortable wearing, possibly restricting their social or leisure activities, and the symptoms can have adverse effects on their relationship. The relationship effects can be twofold: women may discourage their partners from being intimate as they are embarrassed about the discharge or bleeding and, conversely, their partners may become scared to instigate intimacy because they correlate sexual activity with bleeding.

Although, as we have established, the ectropion is not a physically harmful problem, the effects can be detrimental; hence treatment can be offered and undertaken quickly and simply in an outpatient colposcopy clinic.

3.6.4   Infection, Inflammation and Cervicitis

Infection is a very common cause of cervical and vaginal discomfort.
Common infections to affect the cervix include:

- Chlamydia
- Genital herpes
- Gonorrhoea
- Trichomonas

The above infections can cause pelvic and vaginal symptoms such as abdominal pain, discharge, vaginal odour, painful intercourse and vaginal itching, all of which can be embarrassing to discuss. This may give rise to women allowing their problem to worsen through anxiety around seeking help (see Chap. 13).

Infection of the cervix can be caused by bacteria or viruses, leading to inflammation or cervicitis. Cervicitis is a common condition, which can also be caused by allergies, childbirth or trauma to the cervix. In some cases symptoms may be absent, but when symptoms do occur, they may include:

- Low back pain
- Abdominal pain
- Pain during intercourse
- Vaginal itching
- Burning during urination

In women presenting with these combined symptoms, cervicitis should be considered, as well as the possibility of individual stand-alone conditions, because if left untreated, infectious cervicitis can develop into pelvic inflammatory disease and potentially cause infertility, increased risk of contracting additional pelvic infections, or the infection travelling to the uterus (womb). Treating cervicitis is usually using antibiotic therapy, however in severe cases, this may necessitate surgery, however this is far less common.

3.6.5   Nabothian Follicles

Nabothian follicles are benign mucus-filled cysts found on the outer surface of the cervix. In most cases women won't know they have Nabothian follicles until they are noticed on a cervical examination, as seen in Fig. 3.6. These small cysts usually measure anything from a few millimetres to a few centimetres and are a normal finding on cervical examination. They usually don't require treatment unless they are unusually large. Women may not know about Nabothian follicles, so the role of the health professional when noting these as a finding on cervical examination is to reassure the patient with full explanation that they can understand.

Fig. 3.6 Nabothian follicles

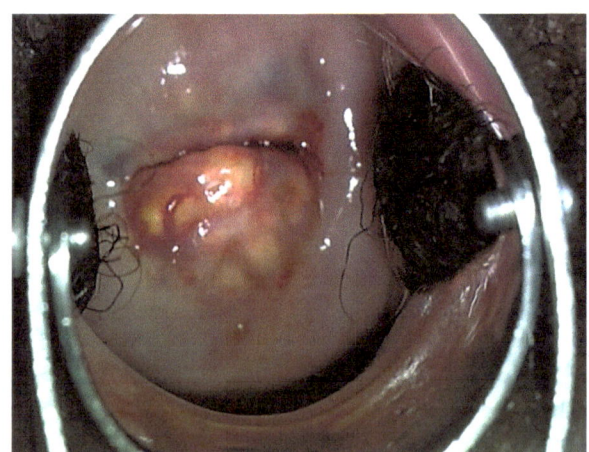

3.6.6 Endometriosis

Endometriosis is a debilitating gynaecological condition affecting many women of reproductive age. Symptoms can vary from mild discomfort to extreme disabling pain and heavy bleeding associated with back pain, bowel disturbances, leg pain and fatigue. Endometriosis occurs when cells from the lining of the womb (endometrium) can be found outside of the womb. These cell deposits occur frequently in the pelvic area but can also be found as far away as the lungs in some cases. Many women who have suffered with symptoms for years may have been incorrectly diagnosed with irritable bowel syndrome initially. In women where endometriosis is suspected, early referral to a specialist centre can reduce the effects this can have on a woman's lifestyle and future childbearing ability. Although not very common, endometriosis can manifest itself on the cervix. This may appear as black or purple spots on the surface of the cervix, which may bleed to touch. This can be painful for the patient and can cause concern for healthcare practitioners if they are not familiar with the appearance of endometriosis on the cervix. If in doubt, always refer to a gynaecologist (see Chap. 5).

3.7 Cervical Polyps

These are tissue growths which can form either on the surface of the cervix or inside the cervical canal. These can be seen via speculum examination and via colposcopy (see Figs. 3.7 and 3.8). Cervical polyps are predominantly non-cancerous and can

Fig. 3.7 Cervical polyp via colposcope

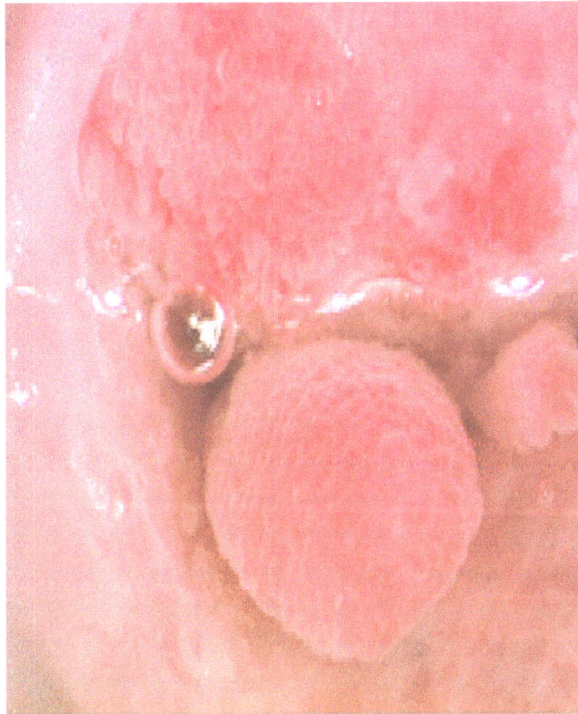

Fig. 3.8 Cervical polyp as seen via speculum

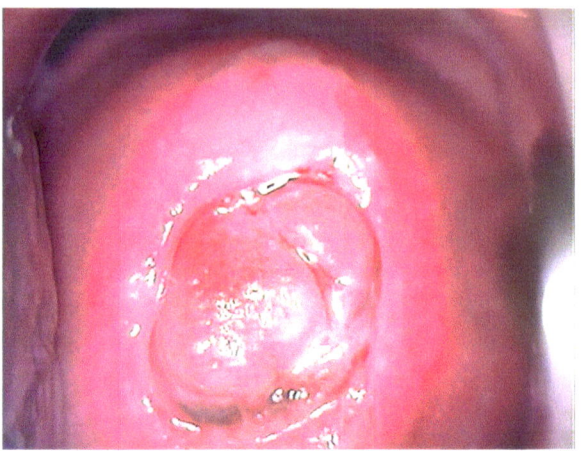

be removed easily in an outpatient clinic. All polyps that are removed should routinely be sent for histological analysis to enable the patient to be reassured that they are harmless. Many cervical polyps will go unnoticed until a cervical screening appointment; however some may cause post-coital bleeding or irregular bleeding. Polyp removal benefits your patient because removal offers reassurance, reduces or eradicates irregular bleeding and assists in getting an adequate cervical screening result as this assists full sampling of the entire transformation zone (see Chap. 2).

This chapter has demonstrated some of the conditions that can affect a woman's cervix. Many women of all ages are reluctant to discuss these sensitive issues with their health professional; effective communication is essential to offer reassurance to patients and families who encounter any of the cervical problems discussed.

References

1. WHO (2014) Comprehensive cervical cancer control. A guide to essential practice, 2nd edn
2. Marshall G (1995) Medical screening—principles and practice. Radiography 1(2):105–113
3. (2016) NHS Cervical Screening Programme: colposcopy and programme management. NHSCSP publication number 20, 3rd edn
4. Schiffman M et al (2007) Human papillomavirus and cervical cancer. Lancet 370:890–907
5. Castellsague X, Muñoz N (2003) Cofactors in human papillomavirus carcinogenesis—role of parity, oral contraceptives, and tobacco smoking. J Natl Cancer Inst Monogr (31):20–28
6. Lu B et al (2011) Efficacy and safety of prophylactic vaccines against cervical HPV infection and diseases among women: a systematic review & meta-analysis. BMC Infect Dis 11:13
7. Department of Health (2018) UK national screening programme. www.gov.uk/government/groups/uknational-screening-committee-uk-nsc
8. WHO (2014) Human papillomavirus vaccines: WHO position paper . http://www.who.int/wer/2014/wer8943.pdf?ua=1. Accessed Oct 2014
9. McIndoe WA, McLean MR, Jones RW, Mullins PR (1984) The invasive potential of carcinoma in situ of the cervix. Obstet Gynecol 64(4):451–458
10. (2017) HPV testing with abnormal cervical cytology speeds up diagnosis of cervical disease. BMJ 357:j3070. Published 26 June 2017

Suggested Reading

(2006) An easy guide to cervical screening. www.cancerscreening.nhs.uk

BSCCP website (2018) Educational resources. https://www.bsccp.org.uk/colposcopy-resources/category/downloadable-documents

Department of Health (2016/17) Responding to domestic abuse—a handbook for health professionals. Department of Health, London

Guidance for good practice in cervical screening, 4th edn. http://www.cervicalscreeningtraining.co.uk/wp-content/uploads/2016/06/Guidance-2014.pdf

National Screening Committee (2000) Second report of the UK National Screening Committee. Department of Health, London

NHS Cancer Screening Programmes. www.cancerscreening.nhs.uk; http://cancerhelp.cancerresearchuk.org; www.who.int/cancer/en

NHS Cancer Screening Programmes (2004) Guidelines on failsafe actions for the follow-up of cervical cytology reports. Publication no. 21. NHSCSP. www.cancerscreening.nhs.uk/cervical/publications

NHS Cancer Screening Programmes (2006) Taking samples for cervical screening—a resource pack for trainers. Publication no. 23. NHSCSP. www.cancerscreening.nhs.uk/cervical/publications

NHS Cervical Screening Programmes (2006) Publications no. 5 and 6. NHSCSP, Sheffield

NHS Cancer Screening Programmes (2006) Cancer screening series no. 2: equal access to breast and cervical screening for disabled women. www.cancerscreening.nhs.uk/publications

NHS Cancer Screening Programmes (2009) Information security policy. NHSCSP. www.cancerscreening.nhs.uk

NHS Cancer Screening Programmes (2011) Confidentiality and disclosure policy, version 4. www.neyhqarc.nhs.uk

NHS Cancer Screening Programmes (2012) Achievable standards, benchmarks for reporting, and criteria for evaluating cervical cytopathology. Publication no 1. www.cancerscreening.nhs.uk/cervical/publications

NHS Cervical Screening Programme (2012) Leaflets and booklets available at www.cancerscreening.nhs.uk including: cervical screening—the facts. www.cancerscreening.nhs.uk

NHS Cervical Screening Programme (2012) What your abnormal result means. www.cancerscreening.nhs.uk

Nursing and Midwifery Council (20) The code

Royal College of Nursing (2016) Female genital mutilation—an educational resource. Royal College of Nursing, London

Royal College of Nursing (2016) Genital examination in women: a resource for skills development and assessment. Royal College of Nursing, London

The Colposcopy Examination (2012) www.cancerscreening.nhs.uk

Adolescent Gynaecology

4

Louise Williams

4.1 The Role of the Clinical Nurse Specialist (CNS) in Adolescent Gynaecology

The World Health Organization defines adolescence as a unique time of rapid development where biological maturity precedes psychosocial maturity and that the unique nature and importance of adolescence mandate explicit and specific attention in health policy and programmes [1]. Paediatric and adolescent gynaecology (PAG) is a recognised speciality and includes a wide range of conditions ranging from simple menstrual problems to complex congenital developmental anomalies.

In order to manage the range of conditions seen in this age group, the gold standard is to provide multidisciplinary care. A key member of the multidisciplinary team is the clinical nurse specialist. Other team members will include gynaecology consultants, endocrine consultants, a urologist, a psychologist and a specialist consultant radiologist. The role of the CNS is to help patients to navigate different services and provide specialist clinical advice and information. Most MDTs will have close links with other specialist centres in order to encourage research, service development and ultimately improvement in care standards. The national organisation for PAG is the British Society for Paediatric and Adolescent Gynaecology (BritsPAG) who holds annual updates for clinicians working in the speciality and those with an interest.

L. Williams (✉)
Paediatric and Adolescent Gynaecology, University College London Hospital, London, UK
e-mail: louise.williams21@nhs.net

© Springer Nature Switzerland AG 2019

D. Holloway (ed.), *Nursing Management of Women's Health*,
https://doi.org/10.1007/978-3-030-16115-6_4

4.2   Puberty

Normal pubertal development in girls follows a pattern described by Tanner based on external primary and secondary sex characteristics, such as the size of the breasts, genitals and development of pubic hair [2]. Breast development is usually the first sign of pubertal development; pubic and axillary hair usually develop around 6 months later. Menarche occurs late in puberty, normally around a similar time to the end of the growth spurt. Puberty usually takes around 18 months to complete [2].

The age of puberty has been in decline over the last century, mainly due to improvements in nutrition and health. In the UK the age of menarche has fallen from 15 years in 1860 to 12.3 years in the 1990s [3].

The internal and external structures also develop in puberty, the inner labia can grow and become more visible, the clitoris and clitoral hood become more prominent and hair grows on the outer labia. Internally the ovaries become larger, and the uterus steadily grows [4].

There may be several factors affecting whether a young person will start their periods early; it has been found that low birth weight, maternal preeclampsia, maternal smoking, raised height or weight and reduced exercise as a child can all cause early onset of menarche [5]. One should investigate if there is development of secondary sexual characteristics before the age of 8 years.

Primary amenorrhoea is defined as the absence of menarche by the age of 15 if the patient has normal secondary sexual characteristics. If there are no secondary sexual characteristics, a diagnosis of primary amenorrhoea can be made by the age of 13 [6].

4.3   Gender and Sexuality

The Government Equalities Office recognises that in order for society to work for everyone, we must strive to remove barriers which may prevent someone who identifies as lesbian, gay, bisexual or trans+ (LGBT+) from reaching their full potential [7]. A way in which this is possible is by raising awareness of LGBT+ issues and being sensitive to specific needs when people are accessing healthcare.

An important place to begin is by looking at the definition of gender, sexuality and biological sex.

LGBT empowerment charity Stonewall defines gender as:

'Often expressed in terms of masculinity and femininity, gender is largely culturally determined and is assumed from the sex assigned at birth' and of gender expression as 'How a person chooses to outwardly express their gender, within the context of societal expectations of gender' [8].

Sex, or biological sex, is assigned to a person on the basis of primary sex characteristics (genitalia) and reproductive functions. Sometimes the terms 'sex' and 'gender' are interchanged to mean 'male' or 'female'.

Sexuality is defined as a person's emotional, romantic and/or sexual attraction to another person.

The Government Equalities Office has released data for 2018 which asked people of different age groups how they would define their gender and sexuality; it's estimated that around 2.5% of the population define themselves as gay, with young people more commonly than older people likely to define themselves as bisexual, pansexual, asexual or queer or to describe their sexual orientation as 'other'. They were also more likely to identify as (gender) non-binary than older respondents.

It is therefore important to be sensitive to the fact that young patients may be exploring what both gender and sexuality mean to them (if anything) and avoid using heteronormative language, whereby heterosexuality is assumed. If a young person would like to speak to you or they have concerns, you may consider sign-posting them to helpful websites such as Stonewall or Brook.

If a young person self-identifies as another gender or no gender, it would be sensible to ask which pronouns they would like you to use—you may ask 'would you like me to use he/him or they?' Or use the person's preferred name. If you can, make a note on the patients' records, so next time they attend for an appointment, the information is available for the clinician/administration team.

Patients who identify as trans should be nursed as an inpatient with other young people of the same gender which they identify as, or if they do not identify as either gender, ask them which they would be more comfortable. When seeing young trans men in the community, care should be taken as to which services they should be referred to; specialist gender identity clinics or endocrinology specialists are better placed to manage gender dysphoria than gynaecology settings, which may be upsetting and stigmatising to attend for a person who does not identify as female.

4.4   The Clinical Consultation: History and Examination

When seeing a young person for a consultation regarding a gynaecological complaint, it is wise to begin with the parent or guardian in the room and then let them know there will be some time to talk alone in order for any confidential information to be shared. During this time a young person should be reminded of their right to confidentiality and the limits (that if they had thoughts of harming themselves or someone else, that information would need to be shared); this is important as it gives a young person some time to disclose any difficult information which may help to consider possible causes for symptoms (such as pregnancy for secondary amenorrhoea). Should a young person disclose sexual assault at this point, detailed questioning should stop and a referral made immediately to children's social care.

It can also be helpful to start by asking the young person what they were expecting from the consultation; they may assume that they have to be examined and feel nervous about it—you can let them know that it may be useful to examine them if required, but if they don't want to be, then they don't have to. It may help to specify what happens during an examination—if you are looking at the skin on the outside, then let them know you will not be using a speculum, or if you need to do a swab test, you can let them know they can do it themselves if they choose to.

4.5 When to Examine?

Build general rapport with a young person by asking them a few questions about themselves and if they know why they've come for an appointment today.

Examination should be conducted by a nurse who is experienced in examining female anatomy; they should be aware that during pubertal development, the vulva can look different to when puberty is complete. For example, the inner labia can look quite asymmetric initially—sometimes with one side developing before the other. It is important to bear this in mind before any normal variation in development is pathologised. Sometimes young people will present feeling as though they suddenly have a lump or growth down below; upon examination this may show to be a normal labial development.

When asking about the presenting concern, gauge the language they are using— only 6.1% of children learn the correct terminology for female anatomy [9]. Studies have shown the girls do not know full vocabulary of genitalia until 15.6 years. They may have words they use at home (minny, flower, etc.) you may wish to clarify which parts they are talking about with them using a diagram or a photograph from online resource 'labia library'. If they refer to their 'vagina', do they mean the part inside, or are they referring to a part of the vulva? And if so, where exactly? Let them know that while it is okay to use the words they feel most comfortable with, it is important that you can understand what they are talking about.

The consultation should be non-judgemental and friendly, so that should you need to ask more intrusive questions, you have built a trusting relationship.

Young people may be seeking reassurance that their development is 'normal'. There are few images in the media showing diversity; however the website labia library [10] is a helpful resource to look at together the spectrum of normality with regard to female anatomy. The British Society for Paediatric and Adolescent Gynaecology (BritsPAG) has also produced a booklet, available online titled *So what is a vulva anyway?* which uses illustrations to show genital diversity; this can be seen in Fig. 4.1.

A young person being sexually active does not mean they necessarily need to be examined; chlamydia and gonorrhoea swabs can be self-taken if the young person is happy to do it or by a first-catch urine (FCU).

If a young person consents to an examination, the clinician should always have a chaperone and ask the patient if they would like to have their parent or carer in with them. Carefully explain everything you are going to do and what you are looking at. This can be an excellent opportunity to educate young people about their bodies and discuss hygiene.

Fig. 4.1 BritsPAG/brook
publication

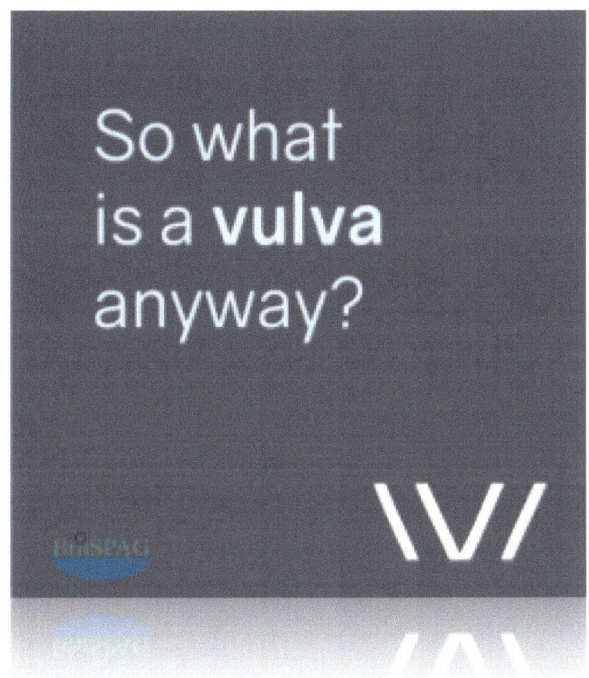

4.6 Safeguarding

Safeguarding is the responsibility of everyone; all children and young people have a right to protection from all forms of physical and mental violence, injury or abuse, neglect and maltreatment or exploitation, including sexual abuse, while in the care of parent(s), legal guardians or another person who has the care of the child [11].

The World Health Organization (WHO) classifies child abuse into four categories, physical, which includes female genital mutilation (FGM), emotional or psychological abuse, sexual abuse and neglect.

Being a nurse working in gynaecology means you may be particularly likely to encounter the signs and symptoms of abuse. It is your duty to report abuse and to know what to do if you receive a disclosure or suspect child abuse. Table 4.1 shows the potential presentations of abuse to gynaecology.

Your local area will have safeguarding guidelines and should have a named lead for safeguarding who can be contacted for advice. You should be up to date with safeguarding training. There may be several ways in which a young person may present in the outpatient setting or accident and emergency.

Table 4.1 Potential presentations of abuse to gynaecology

Disclosure	A patient may tell you about an allegation of current or past abuse
Symptoms	Abnormal vaginal discharge, soreness, bleeding, STI
Signs	Unexplained bruises, bite marks, burns, pregnancy, unkempt
Behaviour	Being quiet or withdrawn, allowing a parent or boyfriend to speak for them

Table 4.2 HEADSS mnemonic

Home	Who do they live at home with? Do they have their own room? Is it cramped?
Education	Any learning disabilities? Do they go to school/college?
Activities	What do they do outside of education?
Drinking/drugs	Do they use either?
Sex and sexuality	Do they identify as gay/straight/bisexual/queer? Do they practice safe sex? Ever had a sexual experience they didn't want to happen?
Suicidality and mental health	Do they experience low mood? If so how do they deal with those feelings? Have they ever felt suicidal?

If there is a suspicion of maltreatment, this needs to be reported to social services. Many practitioners are worried about how to discuss the topic of referring to social services; if you are conducting a referral, you should be as transparent as possible with the young person and/or their family unless you feel as though letting them know may compromise the young person's safety further. You should explain your concerns and that you will be referring to paediatric and social service colleagues so that they will be able to offer further support. You should remember that the welfare of the young person is paramount. If you have immediate concerns regarding a young person's safety, you should call the police.

When considering social history, the 'HEADDSS' mnemonic can be a useful tool when assessing a young person; this is shown in Table 4.2.

It stands for:

Carefully document in the notes issues which have been discussed, and act upon any concerning features.

4.7   Sexual Abuse

Childhood sexual abuse may be acute or historical and involves forcing a child or young person to take part in sexual activities. A young person may disclose months or years later. In the majority of cases, the abuser is an older male family member including father, stepfather or older brother.

If the abuse disclosed is acute, no examination should be conducted but rather an urgent referral to a sexual assault referral centre (SARC). Ideally evidence is collected within 12 h in order to provide an optimum sample.

Physical signs of acute sexual assault or rape may include genital redness, swelling, bruising or abrasions to the hymen and posterior fourchette.

4.8 Childhood Sexual Exploitation (CSE)

CSE is a form of child abuse whereby a young person receives something such as gifts, money or affection as a result of performing sexual activities or others performing sexual activities on them [12].

The young person may not be aware that exploitation is taking place or may feel unable to speak about it.

CSE does not necessarily have to involve physical contact; young people may be encouraged to send explicit images via text or online in return for money or gifts. These images may then be used to manipulate the young person into sending more.

For more information, search online for CEOPs (Child Exploitation and Online Protection Command).

4.8.1 Female Genital Mutilation (FGM)

Female genital mutilation (FGM) is defined by the World Health Organization as procedures which remove or damage the external female genital organs for no medical reason [13]. It is a cultural and not religious practice carried out for a number of reasons including it being a rite of passage, perceiving it as making the girl more marriageable or people believing erroneously that it is religious requirement. It is conducted across many counties in Eastern, Central and West Africa, parts of the Middle East, Indonesia and Malaysia.

It is unclear about the prevalence of FGM in the UK; however estimates made by looking at diaspora communities suggest there may be 137,000 women and girls living with FGM. It is possible that there may be 60,000 girls born in the UK to mothers from FGM-affected countries [14].

FGM is usually carried out on young girls between infancy and the age of fifteen; it is illegal in the UK and is child abuse. It is also illegal for a child to be taken out of the country and to have FGM, and now parents can also be held accountable if FGM is conducted while a child is in the care of someone else.

FGM can cause both physical and psychological symptoms; a young person may present to primary or secondary care with symptoms which may include:

- Recurrent urine infections
- Menstrual issues
- Vulval pain
- Flashbacks
- Anxiety

As a nurse, it is therefore important that you have a good knowledge of FGM and the safeguarding procedures to follow if you see a girl who has undergone or suspected to have undergone FGM.

Acute presentations are very rare; it is more likely you would see a patient who has had FGM historically.

Table 4.3 Department of Health suggested questions to ask regarding suspected FGM	(1) Do you, your partner or your parents come from a community where cutting or circumcision is practised?
	(2) Have you been cut? It may be appropriate to use other terms or phrases

Types of FGM (WHO definition):

- *Type 1*: Often referred to as clitoridectomy, this is the partial or total removal of the clitoris (a small, sensitive and erectile part of the female genitals) and, in very rare cases, only the prepuce (the fold of skin surrounding the clitoris).
- *Type 2*: Often referred to as excision, this is the partial or total removal of the clitoris and the labia minora (the inner folds of the vulva), with or without excision of the labia majora (the outer folds of skin of the vulva).
- *Type 3*: Often referred to as infibulation, this is the narrowing of the vaginal opening through the creation of a covering seal. The seal is formed by cutting and repositioning the labia minora, or labia majora, sometimes through stitching, with or without removal of the clitoris (clitoridectomy).
- *Type 4*: This includes all other harmful procedures to the female genitalia for non-medical purposes, e.g. pricking, piercing, incising, scraping and cauterising the genital area.

Starting a conversation with a young person and their family about FGM can feel difficult, as we may fear upsetting patients. However it is our duty to safeguard and also to give young people an opportunity to talk about their experience, which may affect them physically or psychologically, and refer them for help.

The Department of Health has given guidance on the questions to ask if you suspect a young person has been subject to FGM; these can be seen in Table 4.3.

If the answer to these questions is no, it should be documented in the young person's notes that you have had a conversation about FGM and they have confirmed that they have not undergone the procedure. If you had concerns regarding their answers, you may want to discuss with your safeguarding lead.

As with other forms of abuse, a young person should be seen alone to give them an opportunity to discuss sensitive matters.

4.8.2 Mandatory Reporting

Since October 2016 it has been the responsibility of healthcare professionals to alert the police on the 101 number in cases of FGM found in age under 18. Those that you need to report are seen in Table 4.4. There is also best practice guidance from the Department of Health 2016 as seen in Table 4.5.

This is in the case if:

Table 4.4 When to report to the police (101 number)

• A young person has told you they have had FGM
• If you have examined a patient and seen FGM

Table 4.5 Department of Health 2016 recommendations for best practice

• The family must be informed of the law in the UK and the health consequences of practising FGM
• Ensure all discussions are approached with due sensitivity and are non-judgemental
• Any action must meet all statutory and professional responsibilities in relation to safeguarding, the mandatory reporting duty and local processes and arrangements
• Using this guidance does not replace the need for professional judgement in relation to the circumstances presented
• Document all actions in the parent/child healthcare records

4.8.3 Menstrual Dysfunction in Adolescence

Menstrual dysfunction (MD) in adolescence is relatively common; an Australian study found that around 25% of girls had significant menstrual dysfunction affecting life activities and resulting in school absence [15]. Heavy painful or irregular periods are most common in the first few years after menarche and generally settle down into a regular pattern; however this can take up to 7 years in some cases; the variance can be seen in Fig. 4.2.

Serious pathology is uncommon [17]. The main reason for irregularity is the fact that for the first years after menarche, cycles are anovulatory over half the time. Over time the cycle regulates, and as ovulation happens more frequently, the cycle regulates and periods become less heavy.

As a first line, periods can sometimes be managed by reassurance and advice regarding the use of simple analgesia. This can usually be managed in primary care; however if simple measures are ineffective or the patient has a medical condition which may limit the choices available of managing MD, then a referral to specialist paediatric and gynaecology services may be required.

There are several treatments which can help if a young person finds menstrual dysfunction is inferring with their lives.

A full menstrual history should be taken from the patient, including asking whether they are sexually active; this should be asked without the parent/guardian in the room. This information may exclude certain treatments and help you to consider what suggestions to make.

Tranexamic and mefenamic acid should be offered if there are no contraindications. Tranexamic acid has been shown to cause a 50% reduction in blood loss and mefenamic acid a 20% loss. Tranexamic acid is an anti-inflammatory which can be used as pain relief. Both should be taken when a patient feels a period is coming and while bleeding.

After this the first line of treatment in adolescents is often a progestogen, which may be taken cyclically to improve the regularity of the cycle and reduce heaviness

Fig. 4.2 Variation in cycle length in normal adolescence [16]

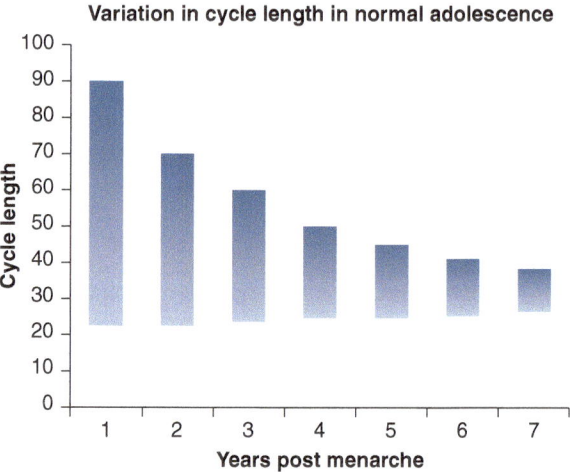

or continuously to defer or delay menstruation, for example, during exam time. An example of this would be norethisterone (NET), which has been shown to reduce blood flow by up to 83% [18]. Patients should be counselled that NET is not licensed as a contraceptive pill and that it is not effective for painful periods and analgesia may still be required. The progesterone-only pill (POP) is also an oral progesterone but in much smaller doses; it can often cause an irregular pattern of bleeding and in some cases prolonged periods and so is not useful in the management of adolescent menorrhagia.

The combined pill (COC) can be an effective first-line treatment for managing periods; a random control trial has found the COC can reduce bleeding by up to 18% and cramping by 50% [19]. Some girls may choose to tricycle packets of their pill in order to time periods in the school holidays.

Once a treatment has been found which works for a patient, they can then stay on this for as long as required, they may after 2 years wish to see what their cycle is like without it, and many find that symptoms are much improved.

Endometriosis is a condition which can start in adolescence; it can sometimes be mistaken for common dysmenorrhoea; however symptoms may be atypical and can include non-cyclical pain, gastrointestinal issues or genitourinary symptoms. For patients who have tried hormonal methods of menstrual control and still continue to have severe pain, a laparoscopy may be considered if endometriosis is suspected (see Chap. 5).

4.8.4 Polycystic Ovary Syndrome (PCOS)

As previously discussed adolescent menstrual cycles are commonly irregular for reasons unrelated to polycystic ovary syndrome. However if an ultrasound scan is performed on an adolescent, the report will often describe 'polycystic ovaries' whereby instead of the usual view of having around 8 cysts (or follicles) on the ovaries being visible, there are 12 or more. PCOS (polycystic ovarian syndrome) relates to a group of symptoms caused by having these extra cysts.

The diagnostic criteria of PCOS from a consensus in Rotterdam are if the patient meets two out of three of the following criteria:

- Infrequent or no ovulation (usually manifested as infrequent or no menstruation)
- Clinical or biochemical signs of hyperandrogenism (such as hirsutism, acne or male pattern alopecia) or elevated levels of total or free testosterone
- Polycystic ovaries on ultrasonography, defined as the presence of 12 or more follicles in at least 1 ovary, measuring 2–9 mm diameter, or increased ovarian volume (greater than 10 mL) [20]

It is important to be cautious when considering a diagnosis of PCOS in an adolescent as all of these symptoms can be present in normal adolescent development [21]. Blood tests may be performed to rule out other issues; however these tend not to be very useful when considering PCOS due the variation of hormone levels throughout the cycle [21]. If a young person has presented with severe hirsutism, this may show a rise in testosterone; if this is the case, a referral to endocrinology should be made for further investigation and management.

If a diagnosis of PCOS is suspected, there are several treatments which may be effective in managing symptoms (see Chap. 2).

4.8.5 Management of PCOS

The patient should have a weight and height conducted in order to work out their body mass index (BMI); being overweight causes insulin resistance which in turn causes the ovary to make testosterone—which can cause acne and hirsutism. Sensible advice regarding diet and increasing activity can be offered, or suggest referral to a local weight loss service for young people.

Treatments for hirsutism include electrolysis and waxing. There is also a prescription-only cream which can be applied to the face to treat facial hair called Vaniqa; this is not always available on the NHS though. An anti-androgen tablet, such as spironolactone, may also be considered.

The combined pill is often the first-line hormonal treatment as it minimises the production of testosterone by the ovary [21].

4.9 Ovarian Cysts

Functional cysts are part of the normal physiological process; they will normally be small but sometimes haemorrhagic. If they cause pain, this can be managed with simple analgesia. If they are seen on ultrasound, a follow-up a few months later will usually show a resolution.

If pain is severe, the cyst is large or a dermoid cyst has been seen on ultrasound, a laparoscopic cystectomy may be performed. Young people should also be counselled on the possibility of an ovarian cyst causing the ovary to tort; if they experience a sudden onset of severe pain, they should attend their nearest A&E.

The incidence of reoccurrence of a cyst depends on the underlying pathology, functional cysts being common in the adolescent age group due to the higher incidence of anovulatory cycles. Menstrual suppression may be considered in order to help prevent a reoccurrence.

Dermoid cysts or teratomas are usually benign; they are germ cell tumours which can appear in the ovaries. They can contain hair, sebum and teeth. Treatment is to surgically remove the dermoid cyst if it is causing pain (see Chap. 5) [4].

4.9.1   Primary Amenorrhoea

98% of young women will have reached menarche by age 15 [4] which means that primary amenorrhoea is relatively rare. Menarche usually happens within 3 years of thelarche or if a young person has no sign of secondary sex characteristics by the age of 13.

If a normal hormonal profile is found on blood test, then anatomical causes of primary amenorrhoea should be considered [4]. An imperforate hymen can be recognised as a bulge of skin at the vulva, which is treated surgically, or more rarely a transverse septum which can be low, mid or high in the vagina. This is usually identified on MRI and requires treatment with a specialist centre and sometimes postsurgical dilation to prevent the septum reoccurring.

As these procedures can take time to arrange with scans and appointments, menstrual suppression should be commenced with advice given regarding analgesia if required.

4.9.2   Mullerian Agenesis

Mayer-Rokitansky-Kuster-Hauser syndrome affects around 1 in 5000 female births whereby there is an absence of the uterus and vagina [22]. Young people present at around 15 or 16 years old with normal secondary sex development but with an absence of periods. It is then discovered on ultrasound or MRI the absence of Mullerian structures. A referral to a specialist gynaecology service should then be made.

4.9.3   Differences in Sexual Development (DSD)

Disorders (or differences) of sex development (DSD) is an umbrella term which describes a group of complex, congenital medical conditions which affect sex development.

DSD may present at birth, when a baby is born with atypical genitalia, or in adolescence with primary amenorrhoea or virilisation at puberty. DSDs are estimated to affect around 1.7% of the population, with some conditions being rarer than others [23].

Historically there have been stigma and shame surrounding these conditions, and as a result many people with DSD had not been told about their diagnoses. This treatment is not acceptable, and openness with families and individuals is now an essential part of their care.

DSD should be managed within a specialist centre which includes an endocrinologist, psychologist, specialist nursing, gynaecology and urology. Psychology should be considered an essential part of patient care.

There are controversies which surround the treatment of DSD particularly relating to early surgeries; girls born with a clitoris that is larger than average may have had a clitoral reduction and/or vaginal surgery. This surgery is considered cosmetic and may cause loss of sexual sensation in the future especially as repeat surgery is often required.

People with a DSD often feel frustrated when their condition is not understood by their GP or clinic nurse. While clinicians cannot be expected to know about all conditions, particularly those which are very rare, it is important to be sensitive when asking about fertility matters and menstrual cycles and should you need to examine someone who has had previous surgery or who may have atypical genitalia.

4.9.4 Contraception and Sexual Health

The age of consent in England and Wales is 16 years old regardless of sexual orientation or gender, as specified by the Sexual Offences Act.

However if you are approached by a young person under the age of 16 for contraception, you may advise them if they meet 'Fraser guidelines' which relate to the case of Gillick vs West Norfolk [24].

The case relates to a mother who did not want contraception to be prescribed to her daughter who was under 16 years of age without her consent. The judge ruled that if a young person met certain criteria of competence, they could receive contraception without the knowledge of their parent or carer. These guidelines are as follows:

1. That the girl (although under the age of 16 years) will understand the advice
2. That a clinician cannot persuade her to inform her parents or to allow them to inform the parents that she is seeking contraceptive advice
3. That they are very likely to continue having sexual intercourse with or without contraceptive treatment
4. That unless she receives contraceptive advice or treatment, her physical or mental health or both are likely to suffer
5. That her best interests require him to give her contraceptive advice, treatment or both without the parental consent

If young people are sexually active under the age of 16, you should use your discretion as to whether they are being potentially exploited or do not have the capacity to consent for themselves. If they do not, you should be transparent with the young person and let them know you have concerns and will need to talk to social care for further advice. If a young person is below the age of 13 years old, a referral to social care is always necessary.

4.9.5 Taking a Sexual History

Discuss with the young person about their right to confidentiality and the reasons you would like to know about the kind of sex they are having. Let them know the reason why it's important to ask certain questions.

Consider your language, and be sensitive to the young person's sexual development; you may consider asking are they sexually active, rather than 'do you have a boyfriend' which may assume sexuality.

Do they have any symptoms? It can be useful to spell out symptoms they may have not considered, for example, lumps and bumps or sores. Have they noticed any change in their discharge that they feel is out of the ordinary? This can be a useful time if a young person has concerns to reassure them about normal physiological discharge and discourage the use of 'feminine hygiene' products which can lead to vaginal infections (such as bacterial vaginosis).

4.9.6 Are They at Risk of Pregnancy and Do They Need a Test?

Conduct a NAAT swab if the history you have taken indicates a young person could have been exposed to chlamydia or gonorrhoea; a young person can take this themselves or provide a first-catch urine if they prefer.

Prevention should be discussed, and young people should be informed about any local services whereby they can gain access to free condoms; the 'C' card scheme now operates in many UK counties whereby a young person can gain access to free condoms every week at pharmacies and GUM clinics.

Discuss contact tracing so that if they are found to have an STI, they know the importance of having any partners they have been in contact with also being treated.

4.9.7 Contraception

A young person may come to you with an idea of what contraception they would like to try. You will then consider what is most appropriate depending on their menstrual history/general health information. It can be helpful to look together at a resource such as the Family Planning Association (FPA) leaflet 'your guide to contraception' which is freely available on their website www.fpa.org.uk/.

It is important to consider with a young person if they feel they will remember to take a pill each day or change a patch on a certain day and what to do should they miss a dose. This may steer you towards a long-acting reversible contraceptive (LARC) method such as the implant or Mirena coil (see Chap. 13).

4.10   Conclusion

Adolescence is a specific period in human development which as nurses we need to have respect for and be able to practice skilful listening skills in order to help support and educate our patients about their gynaecological health. Knowledge in this period of life can set young people up for an empowered future where their health concerns are listened to empathetically and taken seriously.

Young people need to be encouraged to recognise risk and how to keep themselves physically and emotionally safe. Talk about consent within the context of relationships but also practically in the clinic room, letting them know that they have bodily autonomy and should an examination be suggested, they are able to say no if they choose to.

Knowing when and how to seek help is an important skill we can encourage by being open and careful listeners, considering environmental, cultural and sociological circumstances.

References

 1. World Health Organization (2018) Adolescent development. http://www.who.int/maternal_child_adolescent/topics/adolescence/development/en/. Accessed 30 Jul 2018
 2. Marshall WA, Tanner JM (1970) Variations in pattern of pubertal changes in girls. Obstet Gynecol Sur 25:694–695
 3. Graham E, Sugar N, Emans S, Biro F, Herman-Giddens M, Slora E, Wasserman R, Koch G (1998) Secondary sexual characteristics and menses in young girls. Pediatrics 101:949–950
 4. Creighton S, Balen A, Breech L (2018) Pediatric and adolescent gynecology, 1st edn. p 8
 5. Morris D, Jones M, Schoemaker M, Ashworth A, Swerdlow A (2011) Secular trends in age at menarche in women in the UK born 1908-93: results from the Breakthrough Generations Study. Paediatr Perinat Epidemiol 25:394–400
 6. American Society for Reproductive Medicine (2008) Current evaluation of amenorrhea. Fertil Steril 90:S219–S225
 7. GOV.UK. National LGBT survey: research report. https://www.gov.uk/government/publications/national-lgbt-survey-summary-report. Accessed 30 Jul 2018
 8. Stonewall. Glossary of terms. https://www.stonewall.org.uk/help-advice/glossary-terms#g. Accessed 30 Jul 2018
 9. Gartrell N, Mosbacher D (1984) Sex differences in the naming of children's genitalia. Sex Roles 10:869–876
10. Labialibrary.org.au (2018) Home | Labia Library. http://www.labialibrary.org.au/. Accessed 30 Jul 2018
11. Unicef UK. UN Convention on the Rights of the Child (UNCRC)1989—Unicef UK. https://www.unicef.org.uk/what-we-do/un-convention-child-rights/. Accessed 30 Jul
12. NSPCC (2018) Child sexual exploitation. https://www.nspcc.org.uk/preventing-abuse/child-abuse and-neglect/child-sexual-exploitation/. Accessed 2 Aug 2018
13. World Health Organization (2018) Female genital mutilation. http://www.who.int/news-room/fact-sheets/detail/female-genital-mutilation. Accessed 2 Aug 2018
14. Macfarlane A, Dorkenoo E (2015) PP20 estimating the numbers of women and girls with female genital mutilation in England and Wales. J Epidemiol Community Health 69:A61.1–A6A61
15. Parker M, Sneddon A, Arbon P (2009) The menstrual disorder of teenagers (MDOT) study: determining typical menstrual patterns and menstrual disturbance in a large population-based study of Australian teenagers. BJOG 117:185–192

16. Treloar A, Boyton R, Behn B, Brown B (1968) Variation of the human menstrual cycle through reproductive life. Obstet Gynecol Sur 23:80
17. Williams C, Creighton S (2012) Menstrual disorders in adolescents: review of current practice. Horm Res Paediatr 78:135–143
18. Nice.org.uk. Heavy menstrual bleeding: assessment and management | Guidance and guidelines | NICE. https://www.nice.org.uk/Guidance/CG44. Accessed 2 Aug 2018
19. Fraser I, McCarron G (1991) Randomized trial of 2 hormonal and 2 prostaglandin-inhibiting agents in women with a complaint of menorrhagia. Aust N Z J Obstet Gynaecol 31:66–70
20. Revised 2003 consensus on diagnostic criteria and long-term health risks related to polycystic ovary syndrome (PCOS). Hum Reprod 19:41–47
21. Conway G (2016) Polycystic ovary syndrome your medical handbook, 1st edn p 26
22. Nakhal R, Creighton S (2012) Management of vaginal agenesis. J Pediatr Adolesc Gynecol 25:352–357
23. Blackless M, Charuvastra A, Derryck A, Fausto-Sterling A, Lauzanne K, Lee E (2000) How sexually dimorphic are we? Review and synthesis. Am J Hum Biol 12:151
24. Gillick v West Norfolk and Wisbech AHA (1985) UKHL 7 (17 Oct 1985). Bailii.org. http://www.bailii.org/uk/cases/UKHL/1985/7.html. Accessed 2 Aug 2018

Pain and Endometriosis

5

Debra Holloway and Claudia Tye

5.1 Pain

Women present with pain as it is a common problem. The key within women's health is to be able to work out if the pain is gynaecological in origin or from other systems such the bladder, bowels or skeleton, as these can all interact and be hard to distinguish. This chapter links with the previous chapter on bleeding, as the two are often connected, and the chapter on sexual health looking at STI and the impact that they may have on pain owing to adhesions. Adhesions due to previous surgery can also cause pain, normally non-cyclical; therefore, a previous history of surgery needs to be taken into account.

5.1.1 Dysmenorrhea: Period Pain

This is the pain that occurs with menstruation, which can be in the pelvis or lower abdomen [1]. It can also radiate to the lower back, groin and sometimes upper thighs. The pain can be just before and/or with menstruation and is always cyclical in nature. It is difficult to estimate the prevalence, as many women suffer from period pain but do not seek medical help and self-medicate. It can, however, account for time missed from school and work on a cyclical basis.

As menstruation starts, endometrial cells release prostaglandins, which can stimulate myometrial contractions and cause dysmenorrhoea. The severity of dysmenorrhoea depends on the levels of prostaglandins [2]. This can also affect the gastrointestinal (GI) system leading to an alteration in bowel habits.

D. Holloway · C. Tye (✉)
Guys and St Thomas NHS Foundation Trust, London, UK
e-mail: Debra.Holloway@gstt.nhs.uk; Claudia.Tye@gstt.nhs.uk

© Springer Nature Switzerland AG 2019
D. Holloway (ed.), *Nursing Management of Women's Health*,
https://doi.org/10.1007/978-3-030-16115-6_5

Abnormally high levels can be associated with severe dysmenorrhoea, in both primary and secondary types. However, as some women are not responsive to first-line measures, there will need to be different adequate treatments [2]. There have been links with smoking, early menarche, nulliparity and family history [1].

Painful periods can occur by themselves but also with heavy periods (see Chap. 2). There are two types of dysmenorrhoea [1]:

- Primary—which occurs in the absence of any structural pathological condition and normally starts just after menarche.
- Secondary—is associated with identifiable disease, and normally starts in the 30s/40s and can co-exist with heavy periods, irregular bleeding and painful sex, which may suggest a pathological condition.

A good history needs to be taken to try a work out the diagnosis and the investigations needed. Table 5.1 shows some tips for taking a history in women with pain. This should include questions around menstrual history as below.

To diagnosis any pathological condition:

- Carry out an examination, which needs to include: speculum, bimanual and abdominal examinations to look for conditions such as fibroids, indications of

Table 5.1 History-taking in pain

Menstrual cycle	Age at menarche and onset of pain
Onset of pain	Before, with, or after menstruation. Can be relieved by menstrual flow starting such as in endometriosis
Nature of cycle	Days of bleeding, length of cycle, amount of bleeding
Location and intensity of the pain	Abdomen, thighs, spasmodic, cramps, heaviness, congestion Impact of daily activities
What relieves the pain	Include OTC, alternative and heat
What makes it worse	Specific questions on exercise, bowels and bladder
Analgesia used	Type, how much, whether helpful
Associated factors	Headaches, nausea, vomiting, constipation, diarrhoea
Any abnormal bleeding	Refer back to Chap. 2. IMB, PCB, HMB
Other pain	Painful sex – every time, in certain positions, at certain times of the cycle, if deep within the abdomen or superficial in the vagina and on the vulva Pain when passing urine (especially around menstruation) pain with opening bowels (again around periods)
Vaginal discharge or history of STI, PID	Any vaginal discharge
What contraception is being used	Hormonal, intra-uterine.
Other	Any pain with vaginal, speculum examinations. Is this new? Any recent or previous operations, especially gynaecological or pelvic Any nausea or vomiting, backache, diarrhoea

STI sexually transmitted infection, *PID* pelvic inflammatory disease, *OTC* over-the-counter, *IMB* intermenstrual bleeding, *PCB* post-coital bleeding, *HMB* heavy menstrual bleeding pelvic inflammatory disease (PID) and endometriosis, such as a fixed uterus, and any other pathological condition, in addition to trying to pinpoint the location of the pain [3]. During the examination, the nurse needs to look for any masses (fibroids/cysts), a fixed immobile uterus (endometriosis, PID), vaginal nodules (endometriosis) and vaginal discharge (infections).

Further examination is dependent on the history and the examination findings, but would include an ultrasound.

In looking at period pain, it is important to be aware of many differential diagnoses, including [1]:

- Pelvic inflammatory disease
- Ovarian cysts
- Endometriosis
- Fibroids
- Adenomyosis
- Congenital malformations of the reproductive organs
- Copper intra-uterine contraceptive device (IUCD) and misplaced devices
- Return of the natural cycle after being on hormonal contraception
- Previous pelvic or abdominal surgery—causing adhesions
- Psychological problems including sexual abuse
- Cervical stenosis
- Irritable bowel syndrome
- Inflammatory bowel disease

Red flags in pelvic pain should be an acute onset and pregnancy should be excluded because of the risk of ectopic pregnancy, appendicitis, ovarian torsion and acute PID.

Diagnosis of the causes of pain may only be able to be made after the woman has had ultrasound or other imaging such as MRI, hysteroscopy and/or laparoscopy, but in some cases there may be no gynaecological causes found and this should be discussed with the woman [4].

5.1.2 Treatments

Treatments would depend on the cause [1, 2]:

1. Analgesics, such as paracetamol, can be helpful if the pain is mild, and if non-steroidal anti-inflammatory medications (NSAIDs) cannot be taken; they can be combined with codeine if needed.
2. NSAIDs are more effective than paracetamol, as they work by inhibiting or reducing prostaglandin synthesis. If periods are regular, women should be advised to start using them before the onset of the pain. Caution is needed with GI problems and with some asthmatic women.

3. Combined oral contraceptive pill (COCP). This works by ensuring that the endometrium is thin, which results in a decrease in prostaglandin production. Using them as a continuous regime is better than cyclically, but research has not shown any difference in the different preparations.
4. Levonorgestrel intra-uterine system works as above for the COCP and studies have shown that it is as effective at treating period pain as COCP.
5. Anti-spasmodic—these can be used by women to relieve abdominal and period pain as they relax smooth muscle. In combination with NSAIDs, they work better than non-steroids alone.
6. Lifestyle advice—there is some evidence that links smoking, obesity and high fat diets with painful periods. Physical exercise may reduce the pain.
7. Alternative therapies [5]:
   (a) Vitamin B1, vitamin E, dill, fennel, fish oils, zinc (limited or no evidence)
   (b) Heat pads and hot water bottles
   (c) Yoga
   (d) Massage
   (e) Exercise
   (f) Transcutaneous electrical nerve stimulation
   (g) Acupuncture

5.2   Secondary Dysmenorrhea

The treatments for secondary dysmenorrhea depend on the cause, for example, changing a copper IUCD for an intra-uterine system (IUS), removal of fibroids. However, those treatments listed above for primary dysmenorrhea can be used as well. If nothing is effective, the menstrual cycle can be stopped, so that there is no period and therefore no pain. GnRH analogues may be tried for this.

5.3   Dyspareunia

Painful sex is a common problem and one, in common with many other areas of women's health, that women may not talk about. A recent publication by the Department of Health [6] showed that many women have pain with sex, but do not report it. Within any history it is important to talk about sexual issues such as bleeding with sex, painful sex and vaginal issues. Women may present with other gynaecological issues or even in the fertility clinic for a referral for infertility and on closer questioning, it is discovered that they have been unable to have intercourse. It affects about 7.5% of women, but increases in the post-menopausal period with the effects of the lack of oestrogen on the vagina and vaginal dryness [7]. Dyspareunia can be superficial; therefore, on the vulva and vagina, or deep in the abdomen. It can be a symptom of an underlying disease such as a dermatological condition, vaginismus or endometriosis, or of psychological issues, and can cause the woman and the couple great distress. There is often an overlap between the two. However, if a woman presents with severe endometriosis and painful sex, psychological and social issues and problems need to be explored as well [7].

When taking a history, as with most areas of gynaecology, sensitivity is needed, and the use of open-ended and non-judgmental questions, allowing women to talk and tell their stories. For example, it may be a condition related to a traumatic birth, a previous partner's comment on the vagina, etc. All the woman's feelings need to be explored and this may be best done in a psychosexual clinic with the partner as well. In terms of safeguarding, issues around rape, assault and domestic violence need to be explored.

5.3.1 Examination

Some women need to be examined to look for any causes of the pain on the vulva, vaginal and cervix. Table 5.2 show the steps and some of the findings in women with pain. In addition, they may need to have swabs and a cervical screening.

The nurse should be aware of the language that is used, as this may stop the woman from talking, thinking that the nurse does not believe that she has an issue [7].

Management depends on the cause and includes an multidisciplinary team (MDT) approach: treatment of physical causes, perennial massage, removal of anything such as bubble baths that may cause irritation, advice on lubrications and referral for psychosexual counselling [7].

Table 5.2 Examination tips

Vulva and perineum	Tears
	Fissures
	Skin changes
	Candida, herpes
	Dermatosis
	Episiotomy scars
	Lichen sclerosis
	Post-menopausal atrophy
	Atrophy on COCP or when breast feeding
	Bartholin's cyst
	Post-radiotherapy
	Cancer
Speculum	Discharge—swabs
Bimanual	Tenser areas
	Endometriotic deposits
	Vaginal septum
	Cysts
	PID
	Post-cancer treatments
	Pelvic floor problems
	Non-gynaecological

Table 5.3 Types of ovarian cysts

Name	Nature
Functional ovarian cysts	• Largely asymptomatic • Related to menstrual cycle and excessive stimulation by the hormone • Mostly occur in the reproductive age • If they are <5 cm, then they spontaneously resolve [9]; however, if they grow larger they may result in symptoms, such as pain and pressure
Benign epithelial tumours	• Most common tumours and arise from the mesothelium • These include—mucinous cystadenomata, endometrial (endometrioid), tubal (serous), or uroepithelial (Brenner)
Benign germ cell tumours— dermoid cysts	• Generally occur in young women • Mainly benign (3% are malignant) • Develop from the germ cells and may contain elements of all three germ layers and can contain ectodermal (hair, teeth, sebaceous material) endodermal and mesodermal elements • Most are asymptomatic, but as they are dense, there may be a risk of torsion
Borderline tumours	These can be difficult to distinguish on imaging and can appear as simple cysts

5.4 Ovarian Cysts

Ovarian cysts are a common finding in women and are commonly reported on ultrasound reports as incidental findings, more so with some progestogen-only methods of contraception [8]. About 90% are benign, but there are features that make them more likely to be cancerous, and these can be seen on imaging. There are many different types, which can be seen in Table 5.3. The overall incidence of cancer in pre-menopausal women is 1:1000 and 3:1000 after the age of 50 [9]. It can be harder to distinguish between benign and malignant in pre-menopausal women as there is no specific test to use. If there is any suspicion of malignancy, then the women need to be referred under the 2-week wait rule for a blood test and normally MRI to characterise the nature of the cyst. Management of the cysts is dictated by the age of the woman. With ovarian cysts it is important to rule out an underlying malignancy before treating them by monitoring them.

In addition, about 10% of ovarian cysts on ultrasound are found to be non-ovarian in origin. These are: [9]

• Para-tubal cyst
• Hydrosalpinx
• Tubo-ovarian abscess
• Peritoneal cyst

5.4.1 Presenting Complaints of Ovarian Cysts

• Often women have no symptoms, and these are found while undertaking examinations or imaging for other presenting complaints. If the cysts are larger, then there may be pressure symptoms (which may lead to bowel and bladder difficul-

ties), pain with sex, especially on deep penetration, generalised lower abdominal pain and/or discomfort.
- If a woman presents with a sudden onset of acute pain with nausea and vomiting, this may indicate torsion of a cyst and women on conservative management should be warned to look out for these symptoms.

5.4.2 Examination, History and Imaging

In addition to normal questions within the history, and those discussed in the section above on period pain, there are some specific questions to ask:

- Any risk factors for ovarian cancer and/or a family history of ovarian or breast cancer or known BRCA
- Endometriosis symptoms
- Symptoms that may suggest cancer—distension, appetite change, pelvic pain and changes in bowel and bladder function [9]

5.4.2.1 Investigations
1. Abdominal examination may indicate distension if there is a large cyst, and indeed this may be felt on bimanual examination as well. If a cyst is suspected, then ultrasound is   used, normally a transvaginal scan unless it is exceptionally large, in which case abdominal scanning can be used.
2. Pelvic ultrasound—all the cysts have different characteristics on scanning, which aids diagnosis. There are various risk of malignancy models. The most well-known are the Risk Malignancy Index (RMI), as can be seen in Table 5.4, and the International Ovarian Tumor Analysis (IOTA). None of these is designed for pre-menopausal women [9]. Currently, the RMI is suggested by National Institute of Health Care and Excellence (NICE) [10]. If there is any doubt or suspicion, then MRI is used [11].

   An RMI of over 200 or 250 is used to suggest onward referral to a gynaecology oncologist [11].

   The IOTA scan [9] rules suggest the following signs on imaging to indicate malignancy:
   (a) Irregular solid tumours
   (b) Ascites

Table 5.4 Risk of Malignancy Index (RMI) calculation

RMI = U × M × Ca125 [9]		
Ultrasound	Menopause status	Ca125
1 point for: multi-locular cysts, solid areas, metastases, ascetic, bilateral lesions U = 0 for a score of 0, U = 1 (for an ultrasound score of 1) U = 3 (for a score of 2–5)	1 for pre-menopausal 3 for post-menopausal	The value

(c) At least four papillary structures
(d) Irregular multi-locular solid tumours with the largest diameter >100 mm
(e) Strong blood flow
3. Tumour markers—serum Ca125 measurement is used in various risk of malignancy indices [9, 11], but may be elevated in endometriosis, fibroids, adenomyosis etc. It can be used in post-menopausal women and those with complex cysts, but does not need to be taken in all women who are pre-menopausal with simple cysts [9]. It is only raised in epithelial cancers and only in about 50% in the early stages; therefore, normal levels may not preclude ovarian cancer in post-menopausal women [11]. It is suggested by the RCOG [9] that a Ca125 measurement over 200 or rapidly increasing levels would need referral to a gynaecological oncologist.

Other markers that may be used are alpha-fetoprotein (AFP), beta HCG and LDH and these should be measured in all women under 40 with complex cysts, to look for a yolk sac and germ cell tumours [9], but there is no place for them in post-menopausal women [11].

5.4.2.2 Management
Women often fear that they have cancer; therefore, support and explanation are needed. The management of women depends on age, symptoms and the scan/investigation findings.

Asymptomatic Premenopausal Women
Simple benign-looking cysts up to 5 cm can be monitored with ultrasound after 3 months and laparoscopic removal offered if it increases in size or if there is a change in symptoms [9].
Cysts 50–70 mm should undergo annual scanning [11].
In some women, they may be persistent and increase in size; thus, laparoscopic removal should be carried out [9]. Aspiration of cysts is associated with a higher rate of recurrence [11].

Asymptomatic Post-menopausal Women
Simple cysts under 5 cm with normal Ca125 can be monitored with ultrasound. If there is no change in a year, then women can be discharged [11].

1. Symptomatic women
   (a) Women may be admitted as an emergency for laparoscopy if they present with signs of torsion or rupture.
   (b) Otherwise women may consider laparoscopic removal if the cyst is:
       • Over 5 cm
       • Complex
       • Causing symptoms
       • Causing the patient anxiety over cancer

Laparoscopic surgery is suitable for women with a lower RMI 200 and under [11], and unlike in pre-menopausal women, for the management of complex cysts in post-menopausal women the treatment of choice is bilateral oophorectomy [11]. Women with a higher RMI require a laparotomy.

The types of surgery that can be performed are:

1. Laparoscopic aspiration of the cyst, but this is less effective and can lead to reoccurrence [9, 11].
2. Laparoscopic/open ovarian cystectomy is removal of the cyst.
3. Laparoscopic/open oophorectomy if the ovary is distorted with multiple cysts, sometimes including the tube as well. Removal of the ovary should be performed in post-menopausal women [11]. If there is a possibility of removal of the ovaries, then the menopause and fertility need to be discussed (see Chap. 10).

Any suspicion of cancer and women should be referred to an oncology team, as survival rates are improved with the input of an MDT.

5.5 Endometriosis

5.5.1 Introduction

Endometriosis is the second most common gynaecological condition. It is a chronic condition for which there is no definitive cure, the symptoms of which can be debilitating and isolating. It takes an average of 7 years from onset of symptoms to diagnosis, and affects an estimated 1 in 10 women, which is approximately 176 million women [12]. It is difficult to manage and poorly understood. This means that many women suffer, often without help or understanding, for many years of their lives.

This aim of this chapter is to present the current understanding and management pathways for women with endometriosis and to show how multidisciplinary working within a specialist endometriosis centre benefits women, discussing the benefits of the role of the endometriosis clinical nurse specialist [13, 14].

5.5.2 What Is Endometriosis?

Endometriosis is defined as the presence of endometrial glands and stroma outside the uterus, which reacts to the cyclical hormonal activity and results in a usually painful inflammatory reaction [15]. It is a benign condition that is dependent on oestrogen and as such is predominantly a disease of the reproductive years.

With each menstrual cycle, endometriosis has the potential to worsen, with bleeding into cysts (endometriomas), into the fallopian tubes (haematosalpinx), or into the pelvic structures.

Endometriosis appears as superficial endometriosis, ovarian endometriosis (endometriomas) or deeply infiltrating endometriosis (DIE) [16]. Although symptoms can often give an indication of the position and type of disease, it is also the case that individual responses to the disease vary significantly and some women with severe disease can experience only very mild symptoms; in contrast, women with only minimal disease can sometimes experience very severe symptoms.

Although most endometriosis is found in the pelvis, it has in fact been found throughout the body. Therefore, any symptom that is cyclical in nature could be an indication of endometriosis. The presentation and progression of disease varies considerably and is unpredictable.

5.5.3 Classifications and Staging of Endometriosis

Severity of endometriosis is generally classified from stage 1 (mild) to stage 4 (severe). Classification systems are controversial both within the medical profession and the patient population. It is popularly agreed that the extent of the disease does not always correlate with symptoms and it is therefore very important that the patient is not made to feel as though their symptoms are not valid if their disease stage is mild to moderate. Also, the staging tools tend to describe pelvic endometriosis, whereas other sites such as lung endometriosis can produce very severe symptoms and have a highly significant impact on the patient's quality of life.

There is no agreed classification system; however, the most widely recognised is the American Society for Reproductive Medicine (r-ASRM) classification [17]. This can be seen in Fig. 5.1. This system was originally designed to predict fertility outcomes; however, this has not been found to have any predictive value. There are other classification systems, but due to the complexity of the disease, there is no universal agreement on staging and classification [18].

Fig. 5.1 Examples of the classification of endometriosis (Modified from the American Society for Reproductive Medicine)

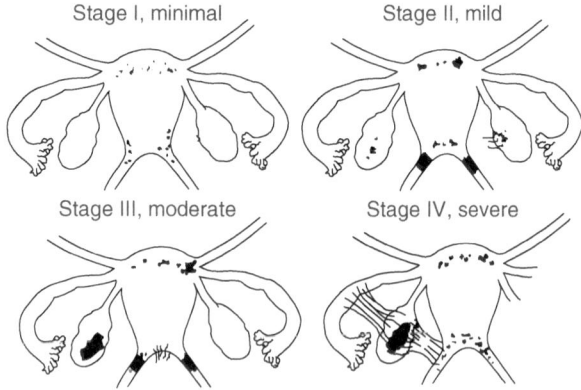

Staging and classification with the American Society [17] tool requires documentation and listing of the appearance, size, location of endometriosis, including endometriomas and adhesions.

- *Stage 1*: minimal endometriosis—describes small superficial peritoneal and adnexal endometriosis up to 3 cm, and filmy adhesions.
- *Stage 2*: mild endometriosis—endometriosis lesions >3 cm, with some deep infiltration.
- *Stage 3*: moderate endometriosis—larger endometriosis lesions, more deeply infiltrating than with mild disease. Partial obliteration of the pouch of Douglas. Dense adhesions.
- *Stage 4*: severe endometriosis—Deep ovarian endometriomas with dense adhesions and obliteration of the pouch of Douglas.

5.5.4 Adenomyosis

Adenomyosis may be defined as the benign invasion of endometrium into the myometrium, producing a diffusely enlarged uterus that microscopically exhibits ectopic, non-neoplastic endometrial glands and stroma surrounded by the hypertrophic and hyperplastic myometrium [18].

Adenomyosis is often associated with endometriosis. In adenomyosis, the endometrial cells are present within the myometrium, usually in a scattered diffuse form and less often in focal cystic form, described as cystadenoma. Again causing an inflammatory response to the menstrual activity and bleeding into the myometrium instead of flowing away with the period. This action causes the uterus to enlarge and become "bulky" [19].

The general opinion is that the most effective surgical management of adenomyosis is hysterectomy; otherwise, the condition should be managed medically. There are, however, some surgical techniques where excision of adenomyosis is performed; this is considered to have greater success when presentation of adenomyosis is focal rather than diffuse. Non-surgical methods such as uterine artery embolisation are occasionally used to treat adenomyosis. Again, these are not widely practiced owing to a lack of outcome evidence support. There is a high risk of uterine rupture in pregnancy after surgery to excise adenomyosis [20].

5.5.5 Common Symptoms

Endometriosis causes pain, but this is just one of the many ways in which the disease can affect a woman's life. It can cause bowel and bladder symptoms, dyspareunia, infertility, and extreme and debilitating fatigue [22].

Symptoms and their severity can vary widely, and do not always correlate with extent of disease. Some women with endometriosis have no symptoms and the diagnosis is incidental, perhaps through infertility investigations or sterilisation [22].

Guidance from the NICE was published in 2017 [22] and suggests that endometriosis should be considered with one or more of these symptoms:

- Chronic period-related pelvic pain (dysmenorrhoea) affecting daily activities and quality of life
- Deep pain during or after sexual intercourse
- Period-related or cyclical GI symptoms, in particular, painful bowel movements
- Period-related or cyclical urinary symptoms, in particular, blood in the urine or pain when passing urine
- Infertility in association with one or more of the above

Pain is usually cyclical and focused on menstruation, resulting in severe dysmenorrhea. It often presents as cramping period-like pains, sometimes worse in the days before the period, lasting throughout the bleeding days and for some days after the period.

Chronic pelvic pain can develop after time, and the patient experiences a continuous pelvic pain that often worsens during her period. Chronic pelvic pain is more challenging to manage as it remains present even when the hormonally influenced activity of endometriosis is suppressed.

If there is bowel involvement, then this can cause dyschezia, irregular bowel habits alternating between constipation and diarrhoea, incomplete emptying of the bowel, and patients often report shooting rectal pain on defecation. Patients with endometriosis are often wrongly given a diagnosis of irritable bowel syndrome. In advanced disease, there may be cyclical rectal bleeding, this should always be fully investigated to exclude any other pathological condition.

With bladder involvement, there may be cyclical haematuria, pain or difficulty emptying the bladder, and incomplete emptying of the bladder. Endometriosis can affect the ureters, causing hydronephrosis, which can reduce renal function; in rare cases, renal failure can occur.

5.5.6 Aetiology

There is no conclusive scientific agreement on the aetiology of endometriosis, its cause, progression and relationship to infertility, although a variety of theories are offered [23].

Popular theories of aetiology include [24]:

- Retrograde menstruation—this normally occurs in approximately 90% of women. Although this is offered as a likely cause of endometriosis, it is not understood why in some women endometrial cells remain within the pelvis and result in endometriosis, while in most instances this is not the case. Some theories suggest inherited properties that affect the peritoneal tissue, predisposing the pelvic epithelium to attachment of the endometrial cells. Immune disorder is considered another possibility.

- Genetic link—sibling studies have shown a genetic link.
- Metaplasia—the transformation of normal peritoneal tissue into endometriosis, theories suggest hormonal or immunological factors influencing this process; however, evidence is unclear.
- Immune response—some women with endometriosis have been found to have an ineffective clearance mechanism, related to immune response. Increased prevalence of immune disorders has been found in women with endometriosis. Women with immune disorders such as rheumatoid arthritis, hypothyroidism and fibromyalgia have been found to have a higher prevalence of endometriosis; however, a conclusive link has not been proven.
- Müllerian rests—cells that are present in the pelvis from embryonic development are stimulated by oestrogen production at puberty.

5.5.7   Endometriosis and Infertility

Endometriosis can have an impact on fertility quite clearly when disease is extensive and distortion of the anatomy occurs. The basic process of ovulation, tubal transportation, fertilisation and implantation can be hampered through ovarian endometriosis affecting ovarian function, reducing ovarian reserve and quality, and also distorted anatomy, which twists or blocks the fallopian tubes.

With severe disease and distortion of the anatomy, there is an increased risk of ectopic pregnancy and therefore early pregnancy ultrasound should be performed to ensure the pregnancy location. The risk of ectopic pregnancy, although rare, is doubled in women with endometriosis [25].

In some women, dyspareunia is so significant that intercourse is not possible at all. Statistically, 50% of women with fertility problems have endometriosis [26], although a large number of these are mild cases. The relationship between the disease and the infertility is not fully understood, although there are several theories. These theories include chronic inflammation, reduced receptivity of the endometrium, reduced ovarian reserve, and distortion of the pelvic anatomy as a result of adhesions [27]. There is ongoing research into stem cell implantation and immune therapy in relation to endometriosis and fertility [28].

Guidance from the NICE [22] recommends that surgical excision or ablation of mild to moderate endometriosis can improve the chances of spontaneous pregnancy. When severe disease is present, discussion about the value of surgical intervention should involve the patient and fertility specialists, including discussion of the risk to the ovarian reserve and the possible impact on fertility if complications arise.

5.5.8   History-Taking

There is great value in allowing the patient to tell her story. Often, she has struggled for years to have her symptoms believed, and may present to a first appointment at a specialist clinic having had unsatisfactory support for their condition in the past. Therefore, the patient should be allowed to explain her symptoms, her priorities and to ask any questions that she might have. The nurse should let the woman know that she has been heard and that she is believed and understood.

Within her story, she will almost certainly volunteer this information; however, these are the important pieces of information that help diagnosis and direct management.

Understanding current symptoms and historical symptoms.

- Pain—type, severity, duration, location, influencing factors, what makes the pain better or worse.
- Bleeding—level of flow, duration of bleeding, regularity of bleeding, any inter-menstrual or post-coital bleeding, an association between bleeding and pain.
- Bowel symptoms—rectal bleeding, constipation, diarrhoea, urgency, bloating, rectal pain, pain on defecation, incomplete emptying of the bowel, any cyclical or dietary pattern to these symptoms.
- Bladder symptoms—haematuria, frequency of urination, difficulty passing urine or pain while passing urine, incomplete emptying of the bladder, any cyclical pattern to these symptoms.
- Dyspareunia—deep, superficial, any alleviating or worsening factors, any psy-chosexual factors.
- Fertility issues.

Gynaecological history

- Age at menarche and onset of current symptoms throughout menstrual life.
- Pregnancy history, parity, deliveries, complications.
- Contraceptive use, which and when, the impact these have had on symptoms, side effects.
- Attempts to conceive, future fertility plans.
- Previous gynaecological surgery, surgical findings.

Pain management history

- What pain management are they currently using? Be specific and find out exactly how they are using any pain relief. For example, do they wait until the pain is extreme before taking any analgesia or do they take a regular dose throughout pain episodes?
- What pain management have they used in the past and to what effect?

5.5.9 Examination and Investigations

Pelvic examination can be useful to a degree. Often, initial visual assessment of the abdomen shows evidence of "erythema ab igne", which is a dermatological response to prolonged and excessive application of heat to the body [29] as seen in Fig. 5.2. In the case of endometriosis, this almost always appears classically as a mottled scarring across the abdomen.

Fig. 5.2 Effect of excess heat on the abdominal skin (https://henrycountywellness.wordpress.com/)

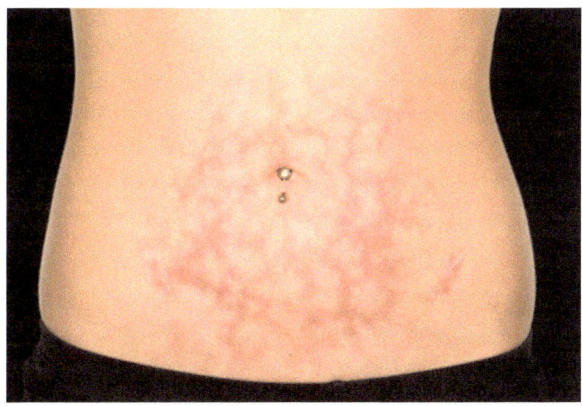

Any palpable masses could indicate ovarian cysts or endometriomas. Vaginal examination can locate palpable nodules or fixed anatomy indicating a "frozen pelvis", and detect any tenderness. A bulky uterus could indicate adenomyosis. There may be visible endometriotic lesions in the vagina or on the cervix.

Transvaginal ultrasound has some value, which differs according to the skill of the person performing the scan. Generally, transvaginal ultrasound is useful for detecting endometriomas and also generally spots any anatomical distortion that is significant and that could indicate severe disease. More specialist practitioners can detect rectovaginal disease, commenting on areas of thickening, assessing the bowel, the bladder and the ureters. These specialist practitioners often combine gentle abdominal palpation to assess the level of mobility of structures within the pelvis and assess any areas of pain.

Magnetic resonance imaging (MRI) should be used to assess the extent and location of disease if severe disease and bowel or bladder involvement are suspected. This allows more detailed assessment of the pelvic structures and detailed imaging discussions within the MDT when planning surgery for women with complex disease [22].

Both transvaginal ultrasound and MRI scans have limitations with regard to the detection of endometriosis, particularly superficial peritoneal disease, which can be extensive and produce highly significant symptoms. Therefore, neither assessment can conclusively exclude the diagnosis of endometriosis, and symptomatic women should be offered a laparoscopy.

Ca125 is not of any value in the diagnosis of endometriosis, as it is often raised with the presence of disease; however, a normal Ca125 result does not exclude the presence of endometriosis [22].

5.5.10 Surgical Management

Diagnostic laparoscopy with histological samples is the gold standard for diagnosing endometriosis. Although negative histology does not confirm the absence of disease.

However, laparoscopic diagnosis is not necessary to initiate medical treatment, indeed in some women the risk of surgery due to comorbidities outweighs the benefit, and their symptoms may be convincing of the disease.

In some cases, imaging and patient symptoms are clear enough to warrant preparation for complex surgery with support from colorectal and or urology consultant surgeons.

If an initial laparoscopy is performed by an specialist surgeon in endometriosis, and minimal disease is found, then usually this is excised during this first-stage operation. If extensive disease is found, involving the bowel or the bladder, then this would not be addressed at this first surgery. In this instance, the patient case would be discussed at the MDT meeting and a second-stage procedure planned with the appropriate MDT present. The patient would be prepared for this surgery with a full discussion of the risks involved, which would usually include a 10% risk of a temporary stoma formation [30].

The woman's fertility objectives would be considered when deciding whether to proceed to complex surgery for endometriosis. The fertility specialists are usually involved in MDT case discussions.

There is current consensus that excision of endometriosis should be performed where possible, in preference to ablation techniques. A systematic review and meta-analysis in 2017 showed that improvement in pain was significantly better when excision was used [31].

The NICE recommends administration of GnRH analogues for 3 months before complex endometriosis surgery [22].

Hysterectomy may be recommended if the patient has adenomyosis or heavy menstrual bleeding, or an accompanying pathological condition such as fibroids. Definitive surgery may also be recommended if the patient has had repeated surgeries with a poor response or return of the disease, depending on age and fertility plans.

5.5.11 Endometriosis After Hysterectomy and Salpingo-Oophorectomy

If hysterectomy is performed, then the woman should be given continuous combined hormone replacement therapy at least until the age of 51 years (see Chap. 10). If the patient receives oestrogen-only HRT (as is common practice for a woman after hysterectomy, as endometrial protection is no longer required), this risks stimulation of any residual endometriosis.

If a patient is obese, they may have higher levels of oestrogen that again could stimulate residual endometriosis, although this is rare.

In some cases, women report continued pain symptoms after definitive surgery for endometriosis. This could be a result of adhesions or chronic pelvic pain, which could be helped by a pain specialist.

5.5.12 Medical Management

When discussing the management of endometriosis, it is important that the patient understands the process of the disease. This understanding helps to explain the principles and rationale behind the recommended or suggested management.

The principle of management is to excise as much endometriosis as possible surgically and then suppress the menstrual cycle with the aim of preventing progression of disease.

Suppression can be achieved with varying success, depending on the individual response to the treatment.

- The Mirena IUS: this is useful as it can be used in addition to the following treatments if the IUS alone is not sufficient to control symptoms and induce amenorrhoea.
- Combined oral contraceptive pill (COCP): the patient should be encouraged to take this continuously with the aim of amenorrhoea. If there are any episodes of prolonged vaginal bleeding, then the COCP should be stopped for 3–4 days and restarted. Some women will need to take a break every 2–3 months.
- Progesterone-only pill—Cerazette: again, this is taken continuously with the aim of amenorrhoea.
- Provera or norethisterone: these higher-dose progestogens can be used if amenorrhoea is not induced with the above methods. They are not recommended for long-term use.
- Depo-Provera injection.
- Progestogen contraceptive implant.
- GnRH analogues such as Zoladex: these are generally recommended for short-term courses of 6 months; however, they are used longer term in rare instances with add-back continuous combined hormone replacement therapy.

5.5.13 Specialist Endometriosis Centres

There are currently, at the time of writing, 51 accredited and 11 provisional endometriosis specialist centres. This accreditation is organised and monitored by the British Society of Gynaecological Endoscopy (BSGE) [13].

Accreditation requirements are [15]:

- A dedicated consultant-led endometriosis service run within a specialist outpatient clinic.
- Each BSGE-listed gynaecological endometriosis specialist consultant within the centre must perform 12 surgical cases of rectovaginal endometriosis that require dissection of the para-rectal space each year. This can include open surgery, but most should be performed laparoscopically.

- A named colorectal surgeon who supports the service and attends surgery with the gynaecologist, when the bowel is involved.
- A named urology consultant and pain management consultant are also listed with the centre.
- All surgical cases of rectovaginal disease where the pararectal space is dissected during surgery are recorded on the BSGE database, and quality of life and symptom questionnaires are completed pre-operatively and at 6, 12 and 24 months post-operatively.
- A named endometriosis nurse specialist is required for each centre.
- Video submission of an operative case where dissection of the para-rectal space is performed is required annually to the BSGE from every centre.

5.5.14 Individualised Care

Endometriosis affects a woman in so many ways, and so differently and unpredictably. It is important for the nurse to manage the patient as an individual and holistically, ensuring that he/she has a full understanding of the symptoms, problems and priorities, to advise and help the patient successfully.

For example, a woman may have dysmenorrhoea and in addition they may have chronic pelvic pain. It is important to address both, as they respond to different treatments. They may also have significant anxiety and depression in relation to their pain, which makes it more difficult to cope with the pain; therefore, talking therapies or cognitive behavioural therapy could be beneficial additions to their care plan.

Women respond differently to hormonal treatments and it is important both to explain the rationale behind any treatment suggested, and to listen to concerns that they may have. This allows any reassurances to be given, while ensuring that the woman retains control of her own care. Any decisions the woman makes about her care, as long as she is fully informed, should be respected by her medical and nursing team.

5.5.15 The Role of the Endometriosis Specialist Nurse

The endometriosis specialist nurse is a relatively new phenomenon, becoming a compulsory component of BSGE specialist centre status in 2014. He/she is primarily responsible for ensuring that all the necessary components of the specialist service are fulfilled within the necessary timeframe, liaising with the wider team to ensure coordination of care pathways and accurate follow-up for complex patients, as required by the BSGE.

The RCN have worked closely with the BSGE and endometriosis charities to produce both a fact sheet on endometriosis for patients and a guide to the role of the endometriosis specialist nurse [14].

The main responsibilities of the endometriosis specialist nurse, as defined by the RCN, are to:

- Lead and develop services
- Ensure that services are linked to primary care
- Support a better understanding of this condition among all nurses coming into contact with endometriosis patients

The RCN also offers guidance on the qualifications and skills of an endometriosis specialist nurse [14]:

- Extensive experience working within a women's health care setting
- Master's level education, critical thinking and decision-making
- Insight into the condition
- Insight into all areas of management, including the wider social political factors

The endometriosis specialist nurse is usually someone with a lot of women's health nursing experience, therefore each background has a slightly different element and skill that bring something unique to the role. Counselling skills are extremely useful, while some nurses may have imaging skills, or perhaps a fertility background. Each skill has value and should be utilised to its fullest.

The most important skills for the specialist nurse are the ability to show true empathy with the patient, whatever their story and whatever their priority; to be the patient's advocate; to listen to the patient and support them through their journey, whatever their choices may be. The experience of the endometriosis patient is as varied as the disease itself, and it is absolutely crucial to understand the subtlety of each individual experience; to ensure that all patient decisions are truly informed choices, that the woman is given clear information and insight into the medical advice from the team, explained in whichever way is necessary for them to really understand the information they are being given; to ensure that they are given the opportunity to talk through their concerns, voice their questions, whatever they are; to give all their concerns weight and value, and to ensure that the woman feels empowered and in control of their choices throughout all elements of their care, while they are the nurse's responsibility.

The endometriosis nurse should educate widely, both throughout primary and secondary care; supporting the supporters, working with charities and support groups; linking with in-patient wards, GPs, pharmacy groups, fertility teams and midwives; educating and supporting practice with enthusiasm and accessibility. Networking nationally is also an important part of the nurse's role, ensuring that care is standardised to the highest level, that best practice is shared and that colleagues are supported.

The endometriosis nurse must understand the disease, and explore all possible ways in which each woman can be helped along their journey, whatever the journey choices the patient may take, recognising that these choices can, and often will, change.

The endometriosis specialist nurse will be able to see a new patient at their first visit to the service, take a good and thorough history and gain a good understanding of their priorities and symptoms. The nurse will be able to order imaging or other investigations, and start medical management if appropriate (non-medical prescribing is a very useful qualification for the endometriosis specialist nurse). Referrals can be made to appropriate MDT members, and the case can be brought for discussion at the multidisciplinary meeting.

The endometriosis nurse should be an approachable, empathetic and non-judgemental point of contact for the woman throughout her journey.

5.5.16 Multidisciplinary Approach

The location of the patient's disease indicates which surgical team is needed and whether the colorectal and/or urology consultant surgeons should be involved during surgery.

The patient's fertility plans must be understood, for the immediate and for the more distant future. It may be necessary to involve the fertility specialists for a consultation about fertility implications, or the patient may need a direct referral for IVF.

The specialist service must include support from a pelvic pain specialist who can utilise a variety of specialist skills to help to address and manage long-term pain.

Women's health physiotherapy should be available.

Some services have access to additional support, such as nutrition and dietetics, counselling or cognitive behavioural therapy courses.

Regular multidisciplinary meetings should be held that are attended by the colorectal, urology, gynaecology and fertility consultants. Radiographic imaging should be presented and discussed with the guidance of a radiology consultant, and forward management plans for complex cases should be discussed and documented.

5.5.17 Alternative Therapies

Women with endometriosis have often explored alternative therapies widely. There are many claims of "miracle cures", and it is important to ensure that patients have correct information from the specialist teams to avoid exploitation.

However, many women find benefit from different therapies and, as long as they are aware of the lack of supportive evidence for most of these, the general opinion is that if something is benefitting the woman, then this is a positive.

Popular activities may include gentle yoga or stretching exercises, meditation, or swimming.

Some women find benefit from therapies such as acupuncture, reiki or reflexology. Women should always be advised that there is no medical evidence that these therapies benefit endometriosis, and encouraged to ensure that any practitioner they approach is appropriately qualified within their particular field.

5.5.18 Endometriosis Diet

There are a wealth of claims and theories about diet and endometriosis. It is important that women know that most of these claims are not evidence-based. There is no evidence that an oestrogen-heavy diet stimulates endometriosis, for example. If a woman asks about this, it is important, again, to educate with the known principles of the action of endometriosis.

However, there are links to diet and symptoms that the woman with endometriosis, particularly where the disease involves the bowel, experiences. For example, it is well known that wheat and gluten can generally cause bloating; therefore, if the digestive system is less efficient because of endometriosis, this symptom is likely to be more extreme.

Some women may benefit from adopting the fermentable oligo-, di-, monosaccharides and polyols diet, devised for irritable bowel sufferers.

When women ask for advice about diet, they can be advised that some women notice that certain foods trigger their symptoms; however, there is not any set guidance as to which foods affect which woman. Therefore, it should be suggested that they try eliminating one thing at a time, to see if there is any benefit, rather than eliminating several things at once, which is far more difficult to sustain and confusing for evaluation of the effect.

5.5.19 Support Groups

Support is available for women with endometriosis, usually arranged through charities, particularly the charity Endometriosis UK. Several hospitals hold support groups alongside Endometriosis UK and their volunteers.

Endometriosis UK also offers telephone support helplines. There are occasional live webchats, again through charities, and sometimes through the NICE.

Endometriosis UK also organises information days for women and their friends and families.

There are also online forums and groups available.

References

1. BMJ Best Practice in Dysmenorrhoea (2018) Accessed 14 Aug 2018
2. Oladosu F, Frank F, Tu D, Hellman K (2007) Nonsteroidal anti-inflammatory drug resistance in dysmenorrhoea: epidemiology, causes and treatment. Am J Obstet Gynecol 218(4):390–400
3. https://www.rcn.org.uk/professional-development/publications/pub-005480
4. Brichant G, Denef M, Tebache L et al (2018) Chronic pelvic pain and the role of exploratory laparoscopy as diagnostic and therapeutic tool: a retrospective observational study. Gynecol Surg 15:13
5. Pattanittum P, Kunyanone N, Brown J et al (2016) Dietary supplements for dysmenorrhoea. Cochrane Database Syst Rev 3: CD002124
6. Public Health England (2018) What does the data tell us? Women's reproductive health is a public health issue. https://app.box.com/s/2nrbo3bxddkf685ifu4y6vjpyy2blumj
7. Lee N, Jakes A, Lloyd J, Frodsham L (2018) Dyspareunia. BMJ 361:k2341
8. https://www.fsrh.org/standards-and-guidance/documents/ceuguidanceintrauterinecontraception/
9. RCOG/BSGE (2011) Management of suspected ovarian masses in premenopausal women. Green Top Guideline no. 62. RCOG
10. National Institute of Clinical and Health Excellence. https://www.nice.org.uk/guidance/CG122

11. RCOG (2016) The management of ovarian cysts in postmenopausal women. Green Top Guideline no. 34
12. https://www.endometriosis-uk.org/. Accessed 8 Sept 2018
13. https://www.bsge.org.uk/. Accessed 8 Sept 2018
14. RCN CNS endometriosis (2015) https://www.rcn.org.uk/professional-development/publications/pub-004776
15. RCN endometriosis factsheet (2015) https://www.rcn.org.uk/professional-development/publications/pub-004777
16. Cirstoiu M, Bodean O, Secara D, Munteanu O, Cirstoiu C (2013) Case study on a rare form of endometriosis. J Med Life 6(1):68–71
17. American Society for Reproductive Medicine. https://www.asrm.org. Accessed 8 Sept 2018
18. NHS England (2013) https://www.england.nhs.uk/commissioning/wp-content/uploads/sites/12/2014/04/e10-comp-gynae-endom-0414.pdf. Accessed 8 Sept 2018
19. Leyendecker G, Wildt L, Mall G (2009) The pathophysiology of endometriosis and adenomyosis: tissue injury and repair. Arch Gynecol Obstet 280(4):529–538
20. Farquar C, Brosens I (2006) Medical and surgical management of adenomyosis. Best practice and research. Clin Obstet Gynaecol 20(4):603–616
21. Grimbizis GF (2014) Uterus sparing operative treatment for adenomyosis. Fertil Steril 101(2):472–487.e8
22. National Institute of Clinical and Health Excellence. https://www.nice.org.uk/guidance/ng73
23. Haney AF (1991) The pathogenesis and aetiology of endometriosis. In: Thomas EJ, Rock JA (eds) Modern approaches to endometriosis. Springer, Dordrecht
24. BMJ Best Practice. Endometriosis—symptoms diagnosis and treatment. https://bestpractice.bmj.com/topics/en-gb/355. Accessed 8 Sept 2018
25. European Society of Human Reproduction and Embryology Management of women with endometriosis. https://bestpractice.bmj.com/topics/en-gb/355. Accessed 8 Sept 2018
26. Fadhlaoui A, Bouquet de la Joliniere J, Feki A (2014) Endometriosis and infertility: How and when to treat? Front Surg 1:24
27. Bulun MD, Serdar E (2009) Endometriosis. N Engl J Med 360:268–279
28. Macer ML, Taylor HS (2012) Endometriosis and infertility: a review of the pathogenesis and treatment of endometriosis associated infertility. Obstet Gynecol Clin North Am 39(4):535–549
29. Gianfaldoni S, Gianfaldoni R, Tchernev G, Lotti J, Wollina U, Lotti T (2017) Erythema ab igne successfully treated with mesoglycan and bioflavonoids: a case report. Open Access Maced J Med Sci 5(4):432–435
30. https://www.endometriosis-uk.org/sites/default/files/files/Information/endometriosis-bowel.pdf. Accessed 8 Sept 2018
31. Pundir J, Omanwa K, Kovoor E, Pundir V, Lancaster G, Barton-Smith P (2017) Laparoscopic excision versus ablation for endometriosis-associated pain: an updated systematic review and meta-analysis. J Minim Invasive Gynecol 24(5):747–756

Suggested Reading

https://www.bsge.org.uk/requirements-to-be-a-bsge-accredited-centre/
https://www.endometriosis-uk.org/endometriosis-facts-and-figures
https://www.endowhat.com/
https://www.england.nhs.uk/commissioning/wp-content/uploads/sites/12/2014/04/e10-comp-gynae-endom-0414.pdf
https://www.nice.org.uk/guidance/ng73/chapter/Recommendations#diagnosing-endometriosis
https://www.nice.org.uk/guidance/ng73/resources/endometriosis-diagnosis-and-management-pdf-1837632548293
https://www.rcn.org.uk/professional-development/publications/pub-004776
https://www.rcn.org.uk/professional-development/publications/pub-004777

Fertility

Wendy Norton

6.1 Introduction

For many people, having children is an essential aspect of their life plan. It is estimated that over 80% of heterosexual couples in the general population will conceive within 1 year if the woman is aged under 40 years and regular unprotected sexual intercourse is taking place [1]. Sexual intercourse every 2–3 days optimises the chances of pregnancy [2]. Of those who do not conceive within this time frame, about half will do so within the second year (cumulative pregnancy rate over 90%) [1]. In the UK, infertility is experienced by around 1 in 7 couples or approximately 3.5 million people [1]. Infertility can be primary (conception has never occurred) or secondary (in those who have conceived before but do not necessarily have a child). Women of reproductive age, who have not conceived after 1 year of unprotected vaginal sexual intercourse, in the absence of any known cause of infertility, should be offered clinical assessment and investigation along with her partner.

Over the past decade, there has been a significant trend in delaying parenthood [3] which has potential implications on fertility [4]. An earlier referral should be offered where the woman is aged 36 years or over, as there is a more noticeable decline in female fertility after the age of 35 [5] and/or there is a known clinical cause of infertility or a history of predisposing factors for infertility [1].

W. Norton (✉)
The Leicester School of Nursing and Midwifery, De Montfort University, Leicester, UK
e-mail: WNorton@dmu.ac.uk

© Springer Nature Switzerland AG 2019
D. Holloway (ed.), *Nursing Management of Women's Health*,
https://doi.org/10.1007/978-3-030-16115-6_6

6.2   Causes and Risk Factors

There are many causes for infertility which makes it difficult to ascertain true figures. Infertility may be caused by a range of medical conditions as outlined in Table 6.1. It is estimated that the main causes of infertility relate to ovulatory disorders (25% of couples), tubal damage (20% of couples), male infertility (30% of couples) and uterine disorders (10% of couples). For 25% of couples, there is no identifiable cause of infertility, referred to as 'unexplained infertility'. Many couples (40%) will have more than one cause [6].

Other risk factors relate to environmental issues, e.g. exposure to chemicals and pesticides [11], and lifestyle behaviours, e.g. smoking and obesity [12].

6.3   Fertility Management in Primary Care

Primary care services are usually the first point of contact for couples having difficulty conceiving. Fertility management should be in line with the agreed local care pathway. The first contact provides an opportunity to give the couple information and make an initial assessment. It is important to include both partners in the assessment process, so they both have an opportunity to ask questions and are involved in any care and/or referral decisions being made. Some people may find this topic difficult to discuss; therefore it is imperative that they receive sensitive, appropriate

Table 6.1 Possible causes for infertility in men and women

Female	Male
• Hormone imbalance • Ovulation problems • Genetic condition, i.e. Turner syndrome • Hyperprolactinaemia • Hypo-/hyperthyroidism • Premature ovarian failure • Polycystic ovarian syndrome (PCOS) • Pelvic inflammatory disease (PID) • Sexually transmitted infections (STIs) • Endometriosis • Tubal blockage • Previous tubal ligation • Uterine problems • Uterine fibroids • Age-related factors • Exposure to gonadotoxins [7]	• Anatomical abnormalities, e.g. obstruction of spermatic ducts; varicocele; undescended testes; congenital absence of the vas deferens • Previous vasectomy • Genetic condition, i.e. Klinefelter's syndrome • Hormonal abnormality, e.g. hypogonadotropic hypogonadism, pituitary tumours • Systemic or neurological diseases • Infections—epididymitis; mumps • Testicular trauma/injury • Iatrogenic causes—steroids, radiotherapy/chemotherapy • Exposure to gonadotoxins • Antisperm antibodies • Erectile or ejaculation dysfunction • Retrograde ejaculation • Prostate surgery [8, 9] No identified cause in 30–40% of cases [10]

and accurate information about investigations and support that can be offered within primary care. Taking a patient history and performing a physical examination will highlight possible risk factors, provide health promotion opportunities to discuss modifiable factors (e.g. obesity and smoking) and identify the need for more urgent referral to specialist services.

6.3.1 Initial Assessment

History taking is a key component of patient assessment that enables care priorities to be identified, and the most appropriate interventions commenced to optimise patient outcomes [13]. Good communication skills and a private environment are essential prerequisites for gathering a detailed history from both partners. Nurses must adopt a sensitive and non-judgemental approach to elicit information whilst being mindful that individuals may be reluctant to disclose information that their partner may be unaware of (e.g. previous sexually transmitted infections or a previous abortion). Responses to some of the questions outlined will guide the additional diagnostic investigations to be ordered and flag the need for earlier referral to specialist services.

History-taking questions should address the following aspects:

- Age.
- Reproductive history—length of time trying to conceive; previous contraception used/stopped.
- Sexual history—frequency of intercourse; awareness of fertile phase; sexual function, i.e. dyspareunia or erectile/ejaculation problems; history of STIs.
- Menstrual history—cycle length details; any heavy menstrual bleeding, dysmenorrhoea, oligomenorrhoea or amenorrhoea.
- Obstetric history—previous pregnancies and miscarriages (with the same or a different partner); delivery/post-delivery complications.
- Current medical status—ongoing management; prescribed medication.
- Past medical/surgical history—e.g. gynaecological conditions/pelvic surgery; testicular injury/surgery.
- Body mass index (BMI).
- Lifestyle factors—alcohol; smoking; recreational drugs; anabolic steroids; occupation; exposure to chemicals, etc.
- Health promotion opportunities—recording blood pressure is good practice and serves as a baseline; check cervical screening status; consider obesity management; smoking cessation advice.

A physical examination may be indicated based on the information gathered; patients should be offered a chaperone. A pelvic examination may not be necessary if a tubal assessment is requested.

Table 6.2 Initial investigations

Female	Male

• Rubella serology
• Haematology screen
• Anti-Müllerian hormone (AMH) as a marker of ovarian reserve
• Serum FSH/LH (day 1–4)
• Serum mid-luteal progesterone
• Prolactin if ovulatory disorder suspected
• Tubal status (depending on local referral guidance)
   – If no existing comorbidities (e.g. PID; previous ectopic pregnancy or endometriosis), refer for hysterosalpingography (HSG) or hysterosalpingo-contrast sonography (HyCoSy)
   – If comorbidities exist, refer for laparoscopy and dye so that tubal and other pelvic pathology can be assessed at the same time [1]
	• Semen analysis (2–7 days recommended abstinence)—sample to be produced by masturbation and assessed against the World Health Organization parameters [14]
	• If there are poor parameters reported in the semen analysis, e.g. azoospermia or severe oligospermia, then repeat semen analysis (3 months later), and consider testing for FSH/LH/testosterone and prolactin

Assess need for sexually transmitted infection screening of both partners (and treatment offered accordingly)	

6.3.2 Initial Investigations

The preliminary investigations, as outlined in Table 6.2, seek to identify the reported major causes of infertility: ovulatory disorders, male factors and tubal damage.

Further investigations may be requested depending upon clinical presentation, patient history or preliminary test results. Following initial assessment, couples with male factor infertility or suspected/or confirmed tubal infertility should be referred to specialist fertility services for in vitro fertilisation (IVF) or intra-cytoplasmic sperm injection (ICSI) treatments (see later in this chapter).

6.3.3 Preconceptual Care

Nurses play a central role in promoting preconceptual care. The health of both women and men before conception is important, not only for pregnancy outcomes but also for the lifelong health of their children [15]. Therefore, providing health promotion and lifestyle advice is an important aspect of the nurse's role. Public Health England [16] advises women planning a pregnancy to check their measles, mumps and rubella (MMR) status at appropriate opportunities (e.g. when attending a contraception clinic or travel clinic appointment), so if vaccination is required, it can be given before trying to conceive. MMR vaccine is no longer recommended in pregnancy as a matter of caution [17]. Rubella infection in the first 16 weeks of pregnancy is associated with a high risk of major and varied congenital abnormalities, commonly known as congenital rubella syndrome [17]. Measles in pregnancy may also lead to miscarriage, stillbirth or premature birth [16]

A healthy diet and regular exercise are also important for maintaining overall health. A normal BMI of 19–25 kg/m^2 should be advised for both partners [18]. Obesity has been associated with lower live birth rates in women undergoing assisted reproduction [19]. Vitamins are important for foetal growth and development, and all pregnant women are advised to take a daily dose of 10 mcg of vitamin D. A daily supplement of 400 mcg folic acid (vitamin B9) and increasing dietary folates before conception and throughout the first 12 weeks of pregnancy help to prevent neural tube birth defects (NTD) and reduce the risk of heart or limb defects and some childhood brain tumours [20]. Women at high risk of an NTD should take a higher daily dose of 5 mg of folic acid.

The teratogenic effects of alcohol on a foetus have long been recognised; hence the safest option is to avoid alcohol whilst trying to conceive. If couples choose to drink, they should be advised to limit their drinking to the UK Government's guideline of a maximum of one to two units once or twice per week for women trying to conceive and three to four units per day for men [21]. Smoking has been linked to infertility, an early menopause, sperm problems and premature or low birthweight babies [22, 23]. If couples smoke, nurses should provide information about the risks of smoking during conception and pregnancy and give advice and support on local and national smoking cessation programmes [24]. Studies have also suggested that caffeine (e.g. in coffee, tea, soft drinks, chocolate and some medication) reduces the chances of conception or may have harmful effects on the developing foetus [25]. The current data is contradictory; a precautionary limit of two cups of coffee/200 mg caffeine per day is advised [26].

6.3.4 Emotional Support

There is evidence that infertility causes considerable emotional stress and symptoms of anxiety and depression, which may affect many aspects of couples' lives and can result in social isolation [27]. Infertility has also been described as a stigmatised condition which makes disclosure difficult for people [28]. Patients may feel embarrassed, exposed and vulnerable at a time when they are at their most sensitive [29]. Some people may have difficulty discussing infertility either within the relationship or with professionals because of the taboos still associated with some assisted reproductive techniques (ART) and/or for cultural reasons. In some ethnic groups or communities, an inability to have a child or to become pregnant can result in them being ostracised or shunned. Infertility can also be used as grounds for divorce with women disproportionately carrying the burden of infertility, as pregnancy and childbirth are manifested in the woman [30].

Nurses' counselling skills can have a significant impact on individual's emotional well-being. Establishing an effective nurse-patient relationship allows the woman and her partner to feel able to share their feelings and concerns in a supportive, safe and confidential environment. Nurses need to be approachable, non-judgemental, compassionate and sensitive to individual couples' beliefs and needs. In addition, nurses can signpost individuals to fertility support groups, e.g. Fertility Network UK, and therapeutic counselling carried out by trained/accredited counsellors. Since patients' needs may vary at different stages of their infertility journey, counselling should be offered prior, during and after assessment or treatment. This provides an opportunity for people to explore their thoughts, feelings and their relationships in order to reach a better understanding of the meaning and implications of any choices they may make [31]. Counselling facilitates discussion of a variety of issues and concerns in a supportive environment and can help individuals make sense of present challenges and develop coping strategies [32]. Counsellors can be accessed via GP surgeries, private providers and licenced fertility clinics.

6.3.5 Onward Referral and Funding

In the absence of any known cause of infertility, expectant management is advised if the woman is under 36 years of age. Referral should usually be considered if the couple have not conceived after 1 year [1], but referral criterion varies among local health authorities. It is estimated that the National Health Service (NHS) spends £68 m per annum on IVF treatment [33]. However, whilst IVF treatment is consistently NHS funded in Scotland, Wales and Northern Ireland, access to NHS funding in England varies from region to region [34]. Since 2013, NICE has stipulated that women who meet certain criteria should be offered three funded cycles. However, funding is at the discretion of local Clinical Commissioning Groups (CCGs) who decide which treatments are funded and the patient criteria for their local area. As of 2017, only 13.5% (27/200) of England's CCGs complied with the NICE stipulations, whilst some CCGs have cut fertility services altogether [35]. Those couples who are not eligible for NHS funded treatment, or women for whom time is at a premium, will need to seek treatment from the private sector. Nurses should familiarise themselves with their local referral policies and NHS waiting times, as well as the contact details for local private fertility clinics, so they can advise patients accordingly.

6.4 Specialist Fertility Care

Despite the range of fertility treatment options currently available, it is estimated that approximately 50% of infertile couples never seek fertility care, and of those who do, 20% wait for more than 2 years before seeing a specialist [36]. Ethical objections to treatment, personal reasons, relationship problems, financial issues and the psychological burden of treatment (including a fear of failure) have been reported as reasons for not pursuing fertility treatment [37, 38]. Therefore, a range of appropriate interventions should be fully discussed with patients, so they can make informed decisions about what treatment option, if any, they may wish to pursue.

There are three main types of fertility treatment available following investigation:

- Medical treatment—including the use of fertility drugs to promote ovulation (see below).
- Surgical treatment—including tubal microsurgery in women with mild tubal disease or surgical correction of epididymal blockage in men with obstructive azoospermia.
- Assisted reproductive technologies (ART)—a collective name for treatments designed to lead to conception by means other than sexual intercourse.

Medical and non-invasive surgical treatments for infertility should be attempted before considering the option of assisted conception [1]. Alternatively, some couples may decide to seek alternative forms of family-building such as adoption or fostering; nurses can help signpost patients to these local/national organisations for further information.

6.5 Assisted Reproductive Technologies

In the UK, ART should only be carried out in specialist centres that are registered with the fertility regulator, the Human Fertilisation and Embryology Authority (HFEA). The HFEA is responsible for inspecting and licencing clinics; maintains a register of information about donors, treatments and children born from treatments; and provides advice and information to patients, donors, clinics and policymakers. All HFEA-licenced clinics must adhere to the HFEA Code of Practice which ensures professionals working within fertility clinics comply with the Human Fertilisation and Embryology Act 1990 (as amended) and relevant legislation.

6.5.1 Planning an ART Programme

The purpose of the initial consultation is to review the patient and partner histories and any previous investigation results. Further diagnostic tests may be requested to determine the best course of treatment and/or screening for transmissible infections. Screening tests that are required prior to commencing ART programmes include HIV 1 and 2 (anti-HIV 1, 2), hepatitis B (HBsAG/anti-HBc) and hepatitis C (anti-HCV-Ab) [39]. A full discussion is important so that couples can make an informed decision about their care. This information should include:

- Full range of treatment options and the associated benefits/limitations.
- Implications and risks of the proposed treatment programme, i.e. multiple pregnancy or ovarian hyperstimulation.
- Implications of using third-party reproduction and legal parenthood requirements (if applicable).
- Welfare of the child assessment.

- Likely success rates and outcomes of proposed treatment, including the possibility of a poor response to drug regimes or low fertilisation rates.
- Cryopreservation and storage of gametes and embryos.
- Treatment costs and the pros and cons of any 'add-on' options for different treatments.
- Explanation of consent forms and individuals' rights to change or withdraw consent at any time before treatment.

The HFEA [39] stipulates that all patients undergoing treatment must be given appropriate information, verbally and in writing, regarding treatment options. In addition, HFEA-licenced clinics are legally obliged to offer therapeutic counselling. Adequate time should be allowed for patients to digest the information, to have opportunities to ask questions and to seek counselling if desired, before consenting to any treatment. Different types of consents include consent to different treatment types; consent to the use and storage of eggs, sperm and/or embryos; consent to being a legal parent (if using donated gametes and/or embryos and the couple are not married or in a civil partnership); and consent to sharing of personal information with other healthcare providers.

6.5.2 Range of Programmes

ART covers a wide spectrum of treatments as outlined in Table 6.3. Depending on the cause of infertility, the following types of treatment may be suggested:

6.5.3 Third-Party Reproduction

The use of 'third-party reproduction' refers to the use of eggs, sperm or embryos that have been donated by a third person (donor) to enable an infertile individual or couple (intended recipient) to become parents [40]. Annually, around 2500 people in the UK have treatment with the help of a donor [41]. Clinics may also offer 'sharing' arrangements whereby another man or woman who is undergoing fertility treatment donates some of their eggs or sperm in return for discounted treatment, reduced storage costs or decreased waiting times, depending on the clinic's policy. Potential egg sharers must fulfil certain eligibility criteria and be registered with the HFEA as donors. All donors must be screened for infectious and genetic diseases and be offered counselling to consider the implications of their donation [39].

In the UK, people conceived through gamete donation can access identifiable information about their donor once they reach the age of 18. Donors and recipients are not permitted to learn each other's identities, either at the time of donation or subsequently [42]. Only non-identifying information about the donor can be given at the point of treatment. Where third-party reproduction is carried out at an HFEA-licenced clinic, UK law states that the recipient parents, rather than the donor, acquire the legal status of parent, even where they have no biological connection with the child. The donor has no legal rights or responsibilities to any children born with their sperm, eggs or embryos [43]. Under UK law, the woman who gives birth is the legal mother; therefore in surrogacy arrangements, the surrogate will be the

Table 6.3 Spectrum of ART programmes

Treatment	Indications	What it involves
Ovulation induction	• Women who are not ovulating or not ovulating on a regular basis	Ovarian stimulation using oral antioestrogens or gonadotrophins to promote follicular development. Ultrasound follicular tracking helps to identify when optimal follicular size (about 17 mm in diameter) has been achieved. Ovulation is triggered by administering hCG. Sexual intercourse can then be timed to coincide with ovulation
Intrauterine insemination (IUI)	• Women with patent fallopian tubes but who cannot conceive • Mild male factor infertility • Unexplained infertility • When semen has been frozen due to a partner's absence	A sample of prepared sperm is inserted through the cervix and into the uterus at the time of ovulation to increase the chances of conception. IUI is usually combined with an ovulation induction regime (as described above) to produce one or more oocytes. Ultrasound monitoring is important to reduce the risk of multiple pregnancy. Sperm are collected through masturbation and washed in the laboratory, so the best-quality sperm is inseminated. If a pregnancy is not achieved after a series of IUI attempts, treatment may be stepped up to IVF
In vitro fertilisation (IVF)	• Tubal damage/blockage • Previous sterilisation • Step up from IUI with unexplained infertility • Oligospermia	Pituitary downregulation regimes are used to switch off the natural ovulatory cycle. Gonadotrophins are then administered to encourage the development of several follicles. When a sufficient response is observed, hCG is administered to further mature the oocytes ready for collection approximately 36 hrs later. The woman is given intravenous sedation, and the oocytes are retrieved by aspirating the follicles transvaginally under ultrasound guidance. Sperm from the male partner (or donor sperm) is used to inseminate the collected oocytes. If fertilisation occurs and an embryo develops, the best-quality embryo is transferred into the uterus 2–5 days later using a catheter under ultrasound guidance. Progesterone luteal support is prescribed to aid implantation
Intra-cytoplasmic sperm injection (ICSI)	• Severe male factor infertility • Obstructive azoospermia • Non-obstructive azoospermia	In cases of severe deficit of semen quality or non-obstructive azoospermia, ICSI may increase the risk of passing on a genetic disorder or male infertility. Therefore, the male partner's karyotype should be checked and genetic counselling offered if applicable [1] In cases of azoospermia, surgical sperm retrieval can be performed to extract sperm directly from the epididymis or testicular tissue Essentially, ICSI follows the same process as an IVF cycle but involves the direct injection of a single sperm into the inner cellular structure of each oocyte to promote fertilisation

(continued)

Table 6.3 (continued)

Treatment	Indications	What it involves
Donor insemination (DI)	• Obstructive azoospermia • Non-obstructive azoospermia • Severe deficits in semen quality in couples who do not wish to undergo ICSI • High risk of transmitting a genetic disorder to the offspring or woman from the man • Severe rhesus isoimmunisation • Single women and same-sex female couples	Can be carried out in a natural cycle or combined with ovarian induction. The process of DI is the same as described for IUI
Oocyte donation cycles	• Premature ovarian failure • Genetic disorders, i.e. Turner syndrome • Bilateral oophorectomy • Ovarian failure following chemotherapy or radiotherapy • Advanced maternal age	Oocyte donors may be known, i.e. a friend or relative, or unknown. The oocyte donor undergoes a stimulated IVF cycle and oocyte retrieval as described above. The collected oocytes are fertilised with sperm from the recipient woman's partner (or donor sperm). The recipient woman is prescribed oestrogen and progesterone to prepare her endometrium for the transfer of the best-quality embryo
Surrogacy	• Congenital absence of the uterus • Significant uterine pathology • Hysterectomy • Medical reason leading to an inability to healthily gestate a pregnancy • Recurrent pregnancy loss • Repeated IVF implantation failures • Option for same-sex male couples who want to have a family	A surrogate gestates a baby for another person or couple (intended parents) with the intention of relinquishing the baby to the intended parents after the birth. There are two types of surrogacy: • Traditional surrogacy involves sperm from the intended father and an oocyte from the surrogate. Fertilisation is achieved by informal artificial insemination or IUI in a fertility clinic. The surrogate will have a genetic link to the child • Gestational surrogacy follows an IVF programme, using oocytes from the intended mother or an egg donor and sperm from the intended father or a sperm donor. The best-quality resulting embryo is transferred into another woman, the gestational surrogate. The surrogate hosts the pregnancy but will not be genetically related to the child

legal parent until the intended parents are granted a parental order transferring legal rights (for further details, see https://www.gov.uk/become-a-childs-legal-parent).

Intended recipients should be offered counselling regarding the physical and psychological implications of third-party reproduction for themselves and potential children. Counselling provides a safe environment to explore the potential impact of disclosure, legal parenthood considerations and the rights of all concerned [44]. In addition, recipients can be signposted to charitable organisations who can provide advice and support to families with donor-conceived/surrogacy-conceived children (see Resources section).

6.6   Key Steps in ART

Whatever ART programme is undertaken, the following general principles apply:

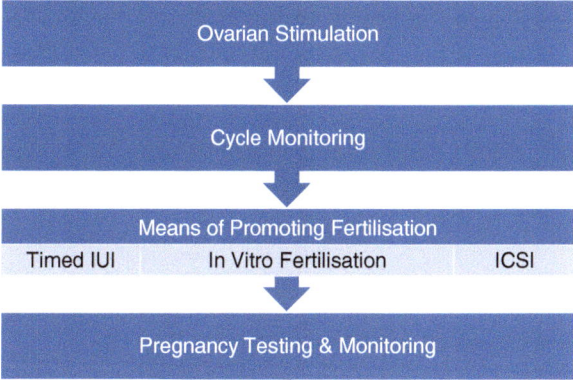

6.6.1   Ovarian Stimulation

Before any fertility treatment, it is useful to measure a woman's ovarian reserve (see Table 6.4). This can predict the likely response to an ovarian stimulation regime. There are three ways to measure ovarian reserve:

- An ultrasound scan of the antral follicle count (AFC) at the beginning of a cycle.
- Measuring the level of anti-Müllerian hormone (AMH) at any point of a cycle.
- Measuring the level of follicle-stimulating hormone (FSH) at the beginning of a cycle.

Table 6.4 Different ways to measure a woman's ovarian reserve [1]

Predicted ovarian reserve	Poor	Good
AFC	≤4	≥16
AMH (pmol/L)	≤5.4	≥25.0
FSH (IU/L)	≥8.9	≤4

There are many different medications that are used within ART, and these can be seen in Table 6.5. When superovulation cycles have been planned, nurses can work alongside the woman and her partner to educate them about the prescribed medications. Nurses need to ensure the couple fully understand their prescription, how these drugs can be obtained, the associated financial costs, drug storage requirements and the mode of action. Women should also be informed of the common side effects of these medications. Where appropriate, nurses can teach the injection

Table 6.5 Common fertility drugs used in ART

Drug	
Clomiphene citrate (Clomid®)	• Oral antioestrogen treatment which induces gonadotrophin release by occupying oestrogen receptors in the hypothalamus, thereby interfering with feedback mechanisms [45] • Used on days 2–6 of the cycle to stimulate and/or regulate ovulation • It is recommended that use is limited to 6 months [1]
Gonadotrophins	• Recombinant or purified urinary FSH ± LH • Acts as a substitute for normal pituitary production to stimulate follicular development. A daily individualised dose is prescribed based on factors relating to age, BMI, PCOS and ovarian reserve • It is recommended that the maximum dose should not exceed 450 IU/day [1]
Gonadotrophin-releasing hormone (GnRH) agonist downregulation/gonadotrophin-releasing hormone antagonists	• Used as part of gonadotrophin-stimulated IVF treatment cycles to avoid premature luteinising hormone surges [1] • A long GnRH agonist protocol, where this drug is taken 2–3 weeks before and during the gonadotrophin injection regime, is usually used in women who have a normal ovarian reserve • A short antagonist protocol, where this drug is started a few days after starting the gonadotrophin regime, tends to be reserved for women who have a poor ovarian reserve or women who have a high ovarian reserve as a means of reducing the risk of ovarian hyperstimulation syndrome (OHSS) (described below)
Human chorionic gonadotrophin (hCG)	• Structurally similar to LH • Administered to mimic the LH surge and trigger ovulation in ART programmes, like IVF, and sometimes used as an adjunct to Clomid • Injection is strictly timed to the schedule of an insemination (IUI cycles) or the egg retrieval (IVF cycles)
Progesterone	• For luteal phase support following IUI or egg retrieval to promote endometrial receptivity • Progesterone supplementation is available in multiple preparations

procedure. Introducing couples to self-injecting can also provide an opportunity to increase the partner's participation in the programme, as well as allowing the couple to retain a greater amount of autonomy by their active involvement. Nurses need to set aside adequate time to demonstrate the injection equipment and procedure and allow the couple to practise the subcutaneous administration technique to develop their confidence.

6.6.2 Cycle Monitoring

Urinary ovulation predictor kits can be used to help detect the LH surge, signalling imminent ovulation. These kits may be useful for women having IUI or DI on a natural cycle or a Clomid cycle where their follicular response has previously assessed via ultrasound. Women start testing their urine daily, approximately 3 days prior to their expected LH surge. Once the LH surge has been detected, some clinics request that patients attend for an ultrasound scan to check the follicular size prior to insemination. Providing the follicular response meets the clinic's treatment criteria, IUI/DI would be carried out on the day of the positive surge and/or the day after.

Whenever gonadotrophin fertility drugs are used, it is important that more detailed monitoring is used to reduce the risk of multiple pregnancy and OHSS. Use of low-dose drug regimens, close monitoring and strict cycle cancellation guidance can reduce these risks. Ultrasound follicular tracking +/− serum oestradiol levels are an integral part of the treatment cycle, providing details of the ovarian response to the drug regime and the thickness of the endometrium. This assessment enables individualised drug doses to be prescribed to safely maximise an individual's response to the drug regime and determine the timing of the insemination or egg collection.

Ultrasound scanning is an advanced level skill often undertaken by nurses working in fertility clinics. In order for nurses to perform pre- and/or post-treatment scanning as part of their role, specialist training must be undertaken. Nurses need to be able to demonstrate knowledge of pelvic anatomy, physiology and pathology of the female reproductive system and undertake supervised practice experience until they have been assessed as competent. Nurse sonographers should audit their ultrasound practice on a regular basis and keep accurate records to document this process [32].

6.7 Additional ART Options

6.7.1 Cryopreservation

The use of ovarian stimulation protocols creates the opportunity for several eggs to be collected and embryos to develop. Supernumerary embryos of suitable quality may be cryopreserved and stored for future use. The advantage of cryopreservation is that these embryos can be warmed to be used in future cycles without having to repeat the first key steps of ovarian stimulation, egg recovery and fertilisation. The standard storage period for cryopreserved embryos is normally 10 years, although in certain circumstances embryos can be stored for longer periods, up to 55 years [39]. A future frozen-thawed embryo transfer (FET) cycle can be carried out on a natural menstrual cycle or using ovulation induction or a hormone therapy drug regime to prepare the endometrium for the subsequent embryo transfer. Embryo cryopreservation can be a highly reliable procedure, particularly since the introduction of vitrification (ultrarapid cooling). Vitrification is now commonly used, rather than the slow freezing technique, and has reduced damage to the internal structures of eggs and embryos, improving the chances of survival. In 2015, birth rates from frozen embryo cycles surpassed those from fresh cycles [46].

6.7.2 Fertility Preservation

Fertility preservation involves cryopreservation and storage of gametes, ovarian reproductive material or embryos for use in a person's future fertility treatment [47]. There are a variety of reasons why someone may want to preserve their fertility:

- Oncology patients—before cancer treatment commences
- Pre-vasectomy—in case personal circumstances change
- 'Social' egg freezing—to delay parenthood
- Armed forces staff—in case of injury
- Transgender people—prior to hormone therapy or reconstructive surgery

Semen cryopreservation (sperm banking) is a well-established practice and has been available for many years. The process involves the male producing samples of semen which are then cryopreserved. Reports suggest that males as young as 13 years (in case of precancer therapy) have achieved successful sperm cryopreservation [48].

In contrast, egg freezing and the use of cryopreserved eggs in treatment cycles are a more recent development. Women wishing to cryopreserve their eggs must undergo a surgical egg collection, but the eggs are cryopreserved rather than left fresh for fertilisation. Since 2010, 471 babies have been born from cryopreserved eggs in the UK, and the number of egg cryopreservation cycles is increasing year on year [46]. Testis and ovarian tissue cryopreservation remain experimental options but are anticipated to become more successful as reproductive technology improves [47].

Nurses need to be aware of the cryopreservation options available in order to discuss fertility preservation with patients inquiring about this service. Accurate information, counselling provision and clear referral pathways are vital to ensure prompt, appropriate access to fertility services to maximise future opportunities. In the UK, storage falls under the regulatory remit of the HFEA. Prior to the gamete cryopreservation, patients must be screened for transmissible viruses to prevent cross-contamination of stored samples. In addition, individuals must give written, informed consent to allow their gametes to be stored and also state how long they wish the gametes to be stored for, what they wish their gametes to be used for and what should happen to these stored gametes in the event of their death or mental incapacitation. The standard storage period for eggs and sperm is normally 10 years, although in certain circumstances gametes can be stored up to 55 years [39]

6.7.3 Pre-implantation Genetic Diagnosis (PGD) and Pre-implantation Genetic Screening (PGS)

PGD and PGS are not methods for treating infertility. Rather, embryos created by IVF are carefully biopsied to enable the extraction of cells to be tested. The embryos are unharmed, and unaffected embryos can then be transferred into the woman's uterus.

PGD is a technique that enables people with a specific inherited condition, or chromosome abnormality, to avoid passing it on to their children. Screening can detect a range of disorders, including cystic fibrosis, haemophilia A, Tay-Sachs disease and Turner syndrome. In the UK, it is illegal to use embryo testing for social sex selection. Over the last 5 years, there has been a 70% increase in PGD, with 712 treatments in the UK in 2016 [46].

PGS is a technique that enables embryos to be tested for any conditions where there might not be the correct number of chromosomes. This condition is known as aneuploidy and is more common in older women. Other patients who might benefit from PGS include women with a previous history of a chromosomally abnormal foetus or women who have repeated pregnancy losses.

6.8   Complications Associated with Assisted Reproduction

6.8.1   Multiple Pregnancy

The most common complication of ART is multiple pregnancy. A multiple pregnancy is associated with preterm birth, foetal growth restriction, pre-eclampsia, maternal pregnancy symptoms and postpartum haemorrhage [49, 50]. Twins are six times more likely to be born prematurely than single babies, which can lead to long-term health problems such as difficulty breathing, cerebral palsy and other physical and learning difficulties. The risk of cerebral palsy is four to six times higher for twins than for singleton babies [51].

In 2007, one in four births in the UK following ART resulted in a multiple pregnancy compared to around 2% in natural conception [46] This most commonly resulted from the routine practice of transferring two or more embryos in an IVF cycle. Since that time, the HFEA launched their 'One at a Time' campaign to tackle the high multiple birth rates following ART, setting clinics a target that only 10% of IVF births should be multiple births. Elective single embryo transfer (eSET) policies were developed. Improved laboratory techniques in selecting better quality embryos, such as culturing embryos for longer to the blastocyst stage and using time-lapse imaging, have been instrumental in reducing multiple pregnancy rates [49]. However, the decision about the number of embryos to be transferred should always be based on the individual, considering the woman's age, the number and quality of embryos and patient's circumstances. In 2016, 11% of births from IVF treatment cycles were multiple births, a substantial decline from the 24% rate in 2008, with no reduction in the pregnancy rate [46].

6.8.2 Ovarian Hyperstimulation Syndrome (OHSS)

OHSS is a potentially serious complication of ovarian stimulation regimes. The incidence of OHSS varies between treatments and patient groups. Mild OHSS has been estimated to affect around one-third of IVF cycles, whilst the combined incidence of moderate or severe OHSS varies from 3 to 8% of cycles [52]. OHSS is characterised by ovarian enlargement and fluid shift from the capillaries to the third space, the non-functional area between cells, as a result of increased vascular permeability, triggered by hCG. Symptoms range from abdominal discomfort, nausea, vomiting and shortness of breath to venous thromboembolism, renal failure and liver dysfunction in more severe cases. OHSS has been associated with maternal death. In most cases, OHSS is self-limiting and requires supportive management and monitoring whilst awaiting resolution [52]. Women with more severe OHSS may require inpatient treatment to manage the symptoms and reduce the risk of further complications. Preventive measures must be incorporated into all clinical protocols to minimise these risks.

6.8.3 Fertility Drugs and Cancer

Concerns have been raised about the long-term safety after using fertility drugs. Whilst some studies have suggested a link between fertility drugs and cancer, it is difficult to establish a causal link from the study results due to a range of methodological limitations. The Practice Committee of the American Society for Reproductive Medicine [53] reported that based on the available data, there does not appear to be a meaningful increased risk of invasive ovarian cancer, breast cancer or endometrial cancer following the use of fertility drugs. However, patients should be informed that infertile women may have an increased risk of these cancers, but using fertility drugs does not appear to increase this risk [53].

6.9 Success Rates

The biggest factor in determining successful fertility treatment is the age of the female, with older women having a lower success rate [46]. According to the latest HFEA figures, there were just over 68,000 IVF treatment cycles carried out in the

UK in 2016, resulting in 20,028 births [46]. The average live birth rate per embryo transferred for women of all age groups was 21%, whilst for women aged under 35 years, the success rate was 29%, which is the highest rate ever reported. The rates can be seen in Figs. 6.1, 6.2 and 6.3.

In 2016, there were also 5447 DI treatment cycles and 8102 IUI cycles performed in the UK. The birth rate for both these programmes is around 12% [46].

Fig. 6.1 IVF birth rates. Key: Birth rate per embryo transferred (PET)—no. of births divided by the sum of embryos transferred for treatment cycles starting in that year. Birth rate per treatment cycle (PTC)—% of treatment cycles started in that year resulting in a live birth

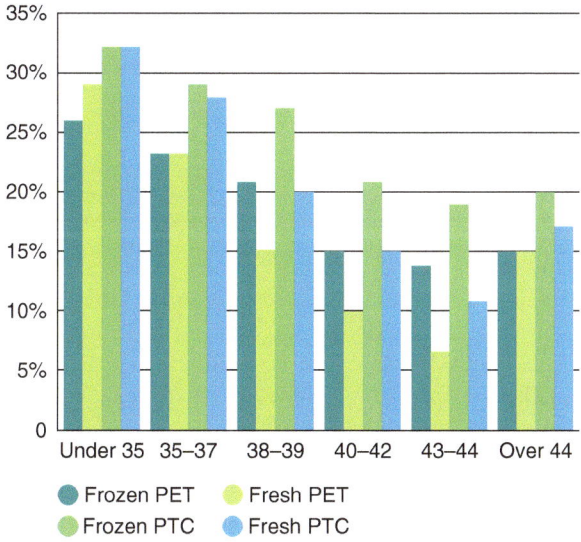

Fig. 6.2 DI birth rates

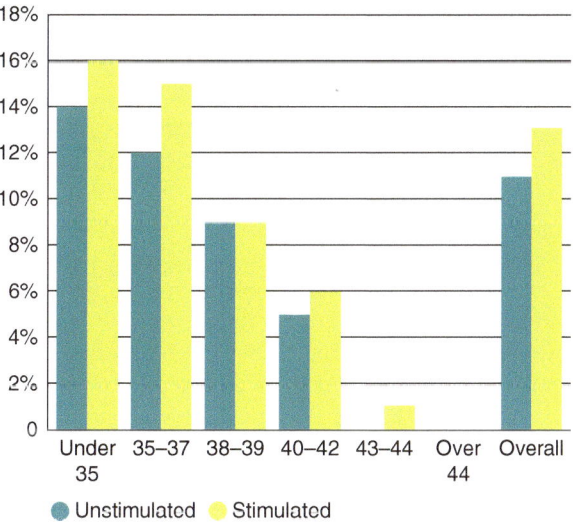

Fig. 6.3 IUI birth rates

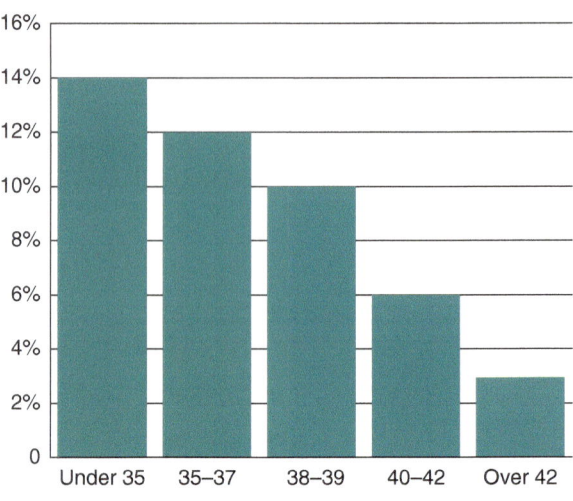

6.10 The Nurse's Role in the Fertility Clinic

The fertility nurse's role is multifaceted and requires excellent communication skills, compassion and empathy. The responsibilities of the fertility nurse within a specialist service encompass:

- Patient assessment.
- Information giving/educating the woman/couple on all aspects of their treatment programme to ensure informed and safe care.
- Providing patient care throughout the treatment cycle from the initial contact to treatment completion.
- Providing ongoing emotional support.
- Ensuring effective communication channels, so the woman/couple are kept fully informed of how their treatment cycle is progressing and can make informed decisions about aspects of their care.
- Maintaining clear, accurate and contemporaneous records.
- Acting as the interface between the woman/couple and other members of the multidisciplinary fertility team to discuss patients' progress.

As a result, the nurse is able to provide the continuity and consistency of care which is paramount to ensuring the patient's, and her partner's, experience before, during and after fertility treatment is a positive one. The provision of care throughout the treatment cycle by a core group of practitioners with whom the patients become familiar is vital to maintain high standards and provide a greater level of empathy and understanding of that individual couple's circumstances. Nurses can also benefit from increased job satisfaction due to greater involvement with couples from the initial contact to treatment completion.

Working within the field of fertility offers career opportunities for nurses to become autonomous practitioners, undertake increased clinical responsibility and utilise advanced level clinical skills. The Royal College of Nursing [32] has developed an Education and Career Progression Framework for Fertility Nursing which outlines ways in which nurses can progress their career and assess and demonstrate their knowledge and competence using the provided progression assessment tool. Role extension opportunities include:

- Pre- and post-procedural care/surgical pathway care.
- Genital/speculum examination.
- Venepuncture.
- Ultrasound scanning.
- Performing inseminations.
- Assisting/performing surgical egg collections.
- Performing embryo transfers.
- Early pregnancy scanning and management.
- Non-medical prescribing.
- Counselling.
- Co-ordinating the day to day organisation of treatment programmes.
- Undertaking nurse-led clinics.

Nurses taking on an extended role must ensure that they have the appropriate knowledge and competence to perform all the required aspects of the patients' fertility programme. Nurses should work in line with written standard operating procedures (SOPs) for all interventions performed within the clinic to ensure quality standards of care are met. SOPs should reflect national regulation requirements and relevant international directives, e.g. for the UK, the HFEA's latest Code of Practice and the European Union Tissue and Cells Directives [54]. SOPs also form part of the unit's overall quality management system and should be regularly updated to ensure they reflect current evidence-based practice.

Fertility nurses are gaining wider recognition of their specialist knowledge and skills and their increasing responsibilities in fertility clinics. The European Society of Human Reproduction and Embryology has launched a certification programme to certify competence and to develop a formal recognition of the quality of healthcare provided by nurses in fertility units [55].

6.11 Conclusion

Infertility has been described as a life crisis affecting as many as 186 million people worldwide [55]. Advances in ART have generated a range of possibilities to assist people to have children. However, many people who have difficulty in conceiving experience feelings of depression, anxiety, isolation, vulnerability and loss of control [56]. Nurses can provide high-quality compassionate care to individuals/couples by ensuring they have timely access to evidence-based information and opportunities to explore their feelings about potential treatment options, to enable them to make informed decisions.

Nurses are at the forefront of patient care and in a unique position to deliver a seamless service from primary to tertiary care. Fertility nurses provide a holistic approach to fertility investigation, treatment and pre-pregnancy care [32]. The field of ART provides an ideal opportunity for nurses to expand their scope of practice and develop their career trajectories. A range of educational and training opportunities and resources are available to facilitate nurses' clinical development and support nurse-led services. However, all nurses have a professional obligation to regularly review and audit their own practice and update their skills and knowledge to ensure they continually work within their level of competency [57].

References

1. National Institute for Health and Care Excellence (2013) Fertility problems: assessment and treatment. NICE guideline [CG156]. Updated Sept 2017. https://www.nice.org.uk/guidance/cg156. Accessed 3 Jul 2018
2. National Institute for Health and Care Excellence (2017) Clinical knowledge summaries: pre-conception advice and management. https://cks.nice.org.uk/pre-conception-advice-and-management#!scenario:1. Accessed 2 Aug 2018
3. Mills M, Rindfuss RR, Mcdonald P, Te-Velde E (2011) Why do people postpone parenthood? Reasons and social policy incentives. Human Reprod 17(6):848–860
4. Balasch J (2010) Ageing and infertility: an overview. Gynecol Endocrinol 26(12):855–860
5. Baird DT, Collins J, Egozcue J, Evers LH, Gianaroli L, Leridon H et al. ESHRE Capri Workshop Group (2005) Fertility and ageing. Hum Reprod Update. 2005;11(3):261–276
6. National Institute for Health and Care Excellence (2018) Clinical knowledge summary: fertility. https://cks.nice.org.uk/infertility#!topicsummary. Accessed 2 Aug 2018
7. Eniola OW, Adetola AA, Abayomi BT (2017) A review of female infertility; important etiological factors and management. J Microbiol Biotechnol Res 2(3):379–385
8. Raheem AA, Ralph D (2011) Male infertility: causes and investigations. Trends Urol Men's Health 2(5):8–11
9. Katz DJ, Teloken P, Shoshany O (2017) Male infertility—the other side of the equation. Aust Fam Physician. 46(9):641
10. Jungwirth A, Diemer T, Dohle GR, Giwercman A, Kopa Z, Tournaye H et al (2015) Guidelines on male infertility, European Association of Urology guidelines. Arnhem
11. Mendiola J, Torres-Cantero AM, Moreno-Grau JM, Ten J, Roca M, Moreno-Grau S et al (2008) Exposure to environmental toxins in males seeking infertility treatment: a case-controlled study. Reprod Biomed Online 16(6):842–850
12. Sharma R, Biedenharn KR, Fedor JM, Agarwal A (2013) Lifestyle factors and reproductive health: taking control of your fertility. Reprod Biol Endocrinol 11(1):66
13. Fawcett T, Rhynas S (2012) Taking a patient history: the role of the nurse. Nursing Standard 26(24):41
14. World Health Organisation (2010) WHO laboratory manual for the examination and processing of human semen, 5th edn. Cambridge University Press, Cambridge
15. Stephenson J, Heslehurst N, Hall J, Schoenaker DA, Hutchinson J, Cade JE et al (2018) Before the beginning: nutrition and lifestyle in the preconception period and its importance for future health. Lancet 391(10132):1830–1841
16. Public Health England (2016) Rubella susceptibility screening in pregnancy to end in England. https://www.gov.uk/government/news/rubella-susceptibility-screening-in-pregnancy-to-end-in-england. Accessed 7 Aug 2018

17. Public Health England (2018) MMR (measles, mumps, and rubella vaccine): advice for pregnant women. https://www.gov.uk/government/publications/vaccine-in-pregnancy-advice-for-pregnant-women/mmr-measles-mumps-rubella-vaccine-advice-for-pregnant-women. Accessed 7 Aug 2018
18. World Health Organisation (2018) BMI classification. http://apps.who.int/bmi/index.jsp?introPage=intro_3.html. Accessed 7 Aug 2018
19. Chavarro JE, Ehrlich S, Colaci DS, Wright DL, Toth TL, Petrozza JC et al (2012) Body mass index and short-term weight change in relation to treatment outcomes in women undergoing assisted reproduction. Fertil Steril 98(1):109–116
20. Royal College of Obstetricians and Gynaecologists (2014) Healthy eating and vitamin supplements in pregnancy. https://www.rcog.org.uk/globalassets/documents/patients/patient-information-leaflets/pregnancy/pi-healthy-eating-and-vitamin-supplements-in-pregnancy.pdf. Accessed 7 Aug 2018
21. Department of Health (2016) UK Chief Medical Officers alcohol guidelines review: summary of the proposed new guidelines. https://www.gov.uk/government/uploads/system/uploads/attachment_data/file/489795/summary.pdf. Accessed 3 Aug 2018
22. Hyland A, Piazza K, Hovey KM, Tindle HA, Manson JE, Messina C et al (2015) Associations between lifetime tobacco exposure with infertility and age at natural menopause: the Women's Health Initiative Observational Study. Tobacco control. tobaccocontrol-2015
23. Public Health England (2018) Health matters: reproductive health and pregnancy planning. https://www.gov.uk/government/publications/health-matters-reproductive-health-and-pregnancy-planning/health-matters-reproductive-health-and-pregnancy-planning. Accessed 7 Aug 2018
24. Public Health England (2015) Health matters: smoking and quitting in England. https://www.gov.uk/government/publications/health-matters-smoking-and-quitting-in-england/smoking-and-quitting-in-england. Accessed 7 Aug 2018
25. Lyngsø J, Ramlau-Hansen CH, Bay B, Ingerslev HJ, Hulman A, Kesmodel US (2017) Association between coffee or caffeine consumption and fecundity and fertility: a systematic review and dose–response meta-analysis. Clin Epidemiol 9:699
26. World Health Organization (2016) WHO recommendations on antenatal care for a positive pregnancy experience. World Health Organization. p 152
27. Rich CW, Domar AD (2016) Addressing the emotional barriers to access to reproductive care. Fertil Steril 105(5):1124–1127
28. Allan H, Mounce G (2015) Managing infertility in primary care. Practice Nursing 26(9):440–443
29. Kendall J (2008) Psychosocial effects of infertility. Practice Nursing 19(2):91–93
30. World Health Organisation (2018) Infertility. http://www.who.int/reproductivehealth/topics/infertility/keyissues/en/. Accessed 9 Aug 2018
31. Quilliam S (2015) British infertility counselling association. J Fam Plan Reprod Health Care 41(2):154–155
32. Royal College of Nursing (2018) An RCN education and career progression framework for fertility nursing. file:///C:/Users/DMU%20USER/Downloads/PDF-006690.pdf. Accessed 10 Aug 2018
33. National Institute for Health and Care Excellence. National Institute for Health and Clinical Excellence (2013) Fertility: assessment and treatment for people with fertility problems (update): costing report: implementing NICE guidance. https://www.nice.org.uk/guidance/cg156/resources/costing-report-pdf-188496685. Accessed 9 Aug 2018
34. European Society of Human Reproduction & Embryology (2017) A policy audit on fertility: analysis of 9 EU countries. file:///C:/Users/DMU%20USER/Downloads/PolicyAuditonFertilityAnalysis9EUCountriesFINAL16032017%20(3).pdf. Accessed 4 Aug 2018
35. Fertility Fairness (2017) Number of CCGs offering 3 IVF cycles has halved since 2013. http://www.fertilityfairness.co.uk/number-of-ccgs-offering-3-ivf-cycles-has-halved-since-2013/. Accessed 9 Aug 2018

36. Boivin J, Gameiro S (2015) Evolution of psychology and counseling in infertility. Fertil Steril 104(2):251–259
37. Domar A, Gordon K, Garcia-Velasco J, La Marca A, Barriere P, Beligotti F (2012) Understanding the perceptions of and emotional barriers to infertility treatment: a survey in four European countries. Hum Reprod 27(4):1073–1079
38. Gameiro S, Boivin J, Dancet E, de Klerk C, Emery M, Lewis-Jones C et al (2015) ESHRE guideline: routine psychosocial care in infertility and medically assisted reproduction—a guide for fertility staff. Hum Reprod 30(11):2476–2485
39. Human Fertilisation and Embryology Authority (2017) Code of practice. 8th edn. HFEA: London. https://ifqlive.blob.core.windows.net/umbraco-website/2062/2017-10-02-code-of-practice-8th-edition-full-version-11th-revision-final-clean.pdf. Accessed 10 Aug 2018
40. American Society for Reproductive Medicine (2018) Third-party reproduction. https://www.asrm.org/topics/topics-index/third-party-reproduction/. Accessed 10 Aug 2018
41. Human Fertilisation and Embryology Authority (2017) Donation. https://www.hfea.gov.uk/donation/. Accessed 16 Aug 2018
42. Human Fertilisation and Embryology Authority. The Human Fertilisation and Embryology Authority (Disclosure of Donor Information) Regulations 2004. (S.I. 2004 No. 1511). http://www.legislation.gov.uk/uksi/2004/1511/pdfs/uksi_20041511_en.pdf. Accessed 14 Aug 2018
43. Nuffield Council on Bioethics (2013) Donor conception: ethical aspects of information sharing. http://nuffieldbioethics.org/wp-content/uploads/2014/06/Donor_conception_report_2013.pdfn. Accessed 26 Jul 2018
44. Joy J, McCrystal P (2015) The role of counselling in the management of patients with infertility. Obstetric Gynaecol 17(2):83–89
45. Joint Formulary Committee (2018) British National Formulary, 75th edn. British Medical Association and Royal Pharmaceutical Society of Great Britain, London
46. Human Fertilisation and Embryology Authority. Fertility treatment 2014–2016. Trends and figures. 2018. https://www.hfea.gov.uk/media/2563/hfea-fertility-trends-and-figures-2017-v2.pdf. Accessed 16 Aug 2018
47. Royal College of Nursing (2017) Fertility preservation: clinical professional resource. RCN, London. file:///C:/Users/DMU%20USER/Downloads/PUB-005986%20(1).pdf. Accessed 10 Aug 2018
48. Anderson RA, Mitchell RT, Kelsey TW, Spears N, Telfer EE, Wallace WH (2015) Cancer treatment and gonadal function: experimental and established strategies for fertility preservation in children and young adults. Lancet Diab Endocrinol 3(7):556–567
49. Chambers GM, Ledger W. The economic implications of multiple pregnancy following ART. In: Seminars in fetal and neonatal medicine 2014. vol 19, no. 4. WB Saunders, pp 254–261
50. Royal College of Obstetricians and Gynaecologists (2016) Green-top guideline no. 51. Monochronic twin pregnancy management. RCOG, London
51. Human Fertilisation and Embryology Authority (2016) Multiple Births: what you need to know. https://ifqlive.blob.core.windows.net/umbraco-website/1315/2017-02-24-multiple-births-leaflet-final.pdf. Accessed 16 Aug 2018
52. Royal College of Obstetricians and Gynaecologists (2016) Green-top guideline no. 5. The management of ovarian hyperstimulation syndrome. RCOG, London
53. Practice Committee of the American Society for Reproductive Medicine (2016) Fertility drugs and cancer: a guideline. Fertil Steril 106(7):1617–1626
54. Human Tissue Authority (2018) Guide to quality and safety assurance for human tissues and cells for patient treatment. https://www.hta.gov.uk/sites/default/files/HTA%20guide%20to%20Quality%20and%20Safety%20Assurance%20for%20Human%20Tissue%20and%20Cells%20for%20Patient%20Treatment%20v2%20April%202018.pdf. Accessed 16 Aug 2018

55. European Society of Human Reproduction and Embryology (2018) ESHRE certification for nurses and midwives. https://www.eshre.eu/Accreditation-and-Certification/Nurses-Midwives-Certification.aspx. Accessed 19 Aug 2018
56. Inhorn MC, Patrizio P (2015) Infertility around the globe: new thinking on gender, reproductive technologies and global movements in the 21st century. Hum Reprod Update 21(4):411–426
57. Rooney KL, Domar AD (2018) The relationship between stress and infertility. Dialog Clin Neurosci 20(1):41

Resources

British Infertility Counselling Association: https://www.bica.net/
Donor Conception Network: https://www.dcnetwork.org/
Fertility Network UK: http://fertilitynetworkuk.org/
Human Fertilisation and Embryology Authority: https://www.hfea.gov.uk/
Multiple Births Foundation: http://www.multiplebirths.org.uk/
National Institute for Health and Care Excellence: https://www.nice.org.uk/
Surrogacy UK: https://www.surrogacyuk.org/

Complications in Early Pregnancy

Fiona Phillips and Flora Saxby

Historically, the role of an early pregnancy nurse (EP) has lacked guidance and structure with variations in skills and practice. The 2017 Royal College of Nursing (RCN) [1] guidelines for clinical nurse specialists (CNS's) in early pregnancy care (EPC) suggest a framework which develops skills and works towards advanced-level practice while acknowledging the diverse range of abilities needed to undertake this role safely and effectively. These include clinical skills, leadership skills, ultrasound skills, data collection and management, service provision pathway managements and co-ordination, early pregnancy care profile development and continued professional development.

Not all nurses will have all of the skills identified within the guidelines, but they recognise the need for continuous personal development to ensure that care is provided safely, effectively and compassionately.

EP nurses undertake extended roles such as:

- History taking.
- Requesting ultrasound examination.
- Speculum examinations.
- Vaginal examinations.
- Swab taking.
- Venepuncture and cannulation.
- Nurse consenting for surgical management of miscarriage (SMM).

Most of these skills are obtained and assessed through in-house teaching, alongside stand-alone courses specific to gynaecology and early pregnancy. Progression to a more

F. Phillips
St Thomas' Hospital, London, UK

F. Saxby (✉)
Relational Integrative Psychotherapy and Counselling, London, UK

© Springer Nature Switzerland AG 2019
D. Holloway (ed.), *Nursing Management of Women's Health*,
https://doi.org/10.1007/978-3-030-16115-6_7

advanced level requires formal training is usually at masters level, such as ultrasound scanning, non-medical prescribing and preforming manual vacuum aspiration (MVA).

The first early pregnancy units (EPUs) were set up over 20 years ago, and currently, there are over 200 units in the UK. In these, women experiencing problems in early pregnancy can expect to access support, advice and treatment. They have resulted in reduced hospital admissions and decreased the average length of stay.

The basic standards for early pregnancy units set by national guidance are as follows:

- Women should be offered the full range of miscarriage managements, supported by written information.
- Any women undergoing the medical management of an ectopic pregnancy should be able to access telephone advice and emergency admission 24 hrs a day and receive written information.
- Guidelines and management should be available for pregnancies of unknown location.
- Serum hCG results should be available on the day of sampling.
- An appropriate environment with a staffed reception area should be provided.
- Access to bereavement counsellors and staff who are formally trained to provide emotional and psychological support.
- Self-referral accesses for a history of recurrent miscarriage, ectopic or molar.
- A direct referral pathway for other health professionals.
- The availability of clear patient information regarding pathology investigations, post-mortem examination and sensitive disposal.
- Both transvaginal and trans-abdominal scans to be available by registered practitioners.

Despite these guidelines, service provision in EPUs across the country varies immensely. Some units provide a walk and wait service, while some require a referral from a GP. Larger city hospitals tend to have longer opening hours and more scanning facilities, whereas some EPUs only open half days, weekdays only. The lack of uniformity in such a vital service means women may need to travel away from their local hospitals for assessment.

Additionally, the care offered can be inconsistent, with different services regarding counselling, miscarriage management and follow-up. In an attempt to standardise service provision, The National Bereavement Care Pathway project is currently being developed. Its objective is to ensure that all bereaved parents are offered equal, high-quality, individualised, safe and sensitive care in any experience of pregnancy or baby loss [2].

7.1   Basic Embryogenesis

An oocyte is released by the ovary and is swept up by the fimbria of the fallopian tube. The oocyte is normally fertilised in the ampulla of the fallopian tube. It is now called a zygote carrying 23 pairs of chromosomes half maternal and half paternal.

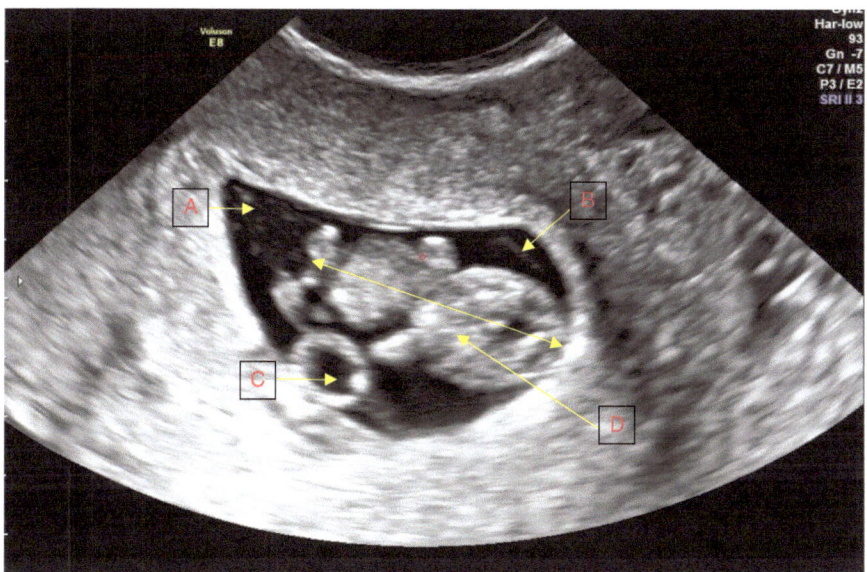

Fig. 7.1 Gestation sac containing structures. (**a**) The chorionic cavity is the first structure seen within the endometrial cavity. Expected growth should be 1 mm per day, and it should be regular in shape. (**b**) The amnion will form around the same time as the yolk sac but is not always seen in early scan. The embryo will develop within this amniotic cavity, and as it grows, the amnion will fuse together with the outer chorion at around 15 weeks. (**c**) The yolk sac is the first structure to be seen within the gestation sac. It is used to confirm an intrauterine pregnancy. (**d**) The embryo or foetal pole can be seen from around 5 weeks on transvaginal scan. It is measured from one end to the other or crown-rump length (double-headed arrow)

The morula stage happens around day 4; the rapidly increasing cells start to organise themselves to outer cells called throblasts and inner cells called embryoblasts. The inner cells clump together in a mass leaving a cavity called the blastocoel. This leads to the formation of a blastocyst around day 5. The blastocyst travels from the fallopian tube via ciliary action and peristalsis to the uterus to implant. It is at this stage that the blastocyst produces human chorionic gonadotropin (hCG) and is detectable in the blood and later urine. The blastocyst will continue to rapidly divide and grow, and around day 15, it is termed an embryo. Foetal heart pulsations can be seen on ultrasound around day 20 post fertilisation. A scan picture showing all of the different structures can be seen in Fig. 7.1.

7.2   Bleeding and Pain

The majority of women who present to EPU's units do so with pain and/or bleeding. They are often upset, stressed, panicked and need their concerns to be validated. It may be their first pregnancy, they may have struggled to conceive or have experienced multiple miscarriages or previous ectopics. Assessment of a woman presenting with bleeding and/or pain in early pregnancy must be undertaken with the utmost skill and the ability to recognise an unwell woman quickly and take appropriate action. An assessment may be part of an initial streaming triage or a full consultation depending on the care setting and the origin of the referral. It is advisable to always complete an independent assessment, with the original referral serving as supporting information.

A full assessment will be guided by all available and relevant investigations including confirmation of an intrauterine pregnancy by transvaginal ultrasound.

When basing care on the report of an ultrasound scan, particular attention should be paid to the clinical indication, date of scan and practitioner. If the report is not in English or incomplete or if doubts are raised as to whether the scan has been undertaken by anyone other than a HCPC-registered practitioner, it is wise to discount it and perform a repeat ultrasound expedity. Information obtained from ultrasound will greatly assist the time poor practitioner in the assessment process but must never outweigh the patient's physical assessment and clinical presentation. The presenting complaints can be seen in Table 7.1.

All physical assessments are to be undertaken with consent, and a chaperone should be offered in line with local policy. Privacy and dignity must be maintained at all times.

Non-English-speaking women should be offered a formal translator, avoiding the use of family members to ensure a thorough and accurate history.

A full gynaecological and obstetric history must be taken including:

- Parity and gravidity including terminations (social or medical reasons).
- LMP including length and regularity of cycle.
- Allergies.
- Natural or assisted conception (if assisted, type, dates of transfer, fresh/frozen cycle, age of donor, reason).
- Date of first positive pregnancy test.
- Management of previous miscarriages/type of termination (expectant, medical or surgical).
- Previous gynaecological and obstetric history (including any past trauma which might make a vaginal examination difficult).
- Female genital mutilation (FGM).
- Contraception history and compliance and dates of any emergency contraception.
- Previous pelvic infections and if they were treated.
- Any mental health diagnosis or concerns, anxiety and PTSD.

Table 7.1 Presenting complaints in early pregnancy

Pain	Bleeding
Onset	Onset
Location	Frequency
Frequency	How heavy (pads per hour)
Duration	Any clots
Pain score	Flooding
Nature (sharp, cramp, pulling)	Postcoital
Efficacy of analgesia	Increases with the pain

- Postcoital or intermenstrual bleeding.
- Drugs/smoking/alcohol intake/nonprescription medications.
- Dates and results of most recent cervical screening and any previous treatment.

7.3 Physical Assessment

- Baseline temperature, pulse, blood pressure, oxygen saturation levels and respiratory rate.
- Urine pregnancy test.
- Height and weight.
- General appearance: pallor, sweaty, clammy, agitated.
- Abdominal examination.
- Guarding/rebound tenderness rigid/soft abdomen.
- Bimanual examination.
- Fundal size.
- Uterine position.
- Any masses.
- Cervical excitation.
- Speculum examination.
- Assess bleeding.
- Assess the cervix and external os (open, closed, ectropion, erosion, actively bleeding). Remove any products and observe for any foetal parts or products of conception.

A provisional diagnosis and possible differential diagnosis must be given following the initial assessment. The provisional diagnosis for women who present with bleeding and/or pain with a positive pregnancy test (PT) should be an ectopic pregnancy until intrauterine pregnancy or miscarriage has been confirmed.

A differential diagnosis would depend on clinical presentation. For instance, a woman with a history of heavy bleeding and large clots that has settled may be a threatened, complete or incomplete miscarriage.

Non pregnancy-related findings must be excluded once an intrauterine pregnancy has been confirmed, and symptoms not attributed to the pregnancy have been ascertained. Pain can be caused by conditions such as appendicitis, diverticulitis, constipation, gastroenteritis or urine infections. In such cases, an appropriate and timely referral must be made.

Women presenting with bleeding and/or pain, who have never had an intrauterine pregnancy demonstrated on ultrasound scan, should be offered a pelvic ultrasound examination to ascertain the location and viability of the pregnancy [3]. If the woman has an intrauterine pregnancy on scan, she must be fully assessed to decide if another scan is required to determine viability and potential cause for the symptoms.

> My level of anxiety was high and I would have really benefited from some time to talk about my experiences and someone to listen. I know the NHS is incredibly stretched

but any nurse or doctor who is able to spend a few more minutes talking and offer some words of comfort really does make all the difference.

Under 10 weeks' gestation, in most cases, a transvaginal scan (TVS) gives the best view of the uterus, ovaries and adnexa. Women must be informed that it is a safe procedure and is considered to be the gold standard assessment tool in ascertaining the location of a pregnancy but that it may cause some discomfort. It is recommended to advise women at early gestations that a single ultrasound cannot be 100% accurate and may not necessarily give a reason for symptoms. She must also be informed that further investigations including blood tests, speculum examination and repeat ultrasound scans may be needed. Women should be advised to empty their bladder before a TVS as this will assist the sonographer and is more comfortable for the woman.

Some women may have had negative past experiences with previous TVS or trauma and request a transabdominal scan. If the practitioner is satisfied that the woman has completely understood the limitations of such a scan, the request must be sensitively respected. It must be made clear to the patient that further investigations may be needed, and there may be a longer wait between rescans. This advice must be clearly documented.

When requesting a scan, it is imperative that the correct information is given on the request form including correct name and date of birth, parity, gravity, LMP and reason for the scan. Often, the practitioner completing the scan has very limited information and is left with no choice but to question the woman and can appear uninformed.

It is good practice to inform the woman the indication, the process of the scan, what will happen after the scan and who will explain the scan results.

7.4   Common Causes of Pain and Bleeding

The majority of nurses working in EPC are tasked with discussing scan reports. The ability to decode the report is an essential skill requiring sound knowledge of the structures detailed on the scan report. Common findings including the presence of a corpus luteum, simple ovarian cysts, fibroids and a subchorionic haematoma (SCH). The EP nurse must be clear that these are normal physiological findings that can cause symptoms. Women found to have simple ovarian cysts must be advised that there is a risk of rupture or torsion. SCH's have been linked to an increased risk of miscarriage, but this is dependent on the size and location of the bleed. In these cases, women must be made aware of the possibility of more bleeding or brown discharge but to return to hospital if heavy or accompanied by pain. Anti-D is required in the cases of rhesus-negative women over 12/40 gestation.

Fibroids can cause pain and bleeding dependent on size and position and have been linked to late miscarriages. Any follow-up should be decided on individual presentation and available service provision. In most incidences, the advice should be to observe but to contact or return to hospital should symptoms escalate. Women should be given a direct contact number to call with any concerns if symptoms are worrying but not urgent.

If no cause for bleeding is found on ultrasound, a speculum examination may be recommended to observe for any cervical pathology such as ectropion, erosion, polyp or trauma. Such cervical pathology is likely to cause some bleeding; however, if there are any concerns on examination, a colposcopy referral may be indicated dependent on clinical presentation and history. Routine smear tests are recommended 3 months after pregnancy; however, if clinically indicated while pregnant, the best time is between 3 and 6/40. Swabs can be taken if there is an offensive discharge or any concern for potential infection. Women must be made aware that they are not having a full sexual health screening and should be directed to local GUM services if they feel this is needed. Women must be able to access the results and treatment if indicated. If Strep B is diagnosed, the woman must be made aware of how important it is to inform her midwifery team, and the result should be recorded in maternity notes.

For ongoing pregnancies, post scan is a good opportunity to ensure women are aware of current recommendations regarding a healthy lifestyle and taking folic acid, they can be signposted to smoking cessation midwives if needed. Women must be aware how and when to commence their antenatal care and provided with contact details should they have any further concerns. This is also a good opportunity to discuss any worries a woman may have. Incidences of domestic violence increase in pregnancy, and the EP nurse is in good position to provide support and advice.

7.4.1 Miscarriage

Unfortunately, bleeding and/or pain can be a sign of a miscarriage. One in four women will experience a miscarriage [4], and for the majority of these women, this will happen within the first 12 weeks of pregnancy. The exact cause of miscarriage is not known; however, there are some known risk factors:

- Age (10% under 30 years, 50% risk at 45).
- Over/underweight.
- Smoking.
- Caffeine.
- Prescription/nonprescription medication.
- Poorly controlled medical conditions like diabetes and hypertension and thyroid conditions.
- Infections (rubella, toxoplasmosis and strep B, German measles), chlamydia, bacterial vaginosis, HIV.
- Genetic.
- Uterine shape (septate/bicornuate).
- Fibroids (depending on location and size more common to cause miscarriage at later stages).
- Hormonal problems, immunological/clotting problems (lupus, antiphospholipid syndrome).

Every woman's experience of miscarriage is different, with even woman who suffer multiple miscarriages recounting different experiences with each loss. The following will discuss the different types of pregnancy loss, but it must be considered that not all women will experience all, if any symptoms.

7.4.2 Threatened Miscarriage

This is a provisional diagnosis when a woman with a previously confirmed intrauterine pregnancy has bleeding and/or pain. Full assessment and ultrasound examination are indicated to ascertain the viability and cause for symptoms.

7.4.3 Complete Miscarriage

This term is used when the uterus is empty, and there is no evidence of previously seen gestation or any retained products of conception. The diagnosis can only be made if a previous intrauterine pregnancy has been established on ultrasound scan or confirmed with falling serum hCG levels. It is recommended that a pregnancy test is taken 2–3 weeks after the diagnosis to confirm miscarriage. If persistent bleeding and a positive pregnancy test are found, a repeat ultrasound serum hCG +/− TVS is recommended to exclude retained products or a molar pregnancy.

Symptoms can vary depending on gestation. Usually, women will experience pain and bleeding commonly heavy with clots. Women can present with period like back pain and lower abdominal pain. This pain may come in waves, and bleeding may correlate with this as the pain is caused by the uterus contracting and dilation of the cervix. Prolonged pain may be due to pregnancy tissue in the cervix preventing it from closing. Women may feel nauseous, dizzy and unwell and have the urge to void.

A clinical decision should made at this point based on the risk of the patient becoming unwell while undergoing a natural process; if the patient is clinically stable, no intervention is required.

> The system turned my loss into a medical problem and ignored the emotional aspect. People were scared because I was crying and they didn't know what to do. I needed someone to ask me how I felt emotionally, as well as whether I was in pain or how much I was bleeding. I could not initiate this, I needed them to ask

Sufficient analgesia, reassurance and privacy must be provided.

A speculum examination may be needed to assess bleeding and the cervix as this can inform decision-making. Prior to this, verbal consent must be obtained, and the practitioner must give a clear explanation for the indication of the examination.

Observations and assessment of bleeding must be undertaken frequently, and assistance should be sorted if pain or bleeding becomes uncontrolled.

At this point, intravenous access and blood sampling, full blood count (FBC) and group and save (G&S), should be considered. If bleeding is uncontrolled, surgical management of miscarriage (SMM) under general anaesthetic may be required.

This can be very traumatic for women and in some cases can develop quickly into an emergency situation. Calmly keeping the woman informed and reassured at every stage is vital.

7.4.4 An Incomplete Miscarriage

An incomplete miscarriage is diagnosed by scan when there is found to be some pregnancy tissue or products of conception (POC) left within the endometrial cavity following bleeding. Women may report that the bleeding has settled or it is still actively bleeding. Treatment depends on clinical presentation, the quantity of tissue retained and level of bleeding.

Challenges arise when a small amount of retained products of conception (RPOC) are found as there are currently no national guidelines or cut-off values for the diagnosis of RPOC. If RPOC is diagnosed on an initial scan, serum hCG is indicated to ensure falling levels to exclude an ectopic pregnancy.

7.4.5 Septic Miscarriage

Women who experience miscarriage and develop clinical features of infection such as flulike symptoms, offensive discharge, pyrexia, tachycardia, hypotension and tachypnoea should be urgently assessed for sepsis. An infection is more likely to spread quicker and be less responsive to treatment in a pregnant woman. A septic miscarriage can lead to organ failure, septic shock and if untreated can be fatal. Prompt recognition and treatment save lives. Frequent observations, blood cultures, FBC, MSU, HVS, appropriate assessment, quick escalation and intervention must be undertaken should there be any indication of infection.

7.4.6 Delayed Miscarriage

This can also be known as a missed miscarriage, silent miscarriage and early embryonic demise, but outdated terms such as an embryonic pregnancy or blighted ovum should be avoided. This is a pregnancy that has stopped developing but has not miscarried. Symptoms may include pain, bleeding or a brown discharge. A delayed miscarriage is diagnosed on scan, and often, women who are asymptomatic are diagnosed at their first trimester screening scan.

> In my first (missed) miscarriage it would have been helpful to have been given more of a warning beforehand that the scan could possibly show a miscarriage. I had gone into the EPU for very light spotting at 11 + 5 wks and was told that spotting at this stage was very normal and very likely nothing to worry about. It was my first pregnancy so I had no idea that the scan I was about to have would show a pregnancy that had ended - I still had all my symptoms, I felt well and very much pregnant. I feel that "playing down" the situation in this case made the shock of revealing no heartbeat so much worse and very shocking.

National guidelines for the diagnosis of a delayed miscarriage on scan are as follows [3]:

- An intrauterine gestation sac with no internal contents with a mean sac diameter (MSD) measures over 25 mm.
- There is an intrauterine gestation sac with an embryo that measures more that 7 mm (from crown to rump), and there is no foetal heartbeat.

7.4.7 Intrauterine Pregnancy of Unknown Viability (PUV)

This term is given to a pregnancy that is seen on a scan in the uterus; however, viability has not been established. This is either because there is a gestation sac, yolk sac and embryo measuring less than 7 mm visualised on scan, but there is no foetal heartbeat seen. Alternatively, there is an intrauterine gestation sac with no internal contents, and the mean sac diameter measures less than 25 mm.

7.4.8 Pregnancy of Unknown Location (PUL)

This is the term given to a situation where a woman is found to have a positive pregnancy test, and the location of the pregnancy has not been ascertained on ultrasound scan. If an initial scan fails to confirm the location of a pregnancy, a serum hCG is taken and repeated 48 h later. If the hCG level is increasing by more than 63%, this is likely to be an ongoing intrauterine pregnancy, but a repeat scan is needed to confirm the location. If the hCG falls by over 50%, it is likely that the pregnancy is failing. In these cases, women should be asked to take a pregnancy test in 14 days to confirm a miscarriage with the advice to return to the unit if the pregnancy test is found to be positive. If the change in value is between a 50% decrease and a 63% increase, women should be reviewed within 24 h post the second hCG result [3]. This is seen as a summary in Fig. 7.2.

It is worth considering that it should be possible to visualise a pregnancy at hCG level of more than 1000 u/ml.

Any woman diagnosed with PUL should be informed of the three likely diagnoses: an early intrauterine pregnancy, miscarriage or an ectopic pregnancy. This should be supplemented with written information, including a contact number for results and advice. The woman should be made aware that if there is any increase in symptoms to seek medical attention. The rationale for taking the hCG should be given. The woman should be made aware of the implications of the results, so if it is bad news, she is prepared. Often, a diagnosis of miscarriage is made by decreasing hCG levels and is given to the woman over the phone. This must be done sensitively, allowing the woman time to process the news and offering to call back if possible when the woman is at home or with her partner. The woman should be advised to take a PT in 2–3 weeks, and by then, all symptoms should have settled. She should

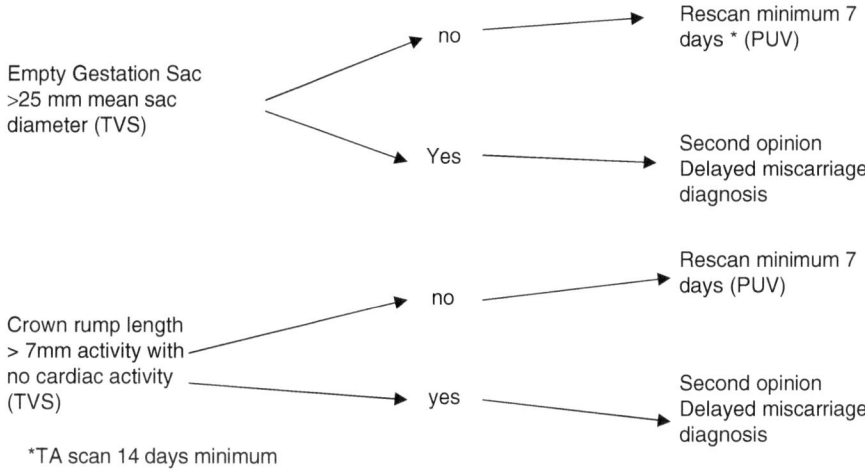

Fig. 7.2 Management of PUV

also be told to expect her period 4–6 weeks post negative PT. All routine antenatal should be cancelled and miscarriage information and leaflets offered. It is good practice to inform women to contact their GP should they have any concerns or if they are finding it hard to cope.

7.5 Hydatidiform Mole/Molar Pregnancy

This is a very rare form of pregnancy loss, only occurring in 1 in 600 pregnancies [5]. More common in women from Asian countries, the Philippines and Japan, there is increased risk with age and with those who have had a previous molar. Women may be asymptomatic or present with bleeding, pain or hyperemesis (due to very high hCG levels). Provisional diagnosis is made on scan (appearing as multiple cystic areas) and confirmed with histology following surgical intervention.

A normal pregnancy has 46 XX chromosomes (female) and 46 XY chromosomes if male (23X from the mother 23Y from the father). A molar pregnancy can be complete or partial. A complete mole occurs when an ovum with no genetic content is fertilised by a sperm (possibly two). This will result in a mass of cells all with paternal chromosomes. There is no embryo.

A partial mole happens when two sperm fertilise one ovum giving too much genetic information (69 XXY). An embryo can be present but will most likely not be compatible with life. Women should be followed up by the National Trophoblastic Screening Centre to ensure falling hCG's. Up to 15% of women develop persistent gestational trophoblastic disease and require further treatment.

> This diagnosis meant any sort of closure on this loss took a long, long time. This had a huge impact on my emotional wellbeing and mental state. I started to panic, wondering, 'Would we ever be able to have children? 'What had I done wrong to cause this?'

Pregnancy avoidance for 6 months from the time urine and blood HCG are negative is advised. Very rarely, an invasive mole, if untreated, can lead to choriocarcinoma however, if caught early, has an almost 100% cure rate [5].

7.6   Management of Miscarriage

Discussing managements of miscarriage requires the practitioner to have emotional intelligence, excellent communication skills and extensive knowledge of all managements including effectiveness, risks, recovery time and what happens if things don't go to plan. All this knowledge should be relevant and evidence based. All available options should be regularly audited, updated and implemented by all staff to ensure consistency and standardised care.

> The nurse who looked after us immediately after we received the shocking news was as professional and supportive as she could possibly have been. It was helpful how calm, compassionate, understanding and respectful she was. The way she acted was matching how we felt. We were able to take all the time we needed to ask all the questions storming into our heads.

All major guidelines advocate the training and support of all staff looking after women who experience pregnancy loss; however, it is often left up to the individual practitioner to seek support and training from such organisations as the Miscarriage Association, The Association of Early Pregnancy Units, Tommy's, and the Ectopic Pregnancy Trust, all of which have excellent online resources and training modules.

Not only hard to hear, the delivery of such information provides challenges for the EP nurse and must be given sensitively but honestly. The incorrect use of language and terminology can have devastating and long-lasting effects on women, whereas information given with empathy and compassion can aid healing and acceptance. The EP nurse is the woman's advocate, enabling informed choice and facilitating a decision that is right for them and their lifestyle, providing support throughout the decision-making process. Unfortunately, the different types of miscarriage management can be seen to provide a horrific choice. Some women require time to choose, while for some women, the thought of having a "dead baby" inside them is appalling so they request immediate action. Managing expectations of these women with a limited and often overstretched service is a formidable challenge. Most hospitals have a system where surgical management of miscarriage can be added on to a daily list, and nurses are undertaking manual vacuum aspiration training to reduce waiting times.

When discussing any managements of miscarriage, clear written and current information about all the options must be provided, and the woman must be given a contact number for advice. Women must be made aware that all managements of miscarriage carry a small risk of infection, uncontrolled bleeding and failure. Surgical managements carry the extra risk of damage to the uterus, cervix and surrounding organs, and if this happens, a laparoscopy is indicated to assess and repair any damage.

All risks and benefits must be reiterated at the point of written consent, including the additional risks associated with having a general anaesthetic. In the case of girls under 16, consent must be obtained in accordance with the Fraser guidelines, and the safeguarding team should be informed in accordance with local policy.

7.7 Expectant Management

It would've been helpful to have been better prepared with information for how the "natural miscarriage" may take place. Being told to expect bleeding like a very heavy, clotting period and to wear thick pads was not enough. I experienced a quite sudden and very painful onset of miscarriage (thankfully on my way home from work), and was terrified by the amount of blood, contraction like pains and the passing of a sizeable pregnancy sac etc. I understand health professionals do not want to scare people, and that all experiences are different, but I feel it is imperative that women are armed with proper, detailed information - even if it is "unpleasant" to have to spell out what could physically happen.

National guidelines recommend using this as the first-line management for all clinically well women for the first 7–14 days [3] for miscarriages under 12/40. The woman must be made aware they may have heavy bleeding with clots (increasing in severity with advanced gestation). Additionally, she should be warned that she may see a sac or an embryo depending on the gestation of the loss, be made aware of what to do if this happens and provided with a way of collecting tissue for genetic testing if required. A discussion around when to take analgesia and antiemetic must be had, and women must be informed that miscarriage can be very painful and how and when to seek help. Expectant management is not indicated for those with any evidence of infection, suspected molar pregnancy, clinical instability, previous history of post-partum haemorrhage, who are unable to receive blood transfusions or who have any clotting disorders. While some women prefer this management choice, wishing to remain at home and reducing intervention, other women decline this management due to the unpredictability and concerns over uncontrolled symptoms. A good support network at home is needed. It is important that a complete miscarriage is confirmed by a pregnancy test or ultrasound scan 2–3 weeks post-miscarriage.

7.8 Medical Management

Medical management is offered to women for both delayed and incomplete miscarriage (individual units will have specific inclusion criteria based on gestation and size pregnancy). FBC and G&S should be taken, and written consent obtained before management is commenced. This management is not indicated if the woman has any evidence of infection and previous history of post-partum haemorrhage, is unable to receive blood transfusions, is on any anticoagulant therapy or long-term glucocorticoid therapy or has allergies to misoprostol.

Misoprostol stimulates the contraction of the uterus and dilation of the cervix. Women must be informed that misoprostol is not licenced for the use in miscarriage but has been used safely and effectively for a long time.

Woman should be instructed to start the process in the morning and to pass urine before inserting the tablets as far into the vagina as possible. They should then be instructed to lay down for an hour after. Bleeding can be expected to start 1–2 hrs after insertion with strong period like pain until the pregnancy tissue passes. Women can have some form of bleeding for up to 3 weeks, but it should not be continuously heavy. If no bleeding happens, women must be advised to contact the EPU as they may require a second dose. It is common for women to experience nausea and/or vomiting, but this should not last for more than 6 hrs. Chills, fever and diarrhoea may happen, and if this lasts longer than 24 h, they must contact the EPU for review.

A pregnancy test should be taken after 3 weeks, but some units will follow-up with a scan to ensure a complete miscarriage has occurred. Women choose this management because it gives them more predictability and control than expectant management but less invasive than surgical managements.

7.9   Surgical Management Under General Anaesthetic

Surgical management of miscarriage (SMM) under general anaesthetic was previously known as dilation and curettage (D&C) and evacuation of retained products of conception (ERPC).

> After the surgery I was signed off very quickly and sent home. I feel this part of the process could have been improved. I wasn't given any written guidance about what to expect in the next few days. The member of staff that discharged me was brief and I was feeling very emotional so I didn't leave with a clear message as to what to look out for. I also wasn't given any suggestions for further emotional support.
>
> I know everyone is different and many people may cope with the experience by themselves but I really struggled with the loss of the baby even though it happened at 10 weeks. I ended up with retained tissues after the first procedure and had painful cramps and bleeding after the operation. I wasn't aware that this was abnormal so didn't return to the hospital.

If a woman has no comorbidities, this is usually performed as a day case. The cervix is dilated, and a ridged suction catheter is placed in the endometrial cavity, removing the contents of the uterus using suction. This is a blind procedure and relies on the skill and experience of the practitioner. In some circumstances, the procedure is undertaken with ultrasound guidance. Women can expect to have light bleeding post-procedure for up to 3 weeks but to report any heavy bleeding or signs of infection. Women must be consented, FBC and G&S and MRSA swabs taken. Women choose this option because it facilitates acceptance, and moving on quickly, they can "schedule" this around their lives, and any tissue recovered can be sent for any requested testing.

7.10 Surgical Management Under Local Anaesthetic Manual Vacuum Aspiration (MVA)

Offered to women with a miscarriage diagnosed on scan under 9 weeks, this equates to a CRL of <22 mm/MSD <33 mm and an incomplete miscarriage with RPOC <5 cm. Often, consultants may undertake this procedure outside these parameters if no other management is possible (the inclusion criteria may differ in diferent units).

The procedure is undertaken as a day case in early pregnancy units either by a doctor or nurse who has under taken MVA training. Women under 25 are offered a swab for chlamydia and gonorrhoea or given oral azithromycin. They must be made aware they will hear a suction sound; some units provide music or headphones for the woman for distraction. Women must be made aware that this procedure can be painful, but supplemental analgesia can be given if needed. MVA is not indicated if any suspicion of a molar pregnancy, any infection, HB under 90 g/l, haemodynamically unstable, any allergy to lignocaine, adrenaline or misoprostol. Women with a large fibroid uterus and post-partum RPOC must be discussed with the consultant for suitability.

Misoprostol is taken sublingually 3 hrs before the procedure, and diclofenac 100 mg is inserted rectally 1 h before the procedure. A speculum is inserted into the vagina; the cervix is cleaned and injected with local anaesthetic. A TA scan is undertaken prior and post-procedure to check there is no remaining tissue.

The cervix is dilated, and a semiridged cannula is inserted into the uterus, and the contents of the uterus are aspirated. The process is repeated until the endometrial cavity is emptied. Women can be discharged after 2 hrs if they are feeling well, passed urine, tolerated food and fluid and have minimal pain and bleeding. They should be advised they may experience some bleeding for up to 3 weeks, but it should not be heavy. Women may choose this management due to the reduced recovery time compared to having a GA.

7.10.1 Anti-D

If a woman is found to have a Rh D (rhesus)-negative blood type, she does not carry the D antigen in her red blood cells. If the blood from a Rh D-positive baby crossed into the blood stream of a Rh D-negative mother, the mother will react to the blood as an unrecognised substance and produce antibodies against it.

This is called sensitisation; sensitising events are any bleeding or trauma. The immunity is permanent, and if exposure to the antigens is repeated, then the antibodies rapidly increase crossing the placenta binding with the baby's RBC which are then destroyed leading to rhesus haemolytic disease. Production of maternal anti-D can be prevented by the administration of exogenous anti-D. This mops up the foetal red blood cells that have crossed the placenta by binding to their antigens and preventing recognition by the mother's immune system. A prophylaxis dose of 250 IU should be offered to all resus-negative women undergoing surgical management for miscarriage or ectopic pregnancy. National guidelines advised not to administer anti-D for threatened miscarriage, complete miscarriage, medical managements of miscarriage and ectopic pregnancy if there has been no surgical intervention.

7.10.2 Sensitive Disposal

> The fact that the hospital offered cremation service was also a huge relief as the 2nd most devastating thought after the lack of heartbeat was: will my baby's remains end up in a medical bin? The nurse explained all the options again and reassured us that remains would be treated with respect.

Any woman who undergoes pregnancy loss has the right to know what is going to happen to the pregnancy tissue. This can bring some comfort at a time of great sadness. This has not always been standard practice, and pregnancy remains were often incinerated with human waste. The term "pregnancy remains" is used in relation to all pregnancy losses that have not exceeded the 24th week including ectopic pregnancy, miscarriage or early intrauterine foetal death. In 2015, the Human Tissue Authority (HTA) published guidelines [6], setting out the minimum standard expected for the disposal of tissue following pregnancy loss or termination of pregnancy which is cremation, burial or incineration in certain circumstances. They also give guidance for staff. This includes informing women of the likelihood of recovering remains following a cremation or perhaps the opportunity for some form of memorialization if burial is chosen. In all cases, the woman should be made aware that there are options for disposal. Verbal and written information about the options should be provided; there should be an opportunity to discuss all options in a sensitive manner, allowing the woman to make the right decision for her. Sensitivity should be shown to the values and beliefs of a wide range of cultures and religions, particularly those of their local community.

If the woman would prefer the hospital to handle the matter, details of who to contact and timescale for this should be provided, should she change her mind.

> When we attended the service, I felt like we could really move on.

Women can choose to have their pregnancy remains returned to them in order to make their own arrangements. This will be at the woman's cost. Accurate documentation, especially if the woman declines, is vital. This should include any consent forms, how and when the remains were disposed of. Trusts should provide training for staff, and all staff should have access to education regarding sensitive disposal and counselling services.

7.11 Ectopic Pregnancy

The ectopic pregnancy rate in the UK is around 1 in every 80 and remains the main cause of death in early pregnancy [7]. Ectopic pregnancy is a pregnancy that implants anywhere outside the uterus, most commonly in the fallopian tubes;

however, implantation can occur in other sites. The fallopian tubes (or oviducts) are hollow muscular tubes lying adjacent to its ovary. The tubes have a delicate mucous membrane lining inside. The diameter of the tube increases as it nears the ovary to form the fimbriae. When the ovum is released at ovulation, it is picked up by the fimbriae fertilised inside the tube and transported to the cavity of the uterus. Damage by inflammation or infection can cause restriction of the transportation of a developing embryo to the uterus resulting in implantation occurring in the fallopian tube. Ectopic pregnancies are reported on scan as either an inhomogeneous mass or a gestation sac (with or without yolk sac and foetal pole).

> I was really scared about what was happening and the nurse who told me what was going to happen and reassured me that I was going to be ok made all the difference.

Risk factors

- Smoking.
- Emergency contraception and progesterone only pill.
- Previous ectopic (7–10%).
- Previous surgery.
- Fertility treatment.
- Intrauterine device (IUD)/intrauterine system (IUS).
- Increase in age.
- Untreated STI.

Other sites for ectopic implantation include:

- Caesarean scar: Implantation occurs in the scar of the uterus from a previous caesarean section. Incidence of this are increasing, most likely due to the impact of elective caesarean section delivery. Dependent on the implantation site within the scar and developing placenta, this type of ectopic pregnancy can result in a live birth, but it carries a high risk of maternal bleeding resulting in a hysterectomy. Management is dependent on individual case. Early treatment options include removing the pregnancy using suction and a cervical stitch or keyhole surgery or using methotrexate injection/s.
- Heterotopic: A twin pregnancy with one implanting in the uterus and the other twin implanting outside the uterus – usually in the fallopian tube. Surgical management to remove the extrauterine pregnancy is usually indicated. It is possible for the intrauterine pregnancy to continue in approximately 30% of diagnosed cases [7].
- Interstitial: A fertilised egg implants in the part of the fallopian tube within the wall of the uterus. This is very difficult to diagnose. As the pregnancy can progress further, it has the potential to cause damage to the fallopian tube and the uterine wall. Management is case dependent but can be surgical or medical, or if the pregnancy is failing, expectant management can be an option. Surgical intervention may impact on future pregnancy as it will weaken the uterine wall.
- Other very rare sites include ovarian, intermural and abdominal.

A woman may present with multiple symptoms including

- LIF and RIF pain.
- Spotting, vaginal discharge and bleeding.
- Abdominal pain.
- Shoulder tip.
- Asymptomatic.
- Gastrointestinal symptoms.
- Dizziness.
- Rectal pressure.
- Feeling faint.
- Nausea.
- Pale.
- Shock.
- Collapse.
- Hypotension (<100/60 mmHg).
- Tachycardia (>100 bpm).
- Pelvic, adnexal and abdominal tenderness on examination.
- Cervical motion tender on bimanual examination.

7.12   Managements of Ectopic Pregnancy

Managements of EP depend on the clinical presentation, location, size of ectopic, presence of foetal heart rate, hemoperitoneum, serum hCG results and potential impact of future fertility. Clear written and verbal information should be given to all women diagnosed with an ectopic pregnancy.

7.12.1 Medical

National guidelines recommend this as the first-line treatment [3] for women who can return for follow-up and have no significant pain, an unruptured adnexal mass < 35 mm, no visible heart rate and serum hCG levels less than 5000 IU/L with no intrauterine pregnancy.

50 mg/m^2 of methotrexate is given as an IM injection, and the medication stops the rapid cell division, but this can take a few days to happen. Success rate varies from 65 to 95% [3] and is dependent on multiple factors including the hCG values and the gestation of the ectopic. Women should be informed to expect mild localised pain at the injection site, abdominal pain, spotting, fatigue, nausea, vomiting and dizziness. The woman must be advised to report any symptoms if concerned and to present to A&E if these are uncontrolled or increasing. Additionally, they should be advised that they still have a chance of rupture, even at low levels of hCG.

Serum hCG should then be taken at day 4, day 7 post-initial injection and then weekly until less than 15 IU/L with an expected decrease of 15%. If a plateau or increase is seen, a review is indicated, and a second dose may be considered if there has not been the expected minimum decrease (+/− uss to exclude FH). Decreased success rates have been reported with an initial higher hCG level; the presence of a gestation sac, yolk sac and foetal pole; and increase in hCG levels between day 4 and day 7. Women will be told to avoid sexual intercourse, alcohol and direct strong sunlight while undergoing treatment. Women are advised to wait 3 months to try to conceive again.

7.13 Surgical Management of Ectopic Pregnancy

This is the first-line treatment for women who have any of the following: moderate pain, significant hemoperitoneum, an adnexal mass measuring over 35 mm, a visible foetal heartbeat and serum BHCG >5000. Standard management is a laparoscopic salpingectomy (removal of the fallopian tube); however, a salpingotomy (preservation of the tube) can be considered if removing a fallopian tube may affect future fertility. Women are usually admitted to the ward with all standard preoperative assessments completed. Often, in these incidences, women can rapidly become unwell especially with a ruptured or live ectopic. The medical team must be informed as a matter of urgency, intravenous access gained, FBC and G&S taken and blood should be cross matched. Any prescribed medication of fluids should be administered. Woman with a ruptured ectopic pregnancy is likely to be in shock, but the sudden appearance of medical staff can be overwhelming and frightening. It is good practice to keep the woman informed at every stage.

Women can usually go home the next day, but a serum hCG must be taken after 7 days if a salpingotomy has been performed. There is no standard follow-up. Women should be advised to take a PT 3 weeks post-surgery and to have a 6/40 reassurance scan at the next pregnancy. They should be advised to contact the unit or their Gp if feeling unwell with any sign of infection or increased pain or bleeding.

7.14 Expectant Management of Ectopic Pregnancy

This may be considered a treatment for women who are compliant with follow-up, have minimal pain, are clinically stable, have an initial hCG <1500 U/l and have static or minimally increasing hCH levels. Women under expectant management will have their hCG levels taken after at regular intervals (usually day 2, 4 and day 7 then weekly) dependent on the decrease. They must be made aware that they may be advised to have another management if clinically indicated and that there is still a possibility of rupture, even at lower levels of hCG hormone.

7.15 Recurrent Miscarriage

Recurrent miscarriage is the term given to three or more pregnancy losses that occur in succession with the same partner. Presently, the NHS will only offer investigations based on this criteria, despite the publications of new guidelines by the European Society of Human Reproduction and Embryology (ESHRE) in 2017 [8].

They recommend diagnosis after two nonconsecutive miscarriages, and women should be offered with antiphospholipid syndrome (APLS) screening, but this will be at the referring clinician's discretion.

> To me (and I'm sure I'm not alone) Recurrent miscarriage has been a devastating, emotional and exhausting rollercoaster that has effected every element of my life because of the mental toll it has taken on me. The pain of the losses and the heartache of yearning so badly for something is with me every day. In the 3 years I have been living this journey, a day hasn't passed where I haven't hurt, thought about my babies and dreamed about having a baby only to then try and stop myself in my tracks as it hurts too much to dream.

Affects 1/100 couples, known causes include:

- Antiphospholipid syndrome (APS) (sticky blood syndrome). It is thought that the antibodies may stop proper implantation.
- Abnormal chromosomes—one partner can carry a chromosomal defect called a 'balanced translocation' that gets passed to baby as an 'unbalanced translocation', i.e. missing or duplicated genetic information.
- Other blood disorders such as factor V Leiden.
- Polycystic ovary syndrome, uncontrolled thyroid and diabetes.
- Cervical weakness.
- Uterine abnormality such as septate uterus.

> Hope is one of the biggest things I think that helps a woman who is dealing with recurrent loss psychologically. That and support.

It is worth noting that around 50% of couples have "unexplained" recurrent miscarriage and approximately 60% of women who have three or more miscarriages will go on to a successful pregnancy. Treatments can include anticoagulant medication, surgery to correct uterine abnormalities and in second trimester cervical stich.

Treatments will be based on any cause of miscarriage.

7.16 Follow-Up After Pregnancy Loss

Follow-up care after any pregnancy loss is dependent on local policy. The majority of EPU's do not routinely provide any formal aftercare (except Molar pregnancy) and advise women to see the GP if they have any concerns post discharge. Women should be informed that their period will return 4–6 weeks post-miscarriage. If further pregnancy is to be avoided, contraception advice should be given, but a woman can resume sexual intercourse when she is emotionally and physically ready. There is variation in advice about when to try for another baby; however, women can be advised to wait until after their first period post-miscarriage, in order to provide more accurate dating. All routine antenatal care should be cancelled as soon as possible. If any cytogenetics testing has been requested, the woman should be informed how she will receive the results and who to contact and a time frame provided. Additionally, women should be advised on how to contact the EPU in the next pregnancy or how to book a reassurance scan.

7.17 Nausea and Vomiting in Pregnancy (NVP) and Hyperemesis Gravidarum (HG)

Persistent vomiting may lead to weight loss, dehydration and electrolyte imbalance. Symptoms include ptyalism (severe saliva production), acute sense of smell, headache, constipation, hypotension, ketosis and hematemesis due small tears in the oesophagus.

> Every hour was dark and intolerable, I was grateful for getting pregnant with this longed-for baby, however the sickness was so bad that it made me think about terminating the pregnancy because I was not sure I could cope with it. It was only through the support of those around me that I got through and am now so grateful to have my baby in my arms

Exact cause is unknown but thought to be hormonal it often runs in families. If HG occurs in the first pregnancy, it is most likely to repeat in subsequent pregnancies. It can affect:

- Homeostasis.
- Electrolytes.
- Kidney function.
- Increased risk of DVT.
- Adverse effects on foetus.
- Psychosocial wellbeing.
- Cultural status.
- Emotional effects.

Around one of seven women experience nausea and vomiting that disappears around the 14th week. Excessive vomiting affecting daily life is widely underreported but thought to be around 1 in every 100. Early treatment is more effective.

A woman presenting with symptoms of HG should be fully assessed including:

- Full history, clinical examination signs of muscle wasting, observations, PUQE score.
- Urinalysis, FBC, U&Es, blood glucose. If previous admission, LFT, TFT, amylase, ABG.
- Ultrasound scan (exclude multiple pregnancy or molar pregnancy).
- Coexisting conditions (UTI, gastroenteritis, neurological conditions).

Treatments will reflect the presentation and severity. Early intervention is linked to increase efficacy, and by the time women present to hospital with NVP, they have tried most of the "home remedies" and require medication and hydration.

Current management includes:

- Hydration IVI (Inpatient Vs Community).[1]
- First-line anti-emetics cyclizing and prochlorperazine.
- IV hydration with assessment of liver and kidney function.
- Second-line anti-emetics such as metoclopramide and ondansetron.
- Third-line obstetric medicine consultant review considering steroid intervention.

Patients with HG have reported negative experiences with health-care staff and were made to feel they were wasting time or a burden in a busy department. This could be attributed to staff's attitude and perceptions of "a bit of sickness" and may be based on personal experience of pregnancy. This rarely happens with any other medical condition. The importance of nursing patients with empathy, understanding and in a non-judgmental manor is fundamental. The potential complications of untreated HG are serious and extremely distressing for a woman. With the EPUs providing hyperemesis clinics and HG being treated in the community, women have now more choice in their treatment.

7.18 Psychological Factors in Early Pregnancy Loss

Please note that the psychological and emotional aspects can also be applied to loss after 13 weeks.

It is important that the psychological consequences of an early pregnancy loss are understood in context. There is often both a bereavement and a traumatic physical event which can be life-threatening. Often, a couple will start dreaming of their child from the initial positive pregnancy test, and the loss dashes these hopes and dreams and can cause a doubt about whether it will be possible for them to have children. With an early loss, there are no accepted and known rituals to manage the grief and often no physical evidence of the loss to mourn, yet the loss is often keenly felt.

There tends to be, as well, a reticence to tell those around about the pregnancy or the loss, so often it is experienced in isolation without the usual support mechanisms in place from family, friends and colleagues that come from a later loss or bereavement.

There is increasing recognition that early pregnancy loss can be traumatic and has significant emotional consequences for both women and men, often resulting in depression, anxiety and trauma or symptoms of post-traumatic stress disorder (PTSD), which can persist for a year or more after the loss.

The most common feelings expressed are isolation, loneliness, denial, distress, devastation, anger, shock, shame, feeling useless and a sense of failure and grief, with women describing their loss as bereavement.

---

[1] Initial assessment in hospital and patient discharged to the community service for continuation of IV hydration and medication.

7.19   Definition of Trauma

Someone is considered to be suffering from trauma when they are plagued in the present by emotions, sensations or memories (often flashbacks) from a past experience in which they were shocked and scared or felt very out of control. There can be a feeling of being trapped/stuck in this experience.

> I would have appreciated more information on seeking counselling at the point when I miscarried as I had no idea about the ongoing effects this would have on my mental health, flashbacks/PTSD like symptoms etc. It was only by chance that after 2 years of emotional suffering, and unfortunately a subsequent miscarriage that I happened to pick up a leaflet for Pregnancy related counselling. By this point I was having regular panic attacks, not sleeping and having disturbing thoughts. If only I'd been told sooner about the psychological impact, maybe I would have sought help earlier and been able to emotionally recover much, much quicker.

In a recent study, Farren et al. [9] have shown that a large number (39%) of women who had experienced a miscarriage or ectopic pregnancy met the criteria for probable moderate to severe PTSD 3 months after the loss. Many were also suffering from moderate to severe anxiety (20%) and some from depression (16% at 1 month and 5% at 3 months after the loss).

The observation that such a significant proportion of women suffer from symptoms of PTSD after losing a pregnancy, and that this is more common than both anxiety and depression, is potentially important and must be considered while nursing women undergoing pregnancy loss.

In other contexts, we know that untreated PTSD has a significant impact on quality of life, relationships, ability to work, suicide risk and physical health. PTSD also has implications for future pregnancies, including poor health behaviour, reduced gestational length and issues with infant bonding.

Other findings were that women with *ectopic* pregnancy suffer from significant levels of emotional distress, with slightly higher levels of PTSD symptoms compared with women who experience a miscarriage, but lower levels of anxiety and depression. As ectopic pregnancy is a potentially life-threatening situation, sometimes the loss of a pregnancy and the potential threat to fertility can be missed as the immediate health needs are attended to.

Recurrent loss: With more losses, the sense of sadness and isolation increases, along with the fear that they might not be able to have their own children. There is often a strong sense of guilt and shame, with the woman blaming herself. There is a hope that they will now get help and investigations, and any information that can be obtained regarding the causes can be helpful, but often there are no answers. It is important to recognise the significance and sadness of each loss, as well as having to go through it again physically.

> Miscarriage is a grief like I've never experienced before. A grieving for a life and so many other things on top of it. Miscarriage affects you (from my experience) mentally and sadly I think mental health is something there is little understanding of among people, so therefore people find it very hard to understand and be empathetic to this type of illness. They

just think you need to pull yourself together and get on- if only it were that easy - hey. They are happy to listen and support for a while, but I think their ability to remain empathetic and understanding of your situation wears thin. That's how it feels to me anyway. One of the consequences of having 5 miscarriages is that all of my relationships have been affected, and I don't know if all of them will recover

The shock of the diagnosis and lengthy follow-up required after a diagnosis of gestational trophoblastic disease (*molar pregnancy*) often resulting in a long delay in being able to try again can increase the sense of anxiety, depression and struggle with sexual desire, with a fear of whether this will mean that they cannot have more children.

Hyperemesis can have a significant psychological effect on the woman and her partner, who can often feel helpless and desperate. It can be a dark time when a woman cannot see her way through, particularly when it is very severe. Understanding, empathy and reassurance are vital during this time to decrease the sense of isolation and desperation.

Nurses can have a vital role in making a difference to the experience during and after the loss and how the woman and her partner, if she has one, recovers. As has been demonstrated in the patient stories, competence and care from health professionals make a significant difference along with the giving of appropriate information about the management options that are available to them, so they are able to be involved in the decision-making process and maintain some sense of control.

What women/couples need from nursing/clinical staff:
Do not assume what they think or feel – ask them.

- Be informed about what the diagnosis is for the patients that you are seeing and what their past medical and pregnancy history is. *Listen to them.*

  I was given an internal examination by a doctor and I was upset and on my own . . . the nurse just watched. She didn't hold my hand or reassure me. Perhaps I wouldn't even remember the moment if she had.

- Women need empathy, compassion, kindness, understanding, reassurance, sensitivity as well as competent care because this shows a recognition of the gravity of the loss. Don't be afraid to provide comfort. The care received significantly affects *well-being and long-term recovery*. An experience of kindness makes a difference to the memories attached to the loss/time in hospital. Unkindness/lack of care can stay with a patient for a long time and increase the negative emotions/trauma attached to the event.

  One partner said: "I am so frustrated because I want to make this better for her and fix it and there is nothing I can do."

- Offer support to the partner, be aware that it is their loss too, but also, they will most likely be concerned about giving support to their partner who is going through it physically, so they may not feel able to express how they feel.
- *Sensitivity* in relation to how they might want the loss to be referred to (baby, foetus, embryo, collection of cells) and an understanding about how important

the care/disposal of the tissue might be, do they want to see the baby – depending on the gestation this may be possible. They may not want to know about this.

You just want the opportunity of having your baby back and nothing else really matters

- Avoid lines like "at least you can get pregnant", "everything happens for a reason", "you are young, you will have another baby" and "this is just one of those things". They are annoying and painful and can seem as though the agony of the present loss is being brushed aside. Do say something like "I am so sorry about your loss". It is very easy to say the wrong thing in these moments, but if there is an air of compassion, this will show through.
- A connection with the nursing staff. *Recognition* of both their *emotional* and *physical* symptoms at the time of the diagnosis and during and after the loss. *NOT* avoidance/distance. Even if you have very little time and you do not know what to say, you can still *ACKNOWLEDGE* what they are going through.
- *Very clear* explanation about what might happen physically with written information, with asking them questions to check that they have understood (they will often only take in very little of what is said on the day) so that they feel they have made their own choice and have a little bit of control over this. They need to know when the bleeding is *too much* and when to come back to hospital, so that they do not come back and sit in A and E waiting for a long time unnecessarily or they do not stay at home too long. With ectopic pregnancy or hyperemesis *how to know when* they should return to hospital. *They are often in shock and not able to ask for things or know what they need.* It is very helpful for them to have a number to call to ask for specialist advice.
- *The opportunity for follow-up* even if this is just a suggestion that they go to their Gp in a few weeks if they are still struggling with anxiety, low mood and flashbacks or feeling as though they are not coping in any way. *Many women will not need this, but if it is suggested, it will help those who do need it to recognise their need and seek support.* Suggesting that they talk to some others about what they are going through to decrease the isolation, especially those who have experienced pregnancy loss themselves, can be helpful. Reassure them that although seeing pregnant friends/new babies may not be possible for a while, this is "normal", and they have not become a bad person. Reassure the couple that some anxiety in a subsequent pregnancy anxiety is to be expected and to seek help if the anxiety feels overwhelming. Easy access to EPC in future pregnancies can really help to reduce the stress and anxiety levels.

References

1. Royal College of Nursing (2017) Clinical nurse specialist in early pregnancy care. RCN, London. https://www.rcn.org.uk/professional-development/publications/pub-006394. Accessed 27 Aug 2018
2. Stillbirth & neonatal death charity (SANDS) (2018) The National Bereavement Pathway. https://www.sands.org.uk/. Accessed 27 Aug 2018

3. (2012) Ectopic pregnancy and miscarriage: diagnosis and initial management. Clinical guideline [cg 154]. https://www.nice.org.uk/guidance/CG154. Accessed 27 Aug 2018
4. The Miscarriage Association (2018) Miscarriage. https://www.miscarriageassociation.org.uk/information/miscarriage/. Accessed 27 Aug 2018
5. The Miscarriage Association (2018) Molar pregnancy. https://www.miscarriageassociation.org.uk/your-feelings/special-circumstances/molar-pregnancy/. Accessed 27 Aug 2018
6. Human Tissue Authority (2015) HTA guidance on the sensitive handling of pregnancy remains. https://www.hta.gov.uk/search?search_api_views_fulltext=sensitive+disposal&sort_by=search_api_relevance&sort_by=search_api_relevance. Accessed 27 Aug 2018
7. The Ectopic Pregnancy Trust (2018) https://www.ectopic.org.uk/. Accessed 27 Aug 2018
8. European Society of Human Reproduction and Embryology (2017) Guideline on the management of recurrent pregnancy loss. https://www.eshre.eu/Guidelines-and-Legal/Guidelines/Recurrent-pregnancy-loss.aspx. Accessed 27 Aug 2018
9. Farren J, Jalmbrant M, Ameye L, Joash K, Mitchell-Jones N, Tapp S et al (2016) Post-traumatic stress, anxiety and depression following miscarriage or ectopic pregnancy: a prospective cohort study. BMJ Open 6:e011864. https://doi.org/10.1136/bmjopen-2016-011864

Additional Resources

Association of Early Pregnancy Units. www.aepu.org.uk/
Child Bereavement UK. https://childbereavementuk.org/
Ectopic Pregnancy Trust. https://www.ectopic.org.uk/
NICE Guidelines. https://www.nice.org.uk/guidance
Royal College of Nursing Guidelines (RCN). https://www.rcn.org.uk/professional-development/publications
Royal College of Obstetricians and Gynaecologists Guidelines (RCOG). https://www.rcog.org.uk/guidelines
SANDS—Stillbirth and Neonatal Death Charity. https://www.sands.org.uk/
The Miscarriage Association—pregnancy loss information and support. https://www.miscarriageassociation.org.uk/
Tommy's Charity—Pregnancy Information and Research. www.tommy's.org

Abortion

8

Amanda Myers and Michael Nevill

8.1 Introduction

It is estimated that 56 million abortions are undertaken globally each year [1], with approximately half of all pregnancies being unintended and half of these ending in abortion [2].

In 2017, the number of abortions carried out on residents of England and Wales was 189,859 [3] and in Scotland, 12,212 [4]. Although both saw slight increases since the previous year, the annual numbers remain relatively stable.

The age profile of women having abortions is changing, with the rate for those aged under 25—and particularly aged under 20—decreasing over the last 10 years and the rate for women aged 30 and over increasing [3].

Ninety-eight percent of abortions in England and Wales were funded by the NHS in 2017, with 70% being performed in approved independent sector places under NHS contract [3]. The vast majority—90%—were performed under 13 weeks' gestation [3].

Abortion is a key aspect of comprehensive reproductive healthcare and an area of practice in which nurses and midwives have developed their roles significantly.

8.2 The Law and Abortion in the UK

It is important that any nurse or midwife working in abortion care has an understanding of the specific legislation relating to abortion, how that affects their practice, and that the legal situation in Northern Ireland is different from that of England, Wales and Scotland.

A. Myers (✉) · M. Nevill
British Pregnancy Advisory Service, Birmingham, UK
e-mail: mandy.myers@bpas.org

© Springer Nature Switzerland AG 2019   153
D. Holloway (ed.), *Nursing Management of Women's Health*,
https://doi.org/10.1007/978-3-030-16115-6_8

In all four countries of the UK, the 1861 Offences Against the Person Act (OAPA) remains in statute and lays down that any woman who attempts to procure her own miscarriage or anyone who assists a woman to procure a miscarriage is guilty of an offence which could result in imprisonment for a lengthy period, including up to a life term.

The Abortion Act 1967 (as amended by the Human Fertilisation and Embryology Act 1990) applies in England, Wales and Scotland but not Northern Ireland and provides a defence against the OAPA, defining grounds upon which an abortion can be undertaken lawfully. Two registered medical practitioners (medical doctors) must agree 'in good faith' that the woman meets one of the grounds for a lawful abortion as listed in the Abortion Act 1967 (see Table 8.1). The doctors' agreement is indicated by their respective signatures on an HSA1 form (HSA2 form in the case of emergency grounds F & G), and after the procedure has taken place, a notification form—HSA4—must be signed by the doctor who takes responsibility for the abortion and sent to the Chief Medical Officer for the relevant country.

In circumstances where an abortion is needed to save a woman's life or prevent grave, permanent injury, only one doctor's signature is required to make the abortion lawful, indicated on the HSA2 form.

In 2017, in England and Wales, 98% of abortions (185,448) were performed under ground C [3].

To be lawful, an abortion must be carried out by a registered medical practitioner. In practice, that means the medications administered for the purpose of inducing the abortion must be prescribed by a doctor, and in the case of surgical abortion, the law, although it has been questioned [5], is currently interpreted to mean the procedure to surgically remove the pregnancy must be performed by a doctor.

In England, Scotland and Wales, abortions must, by law, be performed in an NHS hospital or premises approved by the Secretary of State for Health. England,

Table 8.1 Statutory grounds for legal abortion in Britain

A	The continuance of the pregnancy would involve risk to the life of the pregnant woman greater than if the pregnancy were terminated;
B	The termination is necessary to prevent grave permanent injury to the physical or mental health of the pregnant woman;
C	The pregnancy has *not* exceeded its 24th week and that the continuance of the pregnancy would involve risk, greater than if the pregnancy were terminated, of injury to the physical or mental health of the pregnant woman;
D	The pregnancy has *not* exceeded its 24th week and that the continuance of the pregnancy would involve risk, greater than if the pregnancy were terminated, of injury to the physical or mental health of any existing child(ren) of the family of the pregnant woman;
E	There is a substantial risk that if the child were born it would suffer from such physical or mental abnormalities as to be seriously handicapped.
Or, in an emergency, certified by the operating doctor as immediately necessary:	
F	To save the life of the pregnant woman;
G	To prevent grave permanent injury to the physical or mental health of the pregnant woman.

Scotland and Wales have all recently approved the use of misoprostol in women's homes for the purpose of early medical abortion. This means that the woman can collect the misoprostol when she attends the clinic for the mifepristone, take it home and use it after the agreed interval, allowing women to plan and organise the optimum time to pass the pregnancy in the comfort of their own homes and avoid the risk of pain, bleeding and abortion on the way home when the misoprostol had previously had to be taken within the clinic.

8.2.1 Conscientious Objection

The Abortion Act 1967—which, as noted earlier, does not apply in Northern Ireland—includes a right of conscientious objection, allowing healthcare professionals to decline to take part in abortion procedures [6]. This is interpreted narrowly by the courts, as participation in the abortion meaning 'hands-on' involvement [6]. In addition, in the case of an emergency in relation to a woman's physical or mental health, the right to conscientious objection does not apply [6].

Women seeking abortion should receive evidence-based care provided by well-trained staff who support the woman's right to choose and who will not judge.

8.3 Pre-abortion Assessment

Two key reasons for pre-abortion assessment are to ensure the woman meets the legal requirements of the Abortion Act 1967 and that she is suitable for the type of abortion procedure proposed. However, there is far more involved in providing a holistic and comprehensive service to women seeking abortion, and the role of nurses and midwives in pre-abortion assessment has expanded steadily over recent years meaning they now manage all but those few very specific tasks limited in law to doctors.

- It is important that a woman is seen alone at some point during the pre-abortion assessment. This is to allow the space to make any disclosures (e.g. domestic abuse, female genital mutilation, sexual assault, risk of so-called 'honour'-based violence, trafficking or modern slavery), and to ensure the decision to end the pregnancy is her own and that she is not being coerced.
- Information about the various pregnancy options (parenthood, fostering, adoption, abortion) should be available to the woman should she want them. Most women have already decided that abortion is their preferred option by the pre-abortion assessment, but if she is ambivalent and needs more time or more discussion before she makes her decision, this must be made available to her.
- Full medical and obstetric history and baseline observations should be taken.
- Estimation of gestation should be performed—ultrasound scanning is commonly employed as a method of estimating gestational age [7]. Estimation by last menstrual period (LMP) and/or physical examination may also be used.

- In the case of 'pregnancy of unknown location', clear pathways should be in place to rule out or manage ectopic pregnancy.
- Abortion options available to the woman should be discussed, including respective risks and possible complications, in order that the woman can make an informed choice about her preferred method and provide appropriate consent. In the case of young women aged under 16, an assessment must be made of their capacity to consent to treatment, known as Gillick competence.
- For young women under the age of 18, a safeguarding risk assessment should be carried out to ensure the young person is not at risk of or subject to abuse, including child sexual exploitation, domestic abuse including female genital mutilation and forced marriage, gang violence, so-called 'honour'-based violence and trafficking or modern slavery.
- Information on the various methods of contraception and respective typical use failure rates should be available to women. Access to a preferred method, where possible at the time of the abortion procedure, should be provided. Ovulation can occur as early as 8–10 days post-abortion, so it is important that access to effective contraception for women who want it is made available. It is equally important that where women decline the offer of contraception at the time of abortion, this is respected.
- Women should be offered testing and treatment for sexually transmitted infections, and partner notification should be undertaken where required.
- Prior to any treatment, *two doctors* are required to certify, using the HSA1 form, that they believe 'in good faith' that the woman requesting the abortion meets one of the grounds of the Act, as described previously in this chapter.

8.4 Termination of Pregnancy for Foetal Anomaly

Each year a small but important number of women will end a pregnancy under ground E of the Abortion Act 1967, because of foetal anomaly. These women may have specific needs because it is often, although not always the case, that these are very much wanted pregnancies and the outcome will be felt as a loss rather than a choice [8]. Women and their partners may be in a state of shock or acute emotional distress and may suffer feelings of guilt for the foetal anomaly and for the decision to end the pregnancy [8]. They may also have particular wishes with regard to disposal of the pregnancy remains and mementos.

It is important that these women have access to a choice of abortion procedure. National statistics suggest a disparity in service provision for terminations of pregnancy for foetal anomaly. Seventy-three percentage of abortions for foetal indications (ground E) are performed medically as compared to 65% for all abortions [3]. One reason for this difference may be patient preference, but another explanation may be the limited availability of second-trimester surgical abortion within the National Health Service where most of these terminations are conducted.

8.5   Procedure Preference

Women's preference for type of abortion procedure is dependent upon a number of different factors. Some women may prefer surgical abortion because it is quick, and successful removal of the pregnancy can be confirmed at the time of the procedure, whereas other women may view medical abortion as more 'natural' and would prefer to avoid surgery and anaesthesia. Medical abortion has been shown to be less acceptable to women than surgical, primarily because of the higher level of pain and bleeding with the former [9, 10]. Importantly though, evidence suggests that acceptability of either method is highest when it is the method the woman wants [11].

8.6   Surgical Abortion

In Britain now, there are two primary surgical methods available for abortion. These are vacuum aspiration—either manual or electric—and dilatation and evacuation with the use of forceps (D&E). These methods are largely dependent on the gestational age of the pregnancy, with vacuum aspiration performed to approximately 14 weeks gestation and then D&E procedures performed thereafter to 24 weeks. Where surgical abortion is legal and performed according to modern methods, women can be reassured that it is safe, with major complications and mortality rare across all gestations.

8.6.1   Surgical Abortion in the First Trimester

With the use of a judicious protocol that includes tissue inspection (to confirm removal of the gestational sac), with beta-hCG measurement and prompt referral for evaluation of possible ectopic pregnancy if required, vacuum aspiration can be offered as soon as a pregnancy test is positive [12], with failure rates (continuing pregnancy) between 0.13% and 2.3% [12–14]. Vacuum aspiration is performed using a manual vacuum aspirator or an electric suction machine, with the safety of the two methods being comparable [15]. A cannula is connected to the aspirator, or the electric suction tubing, and is gently inserted through the cervix into the uterus. With the suction action and the gentle manipulation of the cannula inside the uterus, the pregnancy and associated contents of the uterus are drawn through the cannula into the aspirator or suction machine. This procedure is repeated several times until the contents of the uterus are removed, the process taking on average 3–5 min.

The cervix may be primed before vacuum aspiration [16], to soften the cervix and dilate the os allowing the procedure to be undertaken with less need for mechanical dilation, which can be the cause of rare operative complications such as cervical or uterine injury [17]. In the first trimester, the most common agent used for cervical priming is misoprostol. Misoprostol 400 micrograms vaginally 3 hours before surgery, or sublingually 1–2 hours before, has been shown to be effective [17]. There are side effects associated with the administration of misoprostol which include nausea, vomiting, diarrhoea and cramping.

In Britain, first-trimester surgical abortions have commonly been performed using local anaesthetic or general anaesthetic for pain management. It is recommended now though that first-trimester surgical abortion should be provided 'without resort' to general anaesthetic [7, 18], and the use of conscious sedation (a combination of a benzodiazepine and opioid intravenously) for these procedures provides effective pain and anxiety management, and is becoming more commonly used in Britain.

Oral analgesia such as ibuprofen may be given 1–2 hours pre-procedure in the case of local anaesthetic or conscious sedation procedures, followed by local anaesthetic injected intra- or peri-cervically immediately prior to the procedure [19].

In the case of local anaesthetic or conscious sedation, women are likely to experience some abdominal discomfort or pain during the procedure, with cramping particularly as the uterus is emptied and starts to contract. Women should have support and reassurance available during the procedure, employing distraction techniques such as conversation along with an assurance that what they are feeling is to be expected. Procedures under local anaesthesia alone are generally well-tolerated by women who have chosen that option and understand what is involved. They have the advantage of a quick recovery and no restrictions on, for instance driving, afterwards. Procedures with conscious sedation or general anaesthetic have longer recovery times, and the woman should be accompanied from the unit post-treatment and until she has fully recovered from the effects of the sedation or anaesthetic. Clear advice should be provided to women, both verbally and in written form, regarding how to safely and appropriately care for themselves in the post-sedation or general anaesthetic period.

8.6.2   Surgical Abortion in the Second Trimester

Dilatation and evacuation (D&E) is the most commonly performed surgical procedure for abortion in the second trimester, although electric vacuum aspiration can be performed up to 16 weeks gestation. During a D&E procedure, the cervix is dilated sufficiently to allow the passing of forceps into the uterus so that the foetal parts can be carefully removed. Once all of the foetal parts have been removed, vacuum aspiration is used to remove any remaining fluid or tissue.

Pain management for second-trimester surgical abortion procedures can be provided with local anaesthetic, conscious sedation or general anaesthetic. From 18 weeks gestation, it is usual that a general anaesthetic is administered in an operating room setting.

D&E is associated with a low risk of complications and is an acceptable procedure for women [10]. Many women will opt for a surgical abortion in the second trimester in preference to a medical abortion so it is important that both methods are made available [10].

Abortion procedures undertaken in the second trimester will require cervical preparation [7, 20–23]. Pharmacological agents including mifepristone and misoprostol can be used for cervical priming in the second trimester. Mifepristone which must be administered 24 hours prior to the procedure is associated with a more favourable side effect profile than misoprostol.

Alternatively or adjunctively, osmotic dilators are used throughout the second trimester but more commonly from 18 weeks gestation [24]. These dilators are placed directly into the cervical canal 3–24 hours prior to the surgical abortion. Cervical dilators work by absorbing fluid and gently swelling over several hours to dilate the cervix. They also induce the natural release of prostaglandins which leads to cervical softening, making it easier for the operator to insert the forceps through the cervix without causing cervical trauma or uterine injury.

8.6.3 Recovery After Surgical Abortion

During the immediate post-surgical recovery phase, women should have regular post-operative observations undertaken along with assessment of their levels of pain and bleeding. Women generally recover quickly after surgical abortion, and if they have only had a local anaesthetic, they are usually ready to leave the clinic within 30–45 minutes, with aftercare advice. General anaesthetic or conscious sedation increases the recovery time, but after an uncomplicated D&E procedure, a woman will be ready to be discharged 2–3 hours later.

8.7 Medical Abortion

Since the introduction of mifepristone to Britain allowing highly effective medical regimens in the early 1990s, medical abortion has revolutionised abortion care and particularly in the first trimester. In 2017, 65% of abortions in England and Wales were medically induced, almost double the proportion in 2007 [3].

Medical abortion entails the taking of an anti-progestogenic steroid—mifepristone—followed by a prostaglandin analogue, most commonly misoprostol [6]. Mifepristone causes decidual necrosis and softening of the cervix and sensitises the uterus to the action of the prostaglandin, which in turn causes uterine contractions and further softens and dilates the cervix [6]. Use of these abortifacient medications to 70 days gestation is generally termed 'early medical abortion' (EMA), but some medical regimens are effective beyond that gestation, and abortion can be induced medically throughout the course of a pregnancy. The combination of mifepristone and misoprostol is now widely recognised to be the most effective, cost-effective and well-tolerated regimen for EMA [7].

Contraindications

There are not many contraindications to mifepristone-misoprostol, but they include [25–27]:

- Inherited porphyria;
- Chronic adrenal failure;
  Coagulopathy;
- Hypersensitivity to any of the ingredients;
- Known or suspected ectopic pregnancy.

Caution is needed for:

- Long-term use of corticosteroids;
- Conditions that may require steroid therapy for exacerbation, for example, severe or poorly controlled asthma;
- Hepatic or renal failure;
- Malnutrition.

Intrauterine contraception should be removed before medical abortion.

8.7.1 Medical Abortion Regimens

8.7.1.1 Early Medical Abortion (EMA)
The recommended regimen for EMA to ≤70 days' gestation is 200 mg oral mifepristone followed by 800 micrograms of misoprostol 24–48 hours later, vaginally or buccally [7, 28].

Simultaneous administration (misoprostol administered immediately after ingestion of mifepristone) has been shown to be effective, although not as effective as with an interval of 24–48 hours [29]. The simultaneous regimen may be more convenient for women given the legal restrictions in Britain which require women to have both mifepristone and misoprostol administered on licensed premises, potentially resulting in at least two visits to a clinic. The English, Scottish and Welsh authorities have, however, recently permitted home use of misoprostol, thereby facilitating 'single-visit' EMA with the most efficacious EMA regimen. Table 8.2 shows the respective efficacy rates and side effect profiles of simultaneous and interval EMA regimens [29].

Table 8.2 Respective efficacy rates and side effect profiles of simultaneous and interval EMA regimens [29]

	Simultaneous EMA	Interval EMA (24–48 hours)
Possible risks		
Continuing pregnancy	2 in 100	<1 in 100
Retained products of conception requiring further treatment	5 in 100	3 in 100
Surgical procedure required to complete treatment	7 in 100	3 in 100
Side effects		
Nausea	58 in 100	29 in 100
Vomiting	31 in 100	9 in 100
Diarrhoea	35 in 100	5 in 100
Feverishness/chills	69 in 100	15 in 100
Headache	40 in 100	18 in 100
Dizziness	39 in 100	9 in 100

Interval EMA can be extended to 70 days' gestation, with no statistical difference between overall success between 64–70 days and 57–63 days. At 64–70 days' gestation, the continuing pregnancy rate is 3.1% [30].

Most women having EMA in Britain pass the pregnancy at home, which has been shown to be safe, effective and acceptable to women [31].

8.7.1.2 Medical Abortion Beyond 70 Days Gestation

The most evidence-based regimen for medical abortion after 70 days gestation involves 200 mg oral mifepristone, followed 36–48 hours later by hospital/clinic admission and then 800 micrograms of misoprostol vaginally. Four hundred micrograms of misoprostol is then administered vaginally, sublingually or orally every 3 hours, until the pregnancy is expelled.

Around half of women on this regimen can expect to abort within 6 hours [32, 33].

To avoid the risk of a live birth, and the distress that might cause to the woman and those caring for her, feticide by intra-foetal or intra-amniotic injection of a feticidal substance such as potassium chloride or digoxin is recommended from 22 weeks gestation [7].

8.7.1.3 Pain Management

There is little evidence regarding optimal pain management in medical abortion, despite the fact that pain is typical with these procedures, and the severity of the pain increases with gestational age.

In the case of EMA, ibuprofen has been shown to be more effective than paracetamol to manage pain [25], and this may be supplemented by a mild oral opiate.

In the later first and the second trimester, it is common to see the use of a mild oral opiate—or parenteral opioid into the second trimester—alternated with non-steroidal anti-inflammatory drugs [25]. In the second trimester, diclofenac given with the first dose of misoprostol has been shown to reduce the need for parenteral opioids [25].

8.7.1.4 What Women Need to Know

Good advice and information for women undergoing medical abortion is key, particularly in the case of EMA when a woman manages the expulsion of the pregnancy at home.

Women need to know what to expect and be clear about what is abnormal and should alert them to seek medical help.

Pain with EMA is typically described as intense cramping which is most severe for 2–4 hours during expulsion of the pregnancy, after which the pain will generally subside. Most women will experience cramping on and off for about a week after the abortion.

Women should be advised about appropriate use of over-the-counter pain medications and any prescribed pain relief that has been provided.

Bleeding can occur after the administration of mifepristone but is usually light. Approximately 5% of women will abort with mifepristone alone when there is an interval of 24 hours or more between mifepristone and misoprostol.

Most bleeding occurs after misoprostol administration and usually starts within 2–4 hours, although it can be sooner. Bleeding is typically heavier than a period, is likely to include the passing of clots and may increase with advancing gestation.

Bleeding, like a menstrual period, usually continues for 1–2 weeks, and spotting may continue until the next menstrual period. Some women may experience an episode of heavy bleeding 3–5 weeks after the EMA medications and/or have a heavier than normal period with the next cycle. Women can expect their next period within 4 weeks.

Women should be advised that using sanitary towels rather than tampons after the medications may make it easier for them to monitor the level of bleeding.

8.7.1.5 What Women Can Expect to See

As women having EMA will manage the passing of the pregnancy at home, it is important that they are prepared for what they might expect to see.

Up to approximately 7 weeks gestation, the embryo is very small (approximately the size of a peanut) and is unlikely to be seen with the naked eye. Women may see other tissues, including the gestational sac which appears white and fluffy and decidua which looks like brown-red tissue. By 8–10 weeks gestation, women may see the embryo as well as the gestational sac and decidua.

8.8   Disposal of the Pregnancy Remains Post-abortion

It is important that women are given information about how they can manage disposal of the pregnancy remains at home. Some services will agree to dispose of the remains for the woman, if she brings them back to the facility. Some women may wish to flush the remains down the toilet or put them in the bin, and others may wish to bury or burn the remains. Women can also contact a local funeral director if they wish to have the remains formally buried or cremated. There may be a cost associated with this although many funeral services waive the fee.

For surgical abortion and for medical abortion beyond 10 weeks gestation, where women will pass the pregnancy in a medical facility, information about the disposal options available to her should be provided [34]. Those options should include burial, cremation or incineration (burial or cremation only in Scotland). If a woman declines information, or to be involved in decision-making around disposal of the pregnancy remains, that should be respected. Regardless, it should be documented in the medical record that information has been offered and/or provided and what the woman's choice is with regard to disposal, including if she wishes not to be involved in making a decision at all.

Women can take the pregnancy remains away with them for disposal. Clear information and advice on how to appropriately dispose of the remains should be provided.

8.9   Follow-Up After Abortion

Routine follow-up is unnecessary after an uncomplicated surgical abortion at any gestation and where successful medical abortion can be confirmed before a woman leaves the medical facility.

In the case of EMA, most women will manage the abortion at home, and as there is a risk, albeit small, of failure, it is important that successful abortion is confirmed and there is no continuing pregnancy. This can be managed in person or remotely, for example, via a process of self-assessment with the use of a low-sensitivity pregnancy test.

Regardless of procedure type, written information and access to a 24 hour advice service are essential, both for those women seeking reassurance that what they are experiencing as they pass the pregnancy at home during early medical abortion is 'normal' and for those few women who do experience immediate or delayed complications such as excessive bleeding and/or pain or infection. Although not routinely necessary, in-person follow-up should be available to any woman who has concerns post-abortion.

8.10   Advice Post-abortion

Expected pain and bleeding have been covered elsewhere in this chapter.

Excessive bleeding is characterised by soaking two or more maxi-style sanitary towels per hour, for 2 consecutive hours, and this should alert the woman to seek immediate medical advice or to attend A&E.

Women should use over-the-counter medications (ibuprofen or paracetamol) or prescribed pain relief as directed. If the pain cannot be controlled with the correct use of these medications, or the pain persists beyond occasional cramping for a week post-procedure, then medical advice should be sought

Abdominal tenderness, offensive vaginal discharge and/or fever may be suggestive of infection, and the woman should seek urgent medical advice.

Symptoms of nausea, vomiting and fatigue usually stop within 3 days of an abortion procedure, with breast tenderness taking up to 10 days to resolve. In the case of leakage of breast milk after an abortion, the breasts should return to normal after 3–4 days of swelling. Wearing a supportive bra, careful application of cold ice packs to the breasts and appropriate use of ibuprofen or paracetamol may be helpful in managing the discomfort.

8.11   Complications Post-abortion

Where abortion is legal, provided in appropriate environments and according to modern methods, it is safe, and serious complications are rare.

Those complications associated with abortion include continuing pregnancy (failed abortion), incomplete abortion (retained tissue or retained products of conception), infection, haemorrhage and uterine or cervical injury [25].

In the case of first-trimester vacuum aspiration, fewer than one case per 1000 will require hospitalisation [35]. D&E has similar rates of complications; however the risk of a major complication, although it remains small, increases with gestational age [25].

Clinically significant adverse events related to early medical abortion are rare at 1.6 per 1000 cases [36]. In the case of late first- and second-trimester medical abortion, the rate of complications is higher than with surgical abortion, primarily as a result of retained placental tissue and resultant heavy bleeding [10].

Incomplete abortion—often referred to as retained products of conception—is one of the most common complications of both medical and surgical abortion. Women will often present to non-specialist abortion healthcare settings with symptoms suggestive of retained products of conception: prolonged uterine bleeding which may be continuous or intermittent and which is often accompanied by uterine cramping.

Ultrasound is often used in the diagnosis of retained products of conception, but it should be remembered that its main uses post-abortion are to determine whether the gestational sac has been expelled, identify whether a pregnancy is continuing and support a clinical diagnosis of retained products of conception. Several studies have shown that there is no absolute cut-off of endometrial thickness that predicts the need for surgical intervention where the gestational sac has been successfully expelled or removed [37–39]. Thus, while ultrasound can *support* a diagnosis of retained products of conception, the diagnosis should be based primarily on clinical signs and symptoms.

Retained products of conception may be managed surgically, with re-aspiration, or medically with the use of misoprostol. Depending upon the signs and symptoms, if mild, women may choose conservative management as they may expel any remaining tissue with their next menstrual period.

In the case of suspected infected retained products of conception, or where bleeding is excessive or prolonged, an urgent surgical evacuation should be arranged.

Antibiotic prophylaxis is standard for both surgical and medical abortions, but a small proportion of women may present to non-specialist abortion settings with infection post-abortion, most likely a result of a pre-existing infection [7]. Depending upon the severity of the infection, further oral, or in some cases, intravenous antibiotics will be required.

8.12   Psychological Effects of Abortion

It has long been a popular strategy of the anti-choice lobby to peddle misinformation about alleged psychological damage caused to women's health by abortion.

In fact the evidence rejects the notion that abortion increases women's risk of experiencing adverse psychological outcomes [40–42]. The recent Turnaway Study, a 5-year longitudinal cohort study which looked at women's psychological health over 5 years after receiving or being denied an abortion, found that women who had an abortion demonstrated more positive outcomes initially compared with women who were denied [43]. Psychological well-being improved over time such that both groups of women eventually converged, refuting the notion that abortion harms women's mental health [43].

Relief, guilt, sadness, anger and regret are the usual range of emotional responses for women post-abortion [44]. Women most commonly expect to feel relieved and confident post-abortion—63% and 52%, respectively—but 3% of women expect they will struggle to cope [45]. Pre-existing history of adverse mental health is the most reliable predictor of post-abortion adverse mental health issues for those few women who will experience them [7]. It is important therefore that pre- and post-abortion support and counselling are available for those women who want it [7].

8.13 Long-Term Sequelae

Regardless of whether an abortion is performed medically or surgically, there are no proven associations with breast cancer, miscarriage, infertility, ectopic pregnancy or placenta previa [7]. An association but not a causal link has been reported between surgical abortion and subsequent preterm delivery [46].

References

1. Sedgh G, Bearak J, Singh S et al (2016) Abortion incidence between 1990 and 2014: global, regional, and subregional levels and trends. Lancet 388(10041):258–267
2. Bankole A, Singh S, Haas T (1998) Reasons why women have induced abortions: evidence from 27 countries. Int Fam Plann Perspect 24:117–127
3. Department of Health and Social Care (2018) Abortion statistics, England and Wales: 2017. Crown Copyright, London
4. Information Services Division. NHS, National Services Scotland (2018) National statistics. Termination of pregnancy statistics; year ending December 2017. NHS, Newport
5. Sheldon S, Fletcher J (2017) Vacuum aspiration for induced abortion could be safely and legally performed by nurses and midwives. J Fam Plann Reprod Health Care 43(4):260–264
6. Royal College of Nursing (2017) Termination of pregnancy: an RCN nursing framework. Royal College of Nursing, London
7. Royal College of Obstetricians and Gynaecologists (2011) The care of women requesting induced abortion. Evidence-based guideline no. 7, RCOG Press, London
8. Bourguignon A, Briscoe B, Nemzer L (1999) Genetic abortion: considerations for patient care. J Perinat Neonatal Nurs 13:47–58
9. Say L, Kulier R, GUlmezoglu M, Campana A (2005) Medical versus surgical methods for first trimester termination of pregnancy. Cochrane Database Syst Rev 1:CD003037
10. Lohr PA, Hayes JL, Gemzell-Danielsson K (2008) Surgical versus medical methods for second trimester induced abortion. Cochrane Database Syst Rev 1:CD006714
11. Henshaw RC, Naji SA, Russell IT, Templeton AA (1993) Comparison of medical abortion with surgical vacuum aspiration: women's preferences and acceptability of treatment. BMJ 307:714–717

12. Lichtenberg ES, Paul M, Society of Family Planning (2013) Surgical abortion prior to 7 weeks of gestation. Contraception 88:7–17
13. Edwards J, Carson SA (1997) New technologies permit safe abortion at less than six weeks' gestation and provide timely detection of ectopic gestation. Am J Obstet Gynecol 176:1101–1106
14. Paul ME, Mitchell CM, Rogers AJ et al (2002) Early surgical abortion: efficacy and safety. Am J Obstet Gynecol 187:407–411
15. Wen J, Cai QY, Deng F, Li YP (2008) Manual versus electric vacuum aspiration for first-trimester abortion: a systematic review. BJOG 115:5–13
16. Meirik O, Nguyen TNN, Piaggio G et al (2012) Cervical preparation with misoprostol before first trimester induced vacuum aspiration abortion reduces complications: a multicentre randomized clinical trial. Lancet 379:1817–1824
17. Sääv I, Kopp Kallner H, Fiala C et al (2015) Sublingual versus vaginal misoprostol for cervical dilatation 1 or 3 h prior to surgical abortion: a double-blinded RCT. Hum Reprod 30:1314–1322
18. World Health Organisation (2014) Clinical practice handbook for Safe abortion. WHO, Geneva. ISBN 978 92 4 154871 7 (NLM classification: WQ 440
19. Renner RM, Nichols MD, Jensen JT et al (2012) Paracervical block for pain control in first-trimester surgical abortion: a randomized controlled trial. Obstet Gynecol 119:1030–1037
20. Newmann SJ, Dalve-Endres A, Diedrich JT et al (2010) Cervical preparation for second trimester dilation and evacuation. Cochrane Database Syst Rev 8:CD007310
21. Fox MC, Krajewski CM (2014) Cervical preparation for second-trimester surgical abortion prior to 20 weeks' gestation: SFP guideline #2013–4. Contraception 89:75–84
22. Newmann S, Dalve-Endres A, Drey EA, Society of Family Planning (2008) Clinical guidelines. Cervical preparation for surgical abortion from 20 to 24 weeks' gestation. Contraception 77:308–314
23. WHO (2012) Safe abortion: technical and policy guidance for health systems, 2nd edn. WHO, Geneva
24. Hern WM (1994) Laminaria versus dilapan osmotic cervical dilators for outpatient dilation and evacuation abortion: randomized cohort comparison of 1001 patients. AJOG 171:1324–1328
25. Lohr PA, Fjerstad M, DeSilva U, Lyus R (2014) BMJ clinical review: abortion. BMJ 348:f7553
26. EMC. SmPC Mifegyne. https://www.medicines.org.uk/emc/product/3783/smpc. Accessed 4 Aug 2018
27. EMC. SmPC Cytotec. https://www.medicines.org.uk/emc/product/1642/smpc. Accessed 4 Aug 2018
28. Wedisinghe L, Elsandabesee D (2010) Flexible mifepristone and misoprostol administration interval for first-trimester medical termination. Contraception 81:269–274
29. Lohr PA, Starling JE, Scott JG, Aiken ARA (2018) Simultaneous compared with interval medical abortion regimens where home use is restricted. Obstet Gynecol 131(4):635–641
30. Abbas D, Chong E, Raymond EG (2015) Outpatient medical abortion is safe and effective through 70 days gestation. Contraception 92:197–199
31. Ngo TD, Park MH, Shakur H, Free C (2011) Comparative effectiveness, safety and acceptability of medical abortion at home and in a clinic: a systematic review. Bull WHO 89:360–370
32. Hamoda H, Ashok PW, Flett GM, Templeton A (2005) Uptake and efficacy of medical abortion over 9 weeks and up to 13 weeks gestation: a review of 1076 consecutive cases. Contraception 71:327–332
33. Ashok PW, Templeton A, Wagaarachchi PT et al (2004) Midtrimester medical termination of pregnancy: a review of 1002 consecutive cases. Contraception 69:51–58
34. Human Tissue Authority (2015) Guidance on the disposal of pregnancy remains following pregnancy loss or termination. Human Tissue Authority, London
35. Hakim-Elahi E, Tovell HM, Burnhill MS (1990) Complications of first-trimester abortion: a report of 170,000 cases. Obstet Gynecol 76:129–135
36. Cleland K, Creinin MD, Nucatola D, Nshom M, Trussell J (2013) Significant adverse events and outcomes after medical abortion. Obstet Gynecol 121(1):166–171

37. Creinin MD, Harwood B, Guido RS, et al., NICHD Management of Early Pregnancy Failure Trial (2004) Endometrial thickness after misoprostol use for early pregnancy failure. Int J Obstet Gynecol 86:22–26
38. Cowett AA, Cohen LS, Lichtenberg ES et al (2004) Ultrasound evaluation of the endometrium after medical termination of pregnancy. Obstet Gynecol 103:871–875
39. Markovitch O, Tepper R, Klein Z et al (2006) Sonographic appearance of the uterine cavity following administration of mifepristone and misoprostol for termination of pregnancy. J Clin Ultrasond 34:278–282
40. Major B, Appelbaum M, Beckman L, Dutton MA, Russo NF, West C (2009) Abortion and mental health: evaluating the evidence. Am Psychol 64(9):863–890
41. Charles VE, Polis CB, Sridhara SK, Blum RW (2008) Abortion and long-term mental health outcomes: a systematic review of the evidence. Contraception 78(6):436–450
42. National Collaborating Centre for Mental Health at the Royal College of Psychiatrists. Induced Abortion and Mental Health (2011) A systematic review of the mental health outcomes of induced abortion, including their prevalence and associated factors. Royal College of Psychiatrists, London
43. Biggs MA, Upadhyay UD, McCulloch CE, Foster DG (2017) Women's mental health and well-being 5 years after receiving or being denied an abortion. A prospective, longitudinal cohort study. JAMA Psychiat 74(2):169–178
44. Astbury-Ward E (2008) Emotional and psychological impact of abortion: a critique of the literature. J Fam Plann Reprod Health Care 34:181–184
45. Foster DG, Gould H, Kimport K (2012) How women anticipate coping after an abortion. Contraception 86:84–90
46. Shah P, Zao J, On Behalf of Knowledge Synthesis Group of Determinants of Preterm/LBW Births (2009) Induced termination of pregnancy and low birthweight and preterm birth: a systematic review and meta-analyses. BJOG 116:1425–1442

.

Effects of Cancer Treatments

9

Marie Smith, Lorna Lightbody, Ali Allen,
and Michelle Winser

9.1   Role of the CNS in Gynaecological Oncology

The clinical nurse specialist (CNS) uses their expert skills and knowledge in cancer care to support the patient and their relatives throughout their pathway. For women who are diagnosed with a gynaecological cancer, the journey is often complex and involves multiple interventions across the gynaecological multidisciplinary team. All patients will be allocated a CNS at diagnosis who will act as the patient's key worker by providing emotional and practical advice and support, reinforce information and offer written information about the cancer and treatment. The CNS will navigate the patient through their treatment pathway, offering advice and support with financial worries and psychological issues, and will provide advice and support around side effects of the various treatments [1]. At diagnosis the CNS will assess the patient's physical, practical, psychological, emotional, spiritual and social needs by asking the patient to complete a questionnaire that will highlight the patient's most important concerns and allows the CNS to develop a care and support plan around these concerns—this is called a holistic needs assessment [2].

The CNS will act as a patient advocate, communicate between the patient and different teams and increase efficiency in the patient's pathway. They attend the weekly multidisciplinary meetings and are available in clinics and offer support via telephone. The CNS offers an end-of-treatment consultation for patients once they have completed treatment; this is to educate patients on signs and symptoms of recurrence and to direct patients and relatives to various health and well-being events to support patients with survivorship and living with and beyond cancer [2]. The CNS is the point of contact for patients on surveillance and is able to assess signs and symptoms of recurrence and act on this accordingly.

M. Smith (✉) · L. Lightbody · A. Allen · M. Winser
CNS Gynaecology Oncology, Guys and St. Thomas NHS Foundation Trust, London, UK
e-mail: Marie.smith@gstt.nhs.uk

© Springer Nature Switzerland AG 2019
D. Holloway (ed.), *Nursing Management of Women's Health*,
https://doi.org/10.1007/978-3-030-16115-6_9

9.1.1 Post-operative Care in Gynaecological Oncology

Treatment for gynaecological cancers varies depending on the stage and grade of the cancer and the individual's preference. Surgery is often the first-line treatment for earlier stages of gynaecological cancer and can also be performed after chemotherapy.

Hysterectomy is the main surgical treatment for the most common gynaecological cancers, in particular endometrial cancer, ovarian cancer and cervical cancer.

There are different types of hysterectomy; these include subtotal hysterectomy (removal of the womb only), total hysterectomy (removal of the womb and cervix), total abdominal hysterectomy and bilateral salpingo-oophorectomy (TAH/BSO, removal of the womb, cervix and ovaries). Most women that have been diagnosed with a gynaecological cancer will have a TAH/BSO and will often proceed to the removal of the omentum, lymph nodes, para-aortic nodes and any visible disease; this can also be known as debulking surgery or interval debulking surgery if following chemotherapy. Occasionally if there is disease around the bowel, the patient may require a bowel resection which would result in a temporary formation of a stoma or in very few cases the stoma may be permanent. These surgeries are often performed using a midline incision, and the recovery time is usually 6–8 weeks, with approximately 5 days spent in hospital post-operatively for a laparotomy and providing there are no post-operative complications. Many types of hysterectomy can now also be performed laparoscopically (by keyhole surgery) or by robotic surgery. This depends on the primary site of the tumour and the stage of the disease, as well as the consultant's expertise and equipment available. Laparoscopic surgery is frequently performed for women with a higher body mass index (BMI), depending on the stage of the cancer, as it can reduce the risk for post-operative complications, for a patient with an already higher risk. Recovery time for a laparoscopic surgery is usually 4–6 weeks, with approximately 1–2 days spent in hospital post-operatively [3].

Patients with cervical cancer can also be offered a trachelectomy if they have an early stage disease and wish fertility sparing surgery. This involves removal only of the cervix and upper part of the vagina but keeps the body of the uterus intact. This can be performed vaginally or abdominally. Patients with vulval cancer will often undergo a vulvectomy and sampling of inguinal lymph nodes. Regardless of the surgery performed for a gynaecological malignancy, the post-operative care remains largely similar, especially in the immediate post-operative period [3].

The patient will return to the gynaecology ward on the day of surgery, usually after spending 1–2 h in recovery, providing their pain is well controlled and they are clinically stable. Patients with multiple comorbidities and high risk for post-operative complications may spend a night in overnight intensive recovery; this is a provision that would be assessed and organised preoperatively by the consultant surgeons and anaesthetic team. Patients will usually return to the ward with opioid-based analgesia via either an epidural or PCA (patient-controlled analgesia) [4]. A PCA is analgesia delivered intravenously via a pump with a button that the patient controls, usually either morphine or fentanyl delivered as required. The pump has a lock-out period, so the dose of the drug is administered within a safe time frame. The aim of the lock-out period is to prevent opioid toxicity and to ensure the patient is having adequate analgesia. For the duration that the epidural or PCA remains in situ, the patient will require oxygen therapy, as opioids can cause respiratory depression [5]. There will also be an indwelling catheter in situ that will remain until the patient is able to safely mobilise to the bathroom. Intravenous fluids will be running until the patient is able to drink, and the patient may also have an abdominal drain. Occasionally the patient may return with a nasogastric Ryles tube to give the bowel some rest following the surgery. Patients will often be allowed water only by mouth until gut motility returns to lower the risk of bowel ileus.

On the day of surgery, the patient will require hourly observations and monitoring of urine and drain output for the first 24 h following surgery; this can then be reduced to 4 hourly observations, providing the patient is stable. It is imperative in this period that the patient is closely monitored for signs of any post-operative complications. Post-operative complications can include internal post-operative bleeding, dehydration, fluid overload, hematoma, opioid toxicity and related issues such as respiratory distress, pulmonary embolism or deep vein thrombosis, nausea and vomiting, pain, bowel obstruction, sepsis, wound infection and urinary tract infection. As a part of monitoring vital signs, the nursing team will be observing the patient for pyrexia and tachycardia, which may be an indication of internal bleeding, dehydration or infection. Patients will be given prophylactic antibiotics at the time of the surgery, and this may continue for 1–2 days post-operatively also to reduce the risk for the patient. The nursing team will also be monitoring for a blood pressure reading that is outside of normal parameters for the individual patient. The patient will have a baseline set of vital signs at their preoperative assessment for the team to measure against. Altered blood pressure is also an indication of internal bleeding, dehydration and infection. The nursing team must be mindful of other reasons a patient may experience tachycardia or an abnormal blood pressure reading for other reasons such as pain, emotional distress or as a side effect from having an epidural. Urine and drain output should be monitored hourly, and the nurse should be ensuring the patient is passing adequate volumes of urine by using the calculation 0.5 ml/kg/h. A low urine output or high volumes of blood or serous fluid in the drain should be escalated to the medical team for urgent review. Low urine output may indicate signs of dehydration or clinical deterioration, and a high output from the drain may be an indication of a post-operative internal bleed. The wound should also be monitored to ensure there is no bleeding from the incision site, in some cases a pressure dressing may be required to be applied. If a patient experiences respiratory distress due to opioid toxicity, the nursing team would assess the patient and administer naloxone to reverse the opioid effect and then ensure the patient is followed up by their medical team. It is important for the nurse to consider when reversing the effects of opioids that this in turn can increase the patient's pain. The medical team and specialist pain team need to be involved if this occurs. As part of monitoring vital signs, the nursing team will also observe the patients' oxygen saturation levels. Patients can desaturate post-operatively for a multitude of reasons including their position in the bed, respiratory tract infection, hospital-acquired pneumonia, pleural effusion or pulmonary embolism. As with any other abnormal vital sign reading that is of concern in the post-operative period, the nurse will need to increase the frequency of monitoring vital signs and have the patient reviewed by their medical team. It is important to monitor that pain and nausea are well controlled, and some patients may find they suffer with pruritus secondary to the opioids. The anaesthetic team will review the patient before they leave the recovery room to ensure they have adequate analgesia and other necessary medications are prescribed before they return to ward-based care [6].

The enhanced recovery programme is used nationally throughout the United Kingdom for many surgical patients, not just in oncology surgery [7]. The research has shown early mobilisation, and eating and drinking can reduce the risk of post-operative complications. The surgical team will advise when it is safe for a patient to begin drinking oral fluids and when it is safe to commence a light diet; this will be dependent on the extent of the surgery and the patient's recovery post-operatively. The day following the surgery, providing the patient is clinically stable, the patient should mobilise to the chair at the bedside. By optimising and encouraging early mobilisation, this can help to begin to move any secretions on the chest following intubation, preventing chest infection and allowing the patient to maximise the intake of oxygen into the lungs. Deep breathing exercises should also be encouraged and supported by the physiotherapy team. Mobilisation will also encourage the patient's bowels to be less sluggish. It is important for the patient to open their bowels following surgery; this can often take a couple of days. Some patients may develop a post-operative bowel obstruction, which can be known as an ileus. This causes the patient to continually vomit large volumes of dark green fluid. All patients will be seen by the medical team following their surgery and be examined and have their bowels listened to abdominally using a stethoscope. The medical team will also ensure that all patients are taking regular laxatives to encourage gut motility and monitor the patient's bowel movements post-operatively.

Following the recovery period on the ward, the patient will be discharged home with analgesia, laxatives and low molecular weight heparin injections to reduce the risk of developing a thrombosis. The patient will be given wound advice and have district nurses arranged if required. The patient will be given information on what to do and who to contact if they have concerns [7]. The patient will usually be followed up in the outpatient clinic 2 weeks post-operatively for a wound check and the final histology results from the surgery.

In conclusion, surgeries for gynaecological cancers vary, are complex and can carry significant risks for the patient. Therefore, it is vital that the nursing and medical team work together to closely monitor the patient in the post-operative period to reduce the risk of developing a significant complication.

9.2   Post-radiotherapy Symptoms in Gynaecological Cancers

Of the 19,500 women diagnosed with a gynaecological cancer each year in the United Kingdom, it is estimated that approximately 19% of these will receive pelvic radiotherapy, in an adjuvant or neoadjuvant setting [8]. Sixty-seven percentage of these women will survive more than 5 years following treatment [8]. Indications show that over 50% of these women will experience long-term effects following their treatment [9]. Therefore, it is pertinent nurses understand how to support women and their side effects.

9.2.1 External Beam Radiotherapy

Radiotherapy is high-energy X-rays which destroy the cancer cells whilst minimising damage to the surrounding normal cells [10].

Within gynaecological cancer treatment, the radiotherapy treatment can be external or internal or a combination of the two.

External beam radiotherapy (EBRT) is short daily treatments from Monday to Friday with a rest at the weekends. This is normally for a period of 5 weeks.

Radiotherapy is also given to palliate symptoms in advanced cancer. This may reduce the cancer to help control symptoms such as bleeding and improve quality of life [8].

9.2.2 Brachytherapy

Internal radiotherapy, also known as brachytherapy, provides high-dose radiation directly to the tumour or area being treated but only a low dose to the surrounding tissues [11]. This helps to minimise the side effects to the surrounding organs.

A radioactive source is inserted close to the area being treated such as the cervix or womb through the vagina as a targeted treatment [11]. The position of these rods is into the uterus via the cervix with the applicators going into the fornix of the vagina. This is given as a few separate treatments. The treatment delivers the radiation through tubes called applicators placed in the vagina/womb.

9.2.3 Cancer of the Cervix

Radiotherapy for cancer of the cervix can be EBRT, brachytherapy or a combination of the two [11]. It is the main treatment used for larger tumours that are not curable with surgery alone [11]. It is also used after surgery if there is a high risk of the cancer returning [11]. Depending on the stage of the tumour, concurrent weekly chemotherapy 1 day/week is also given. Chemotherapy helps the radiotherapy to be more effective [8]. This may then also followed by brachytherapy.

9.2.4 Cancer of the Endometrium

Radiotherapy may be given to women with womb cancer after surgery (adjuvant) to reduce the chances of the cancer coming back or to relieve symptoms in advanced womb cancers [8]. This is EBRT or brachytherapy or a combination of the two. Women with earlier stage disease are regularly followed up to observe for signs and symptoms [10].

9.2.5 Cancer of the Vulva

Radiotherapy is given to reduce the size of the vulval tumour [8]. Chemotherapy may also be given; this is called chemoradiation [8]. Radiotherapy is given following surgery if the cancer isn't completely removed or if the lymph nodes are positive. It is also used in recurrent vulval cancer [9]. In advanced vulval cancer, radiotherapy is used to palliate symptoms such as bleeding [8].

9.2.6 Vaginal Cancer

Vaginal cancer is rare. Sometimes, cancers which start in the cervix or womb spread to the vagina [8]. Women may have EBRT or brachytherapy or a combination. They will also have chemotherapy. Brachytherapy is dependent on the tumour [8].

9.2.7 Side Effects During Radiotherapy

It is important nurses support women through their treatment and help them understand the side effects of radiotherapy. Side effects may occur during treatment or later, after treatment finishes. These are called late effects [8].

Nurses, alongside the oncologists, provide information and educate women before their treatment to ensure they are fully informed. Women should know where to go for support and have contact details of their specialist nurse.

Initially, side effects may start a week or two into the treatment. Women may not experience all the side effects. Their experience may depend on the type of cancer they have, whether they have had surgery or how they react to their treatment. Psychological side effects must be explored with these women as loss of fertility and sexual function may be affected [8].

9.2.8 Fatigue

Radiotherapy can make women feel tired. This may continue after the treatment has been completed and last a few months. Energy levels improve gradually, but this may vary from patient to patient [11].

Nurses can support women by discussing ways on how to manage their fatigue. Helpful tips are:

Managing work-reducing hours, sick leave and phased return to work.

- Pace themselves, listen to their bodies and don't overdo things.
- Take regular breaks.
- Plan regular physical activity like short walks.
- Ask family/friends to help with children/pets/housework.
- Referrals to local cancer support groups and networks.

9.2.9   Effects on the Skin

Radiotherapy can cause skin reactions to the area being treated. The area may look red, sore and become dry and flaky [10].

Radiographers will perform regular skin checks. If a woman complains about her skin, the radiographer must be informed as they will advise creams or dressings. Sometimes, analgesia is also advised [10].

Skin reactions can be worse up to 2 weeks after treatment has been completed before they improve [8]. Women should be advised this may happen.

Women receiving pelvic radiotherapy may find the hair around the genital area fall out or become thinner. This may be temporary or permanent. To encourage healthy skin, good advice is to bath rather than shower; pat area with clean, dry towel; wear loose clothing; do not shave or wax; and avoid the sun [10].

9.2.10   Bladder Side Effects

Pelvic radiotherapy causes irritation and inflammation to the lining of the bladder. Symptoms include frequency, nocturia, cystitis, urgency, haematuria and incontinence. Avoid alcohol and caffeine as these can exacerbate symptoms. Encourage women to drink at least 2–3 l of fluids per day as this reduces the irritability of the bladder [8]. Refer to the oncology dietician. Doctors may prescribe medications to alleviate symptoms.

9.2.11   Bowel Side Effects

Bowels can be affected by pelvic radiotherapy treatment. These symptoms can include:

- Loose stools, diarrhoea or constipation.
- Feeling to open bowels urgently.
- Crampy, abdominal pain.
- Flatulence.

These symptoms are less common but important to be aware of:

- Tenesmus.
- Passing mucous or blood on passing stool.
- Some bowel incontinence.

Loperamide is often prescribed to alleviate symptoms. Referral to the oncology dietician is useful. Drinking 2–3 l of fluid is advisable to replace lost fluids through diarrhoea [8]. A card called the 'just can't wait' toilet card from Macmillan is helpful as this enables access to toilets in public places without embarrassment.

9.2.12 Vaginal Effects

Radiotherapy to the pelvis can cause the vagina to become narrower, less stretchy and dry [8]. This can make sex and examinations uncomfortable for women. Vaginal dilators help prevent the vagina from narrowing. It is advised that dilators are used 5–10 min, three times per week to prevent vaginal stenosis and adhesions (3). Specialist nurses and radiographers will show women how to use them. A vibrator or regular sex has the same effect. Vaginal dryness can make sex uncomfortable. Nurses can support women by advising vaginal lubricants and creams that may help. Oestrogen creams can help in certain patients, although should be avoided by women with womb cancer [8]. Sometimes referral to a psychosexual counsellor is helpful (see Chap. 10).

9.2.13 Early Menopause

When women receive pelvic radiotherapy, it stops the ovaries from producing the hormones oestrogen and progesterone [8]. This in turn brings on the menopause. When early menopause is brought on by the effects of radiotherapy or surgery, the symptoms can be more noticeable than a natural menopause (see Chap. 10) [8]. Symptoms may include:

- Hot flushes and sweats.
- Vaginal dryness.
- Passing urine more often.
- Lower sex drive.
- Aches and pains.
- Mood swings and poor concentration.

Some symptoms can be treated with HRT [8]. Referral to a specialist menopause clinic can help for assessment of symptoms. Psychosexual counselling is helpful for women to discuss their feelings, and signposting to support groups and charities for peer support is beneficial.

9.2.14 Loss of Fertility

In younger women, pelvic radiotherapy can mean a loss of fertility [9]. The effects of menopause and psychological aspects of loss of fertility can be traumatic for young women. This should be discussed before treatment starts [9]. In some circumstances women can be referred to an infertility specialist to discuss options of storing eggs or embryos for surrogacy later on [8]. This is very distressing, and ensuring the women and their families are getting the right support is vital. The role of the nurse is pertinent to ensure the right support is available. Referrals to either a specialist counsellor or therapist should be offered (see Chap. 6).

9.2.15 Late Effects of Radiotherapy

For most women, side effects from radiotherapy will disappear a few weeks after treatment finishes. However, some side effects persist. Late effects are side effects that don't go away within 6 months or new side effect that develops months or years later as a response to treatment. The risk of developing late effects depends on the type of cancer, the dose of radiotherapy and any other treatments such as surgery [10].

Some late effects will disappear over time, but women may need support to help manage them [8]. The most common late effects following pelvic radiotherapy are changes to the function of the bladder and bowel [8].

Changes to the bowel habits may include:

- Loose bowel movements.
- Urgency.
- Constipation.

Sometimes medication is needed to control these symptoms. An assessment by an oncology dietician is helpful. Occasionally, the oncologist may refer the patient to a gastroenterologist if symptoms are severe [8].

Bladder effects are common following radiotherapy as the bladder can shrink after treatment [8]. Women find they need to pass urine more often or are incontinent. If women are experiencing these symptoms, encouraging pelvic floor exercises is a good place to start. Discuss fluid intake, and avoiding caffeine is also helpful [8]. A referral to uro-gynae CNS may be beneficial for assessment.

Women may experience vaginal bleeding months after treatment has been completed. Following radiotherapy, fine blood vessels may develop in the vagina, lining of the bladder or bowel. This may cause some vaginal bleeding, haematuria or on bowel motions [10]. It is important to reassure women but also ask the oncologist to examine them as on rare occasions it can be due to other reasons.

Lymphoedema occurs in some women. This is a swelling in one or both of the legs [8]. It is more common in women who have had their pelvic lymph nodes removed during surgery [10]. These women must be referred to a lymphoedema specialist team. Refer to Sect. 9.3 for information.

As previously discussed, changes to the vagina can make sex difficult and uncomfortable. This can be an ongoing problem for some women psychologically and physically long after treatment is finished. Refer to sexual function and body image chapter.

9.3   Lymphoedema in Women with Gynaecological Cancers

9.3.1   Introduction

Women with gynaecological cancers can have a risk of getting lymphoedema, so too can those who have treatments for these cancers. It cannot be cured, but if it is diagnosed early, it can be managed effectively [12].

9.3.2   What Is Lymphoedema?

Everyone has small amounts of fluid called lymph in their body tissues, most of this fluid is collected by an arrangement of drainage tubes or channels called the lymphatic system, and it runs alongside the blood vessels.

Lymphoedema is swelling which occurs when there is a build-up of lymph in the limbs due to the lymph not draining out properly. The swelling can accumulate at the end of the evening and go down overnight. If the swelling is not treated appropriately and timely, it can become fixed in the limbs permanently. It is a chronic condition; it can occur in any part of the body and can result in tightness or heaviness of the tissues or limb [13].

9.3.3   Causes

There are benign conditions that can cause lymphoedema; here we are more interested in the type caused by cancer or its treatment. Large gynaecological cancers, such as large tumours in the ovaries or pelvis, can put pressure on the legs and cause swelling. Advanced cancers of the vulva especially ones which has spread to the groin lymph nodes can cause lymphoedema. Treatment in the shape of surgery, radiotherapy or chemotherapy may reduce these tumours and take some of the pressure from the lower limbs and improve the lymphoedema [12].

Lymphoedema can also be caused by certain treatment interventions:

9.3.3.1 Surgery

Removal of lymph nodes during cancer surgery can lead to swelling or lymphoedema in the future. Surgery for endometrial and ovarian cancer often removes some of the pelvic and para-aortic lymph nodes. The risk of lymphoedema occurring from this surgery is thought to be between 5% and 10% [14].

Surgery for cancer of the vulva often involves removal of either unilateral or bilateral groin lymph nodes (though less radical procedures such as sentinel node biopsies are being used when suitable). This surgery increases the risk of getting lower limb lymphoedema; the risk is thought to increase to 20% or more [14].

Though there will be swelling initially after the surgery, this should go once mobility is increased and healing has occurred. It is only called lymphoedema if it occurs again in the future and does not go.

9.3.3.2 Radiotherapy

Women with cancer of the cervix (stage 1B2/2 or more) may have radiotherapy as their radical treatment, often given with chemotherapy. This involves 25 fractions of radiotherapy over a 5-week period. In the long term, this can compromise the lymphatic system in the pelvis. Other women with cervical cancer will have had surgery as their primary treatment but then require radiotherapy as an adjuvant treatment when the stage turns out to be greater than originally thought.

Some women with cancer of the vulva may also require radiotherapy as an adjuvant treatment (after surgery) if they were spread to lymph nodes or small margins free of the disease. Women with endometrial cancer may require radiotherapy (following surgery) if their disease is staged as 1B or more. Though both surgery and radiotherapy can lead a person to have lymphoedema, having more than one treatment (which can happen) can increase the risk.

9.3.4   Measures to Try and Prevent Lymphoedema Occurring in the First Instance

- Women should wear flight socks if going on long-haul flights, drink water and move their legs.
- Keep limbs/skin clean and moisturised.
- Check for abrasions or cuts and keep cuts clean; if there is risk of infection, it is wise to seek advice.
- Avoid having injections into the limbs closest to the surgical interventions or where the radiotherapy was administered.
- Report signs of infection; if cellulitis, people should see their surgeon/oncologist/general practitioner.
- Avoid shaving or waxing limbs that have a risk of lymphoedema; use creams to remove hair.
- Keep toenails short to avoid problems with the feet (cuts) [15].

9.3.5   Should Lymphoedema Occur

9.3.5.1 Treatments for Lymphoedema
This is made up of a combination of elevation, compression bandages or stockings, deep tissue massage, skin care and external pneumatic compression (EPC).

9.3.5.2 Elevation
Whenever the leg/legs are raised, fluid will drain better; it is good to elevate them as high as possible. Elevate the foot of the bed so that the legs are higher than the head [12].

9.3.5.3 Compression Bandages/Stockings
At the beginning compression bandages may be necessary to help squeeze the worst of the fluid out of the affected limbs. Once the fluid is better controlled, stockings can be worn instead of the bandages. Compression can help, particularly when one is standing. The stockings need to be specially fitted and ordered, the usual strength is a 'class II', but sometimes a stronger 'class III' is required. Assessment by a lymphoedema specialist will be necessary to make sure that one gets the best kind of treatment for the type of oedema one has [15].

9.3.5.4 Deep Tissue Massage
There are two types of deep tissue massage: lymphatic drainage therapy and manual lymph drainage. These comprise of applying very light pressure in rhythmic motions to increase the flow of lymph fluid out of swollen tissue. (Visit National Lymphoedema Network Website for a list of professionals and specialist centres.) [13].

9.3.5.5 Skin Care
People with lymphoedema are advised to monitor their skin, moisturise, report cuts or infections and have infections treated. It is wise never to walk around barefooted.

9.3.5.6 External Pneumatic Compression (EPC)
Sometimes despite wearing compression stockings, there is still fluid accumulated by evening time. EPC is a pneumatic boot which inflates to squeeze fluid out of the leg. A doctor would assess if these were necessary. It may be possible to have a trial of these before someone goes out and buys them.

9.3.5.7 How Can the Patient Help Their Lymphoedema
They can look after their skin.

- It is important to elevate the limbs.
- It is essential to wear the stockings/bandages as per instructions.
- Exercise helps and keeping the weight down is useful when trying to control lymphoedema.

- Give up smoking; this will help protect blood vessels.
- Eat a healthy diet, will help with weight and blood vessels.
- People are advised not to walk barefooted [16].

9.3.5.8 Coping with Lymphoedema

Lymphoedema changes the way you look and therefore can have an impact on lifestyle. It can also be a reminder to women that they have had cancer. This can be emotionally challenging for some women to accept. Some women may experience emotions such as low mood, self-consciousness, anger or guilt. As nurses, we should talk to our patients and listen to how they are feeling. Nurses can offer support through listening, referring to support groups or psychological support. Online forums are useful too as it helps women to talk to other people who have lymphoedema [16].

9.4   Psychological Health of Women with Gynaecological Cancers

9.4.1   Introduction

In gynaecological oncology, some women are cured of their cancer and some live with their illness for years. This means that there are a lot of women living with the effects of having cancer and treatment, and they may have many needs that need to be met.

One of the main goals of cancer treatment has been to cure or prolong life; however more recently quality of life has become as important as quantity to a lot of patients and healthcare professionals. This involves considering the psychological well-being to be as important as alleviation of physical symptoms or removal of diseased organs.

9.4.2   When Can Psychological Problems Occur?

9.4.2.1 At Diagnosis

A woman has been experiencing a gynaecological problem, and following referral and investigations, she finds herself with an appointment to see a specialist for her results.

This woman may have been told that she has a suspected cancer or the investigations may not have pointed in that direction.

She may attend the clinic on her own, with a partner, a child, a parent, a friend, or a neighbour.

This woman may notice that for this appointment, a specialist nurse/nurse is sitting in, and this is new.

Table 9.1 This is a range of emotions she may go through

Shock	Tearful	Anger
Disbelief	Waves of sadness	Blame
Panic	Fear	Guilt
Being overwhelmed	Terror	Not hearing
Numbness	Faint	Shaking
Anxious		

Table 9.2 And this is another range of emotions that a woman may display at new diagnosis [17]

Calmness	Denial	Higher being/force
Positivity	Bargaining	Beliefs/faith in a God
Action/agency/ practical		
Resignation/acceptance		

She is told she has cancer. This can cause a range of emotions in women as can be seen in Tables 9.1 and 9.2.

The reactions and emotions will vary as will the woman/sitting in front of the doctor or nurse. Understanding why people react in certain ways is difficult but may be influenced by many factors. It is safe to say that a lot of people are shocked by being told they have cancer; even if there was a strong indication or 'hints' before-hand to suggest it, 'it gets real when it is said out loud'.

What happens next may be influenced by how secure the person is in themselves and their lives, their inner resources, how used they are with dealing with traumas and how experienced they are at it. Another factor is what their social support network is like (friends and family), where they are in life, their financial situation, their work, other life issues, other health issues and any other problems (such as relationship difficulties).

9.4.3 The Healthcare Professional's Response

It is usually a doctor who informs the patient of their cancer diagnosis. This usually occurs with a nurse specialist/nurse in attendance to support the patient and to write information/timelines for future appointments/investigations or treatments.

The healthcare professionals who hold such sensitive sessions are required to complete an advanced communications course or equivalent.

It is difficult to give a patient a diagnosis of a gynaecological (or any) cancer. The professional may feel sad for the patient/their family. The doctor or specialist nurse may feel a little apprehensive about the patient's/relative's reaction whether this is with tears or anger.

It is best for the healthcare professional to be kind and have empathy, to be strong and stable (if you can), and holding and stalwart. It is advisable to take the lead from the patient and give them only as much information as they can take in. The patient can always return for another appointment if necessary.

9.4.4   What All This Means for the Patient/Carer

9.4.4.1 Isolation

Women with gynaecological cancers can feel mentally and physically isolated whilst they and their loved ones get to grips with a diagnosis and treatment plan. It can cause stress on their relationships.

It can be difficult for both parties to express their feelings with each other. Because there is uncertainty and possibly a lot of fear, it may be difficult to know what to say.

Sometimes there seems to be a desire from the patient to protect their loved ones (by keeping worries to themselves) and vice versa. Sometimes there can be a social pressure to be positive and 'fight', which though admirable may not leave room for worries, fears and negativity which are equally valid and important to express [18].

Feelings can manifest in physical symptoms, such as:

• Fatigue.
• Lack of energy.
• Difficulty of sleeping.
• Lack of libido.

Many of these symptoms may be caused by the cancer or the treatment, but some can be caused by worry. This seems like a normal reaction to a cancer diagnosis, and these feelings and symptoms should recede over time [18].

9.4.5   Ways of Coping

'Fight'—getting on with the practical details, following the treatment plan and getting caught up with the actions. This may be automatic and a survival instinct and may feel like there is no choice but to do this.

'Freeze'—person breaking down or collapsing, this too can be an automatic and instinctive reaction to bad news or extreme fear, and one usually can move out of this in time and with support.

'Flight'—someone may want to deny what is happening; someone may want to focus on their life before the cancer, 'I have plans, holidays, etc.'; usually someone moves from this way of thinking; but occasionally someone chooses not to have treatment or conventional medicine and chooses some other path. At the end of the day, the choice should be with the patient [19].

9.4.6   Support

A lot of the support the patient will have will end up coming from their own resolve, more will come from those around them, though at the beginning, both parties may need some assistance/signposting from the healthcare professionals.

It is very important that the patient and their loved ones get to voice their thoughts and emotions, either together or separately with the doctors, nurses or counsellors/ psychologists (if onward referral is desired/deemed necessary). Psychological support should always be offered.

Information provided by the hospital, reputable websites and cancer helplines will help. Patients and their significant others will research information for themselves and should have an opportunity to run this by their oncology team for clarity.

9.4.7   Solutions

There are numerous solutions to psychological issues though it may take some time to discover them.

- It is good to be able to accept the bad days with the good ones so as not to feel under pressure to be okay all the time. A person or their significant other may need permission to be negative as well as positive, so that they can be true to how they really feel [18].
- Having a cancer diagnosis or going through treatment can be a constant battle as the patient may fight to keep control over things they cannot possibly control. Awareness can sometimes help, and focussing on what the person can influence may also be beneficial.
- Complementary therapies can help with energy levels and can relieve stress and symptoms.
- Conventional medications can ease some of the symptoms and when people are feeling better psychically, they may feel better mentally too.
- Gentle exercise can relieve fatigue by encouraging endorphin production and generally improving energy levels.
- It can be difficult to eat well if one is feeling ill or low; it is important to be able to eat small amounts regularly and to drink plenty especially if the appetite is waning [18].
- It is thought that getting up and getting dressed even when someone feels very low can create a little motivation and helps to improve the mood, though is not easy when the person is depressed.
- It can be good to be distracted when a person is psychologically unwell; being around people such as friends and going on days out can take the focus from being ill and the cancer journey. Hobbies can also provide such diversion. Of course, one may need to go against their instinct, as they may prefer to be alone or stay in bed if they feel very low.
- If someone wishes to speak about what is going on for them, support groups can be helpful, as it will be filled with peers (patients) that will have a certain understanding of what it is like to have cancer. Sometimes it is easier to speak with people that are not in one's family or friend groups; there is not the same need to protect them.

- If people don't wish to speak about their psychological problems, they may find relief from writing about them in a journal or diary.
- If someone feels angry or frustrated, it can help to thump a pillow or scream (loud music optional).

9.4.8 Effects Treatment Can Have on Mental Health

9.4.8.1 Surgery

I will list some of the effects of surgery which can influence mental health:

- Loss of fertility, body image issues (scarring), early induced menopause, menopausal symptoms, bone loss, operations put life on hold, prolonged stay in hospital and risk to life.
- Other attacks on mental health are stoma, sexual problems, fear of intimacy, exacerbating existing conditions and complications such as bleeding, infections and clots [20].

9.4.8.2 Radiotherapy

These are some of the effects of radiotherapy that may influence psychological well-being:

- Loss of fertility, vaginal stenosis, bowel problems, cystitis, skin soreness and fatigue [11].

9.4.8.3 Chemotherapy

These effects can influence mental health:

- Infection, nausea/vomiting, hair loss, constipation/diarrhoea, sore mouth and risk of sepsis.

9.4.8.4 Conclusion

Recently psychological well-being is seen as equally important as physical health. Women who are given a diagnosis of gynaecological cancer are automatically trust into a psychological whirlpool, which with time, information and support they should come to terms with.

One cannot underestimate the stress on mental health for the patient and the family/loved ones; also healthcare professionals are not immune to the suffering of their patients and may be affected emotionally by what is happening with their patients.

Communication is very important between the patient and their loved ones and between the healthcare professionals and the patient so that feelings and thoughts are transparent.

There are coping mechanisms and solutions which will take some of the mental strain from the patient, some they will figure out in time and some they can have sign posted for them by the supportive resources in the hospital and self-research.

If patients get support early on in their cancer journey, it will help them in time return to a 'new normal' so that they can have satisfying lives after cancer, and if they do not receive this and do not have the resource to cope, they may continue to suffer psychologically long after they have been treated.

The aim will always be for patients to heal psychologically as well as physically.

9.5   Sexual Function and Body Image Following Gynaecological Cancer Diagnosis

Sexual function, or sexuality, is a multidimensional concept and must be assessed holistically and on an individual basis, in particular following a diagnosis of a gynaecological cancer. Sexuality can involve sexual function, one's perception of their own sexuality and sexual relationships. Sexual function can change following a diagnosis alone of a gynaecological cancer, for example, vaginal or vulval cancer where a woman is physically unable to have intercourse due to pain from a tumour or narrowing of the vagina, and also following treatment for a gynaecological cancer, for example, a surgical intervention.

Surgery for a gynaecological cancer may result in an induced menopause and reduced libido due to lack of oestrogen post removal of both ovaries. These can be treated with HRT or alternatives as discussed in menopause management following a gynaecological cancer. Surgery which involves removal of the cervix or part of the vagina can also result in pain on having intercourse. Abdominal surgery involving removal of the female reproductive organs, laparoscopic or laparotomy, can have an impact on a women's sense of femininity and can therefore affect their perception of their own sexuality and sexual function. Surgical intervention can also have an impact on bladder and bowel function which can affect sexual function, physically and psychologically. Some women require vaginal reconstruction, and this can also cause a reduction in libido but also an altered sensation during intercourse.

Women who go on to have radiotherapy following surgery for gynaecological cancer or as a palliative treatment can also experience vaginal stenosis or vaginal adhesions, and this can make intercourse painful. Therefore, these women are given vaginal dilators to use for a minimum of 5–10 min three times per week to keep the vagina open (see Sect. 9.2.2). Radiotherapy can also cause vaginal dryness, and many women will use regular vaginal moisturisers and lubricants. Women who can have vaginal oestrogen also find this can be very effective. Women treated with brachytherapy, which is internal radiotherapy (See Sect. 9.2.2), for their gynaecological cancer can also struggle psychologically with having intercourse and being examined due to the invasive nature of the treatment.

Women can be referred to psychosexual therapists or support groups for support, as well as to charities for peer support. Women can be offered advice on vaginal moisturisers and lubricants as well as use of dilators or vibrators to help with vaginal adhesions and to boost confidence in their own sexual function. Many women find complimentary therapies useful, for example, aromatherapy which can help women to relax by being touched. Many women also find exercise, in particular those that strengthen the pelvic floor, to be beneficial.

Regardless of treatment, sexual function can be affected by the diagnosis alone of having a gynaecological cancer. It is important for women to feel safe when explaining what is concerning them about their sexual function with their healthcare professional (HCP) and that the HCP seeing them can advise them appropriately.

9.6   Induced Menopause in Gynaecological Oncology Patients

The average age of natural menopause is 51 years old. Therefore any menopause before the age of 51 is considered premature [21]. Menopause is diagnosed as a retrospective event of the cessation of menstrual cycles for a period of 1 year. A woman with a natural menopause spends almost one third of her life in the menopause. A medical intervention or treatment in a premenopausal woman that results in menopause is therefore induced and results in premature menopause or a menopause that occurs before the natural time. This induced menopause therefore results in the woman spending potentially half of her life in the postmenopause phase or longer.

In terms of gynaecological cancers, depending on the age at diagnosis of the woman, undoubtedly she will have an induced menopause if premenopausal at diagnosis or report worsening of pre-existing menopausal symptoms if peri- or postmenopausal at the time of diagnosis. Cervical cancer patients are often the worst affected as there are two peaks in age-specific incidence rates: 25–29 with 19 per 100,000 women and 85–89 with 12 per 100,000 women. The majority of women with cervical cancer are diagnosed between 25 and 64 years old, and therefore many of these women would be premenopausal at the time of diagnosis (see Chap. 10) [22].

Treatments for gynaecological cancers that result in an induced menopause include:

1. Radical surgery involving removal of both ovaries (bilateral salpingo-oophorectomy), resulting in surgical or immediate menopause.
2. External beam radiotherapy or internal brachytherapy.
3. Chemotherapy causing chemical menopause which can cause permanent or temporary ovarian failure.

Symptoms of iatrogenic or induced menopause are often significantly more intense than those of natural menopause due to the age of the woman and the sudden onset of symptoms. However, it is important to base menopause management on each individual woman's symptoms as these can vary amongst women, in severity and duration. Menopause symptoms are categorised as vasomotor, cognitive, uro-gynaecological and involving connective tissue, psychological and sexual. Common menopausal symptoms include hot flushes, night sweats, difficult sleeping (resulting in fatigue and irritability), reduced libido, memory and concentration problems, vaginal dryness and pain, itching or discomfort during sexual intercourse, headaches, mood changes, palpitations, muscle aches and pains, reduced muscle mass and recurrent urinary tract infections. There are also more long-term complications including cardiovascular disease and osteoporosis and dementia, which can have a particular impact on younger women with induced menopause [21]. Many menopausal symptoms are interlinked; the relationship with menopause and cancer treatments is complex, and Fig. 9.1 sets out the interlinked nature of the presenting complaints.

Management of induced menopause in gynaecological cancer patients is vital. It can become more controversial in the literature and amongst healthcare professionals when it comes to treating endometrial and ovarian cancer patients than with cervical, vaginal and vulval cancer patients. Practice is changing constantly with new evidence emerging as a result of research and developments within media sparking debate. The main safety concern amongst many practitioners is often fear of a cancer recurrence due to the link between these cancers and oestrogen dependence. However, it is unclear why this is of such concern as there have been no conclusive studies on recurrence rates in replacing hormones that the woman would have made herself when premenopausal.

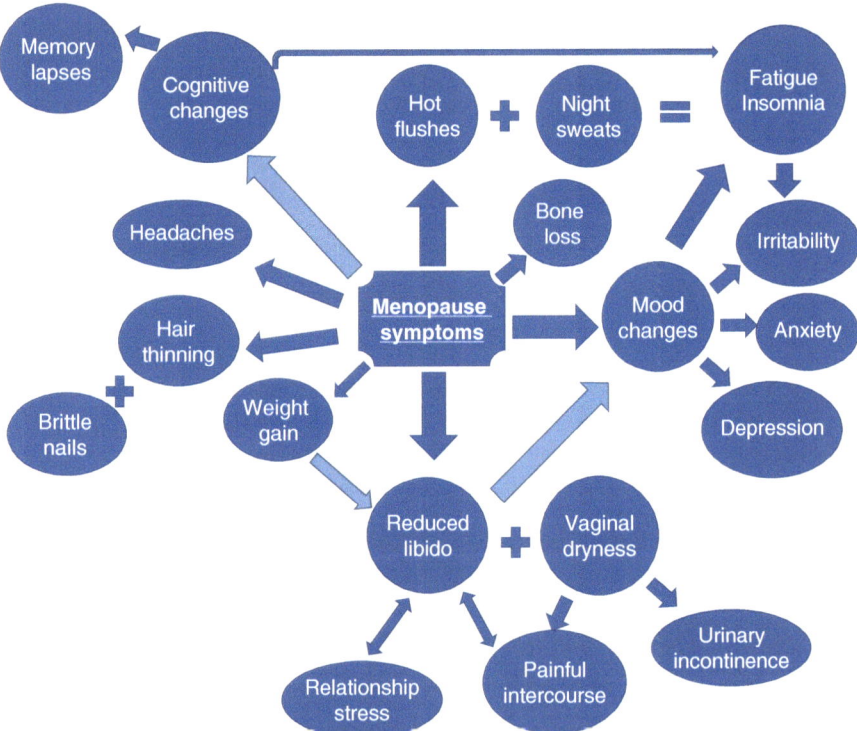

Fig. 9.1 Effects of menopause in cancer

9.6.1 Use of HRT in Gynaecological Cancer Patients [23–25]

In women who have been diagnosed with a gynaecological malignancy premenopause, the effects of hormone replacement therapy (HRT) for management of menopausal symptoms can significantly improve their quality of life reducing many of the vasomotor symptoms and therefore the psychological symptoms. It can also reduce the risk of coronary heart disease, stroke, dementia, osteopenia, osteoporosis and bone fractures. The incidence of these risks is higher in younger women as they experience menopause for a longer period of time than women who have a natural menopause or have a cancer diagnosis at a peri- or postmenopausal age.

Women who have experienced an induced menopause at a younger age should have regular bone densitometry in combination with lifestyle advice around bone health, including diet, calcium and vitamin D intake, alcohol consumption and smoking and regular exercise. Women who have induced menopause at a younger age and are suitable to have HRT should have it as soon as safely allowed as according to NICE HRT is protective of cardiovascular function and bone health and the most effective treatment for vasomotor symptoms and low mood due to menopause [21].

Use of HRT in women who have been diagnosed postmenopause varies on the site of their primary tumour and the evidence-based literature on HRT, on their individual clinician preference around use of HRT and also on the symptoms they are experiencing and the severity of these symptoms.

Women should have individual risk assessment for HRT, particularly women who have been diagnosed with a gynaecological malignancy. Lifestyle advice should be given based on this assessment.

There are few contraindications to having HRT in women with gynaecological cancers and the exceptions being endometrial at later stages, sarcomas and some ovarian. If in doubt, then the women should be referred to a specialist menopause clinic (see Chap. 10).

9.6.2 Alternatives to HRT for Gynaecological Cancer Patients [26]

There are over 200 alternatives to HRT for the management of menopause in the literature with little research evidence. Many of these alternatives are herbal preparations, for example, St. John's wort which has been proven to help with depression but not with hot flushes. Evening primrose oil is also widely used but does not help with menopausal symptoms. Alternative medicines, for example, acupuncture or homoeopathy, are also widely used as well as complimentary therapies, for example, aromatherapy and yoga. Many women use these alternatives for specific symptoms in combination with HRT or other medications, for example, antidepressants.

Alternatives will only treat the vasomotor symptoms and generally do not have a part to play in the other health benefits that HRT brings for this younger population.

Alternatives that have been proven to have some efficacy include:

- Exercise to reduce hot flushes and general well-being.
- Reducing caffeine and alcohol intake which may help with hot flushes and night sweats. Identifying a trigger such as caffeine or some particular alcoholic drinks can be vital for some women in managing their symptoms and planning when they are likely to be worse, for example, after an espresso or glass of red wine.
- Vaginal lubricants and moisturisers including those with oestrogen for topical use help with atrophic vaginitis and therefore have a positive impact on sexual functions. Use of vaginal oestrogen depends on the primary site of the gynaecological cancer, although it can be used following many treatments for a gynaecological cancer diagnosis and the literature states that a minimal amount of vaginal topical oestrogen is absorbed systemically, many healthcare professionals and oncologists will opt to wait a period of time before introducing vaginal oestrogen and will advise use of vaginal moisturisers and lubricants initially.

Other alternatives that are widely available and recommended that require additional research include homeopathy; magnetism; phytoestrogens; dehydroepiandrosterone; chasteberry and herbs such as hops, sage, leaf, liquorice and valerian; vitamin C; progesterone skin creams; and reflexology.

Acupuncture is not currently regulated for menopause symptoms, but it is believed by many women that it can reduce hot flushes and night sweats. Black cohosh also requires more research, but many women find it reduces night sweats and hot flushes.

Non-hormonal medications frequently prescribed by menopause specialists for treatment of symptoms include antidepressants which are used to treat hot flushes and night sweats; however, they are not as effective as HRT, can have an impact on some cancer medications and have some side effects (see Chap. 10).

It is also important to note that many alternatives to HRT for menopause management have been proven to be ineffective by NICE [21] and also are unsafe for use, and these include evening primrose oil, ginseng, dong quai, kava kava, beta blockers and vitamin E.

9.7 Conclusion

Undoubtedly many women suffer with menopausal symptoms; this can often be enhanced in women with an induced menopause as a result of treatment for a gynaecological cancer. Depending on age, site of the primary tumour, treatment modalities and severity of symptoms, these women can be offered a variety of treatments. However these treatments vary on clinician preference and most recent evidence-based research on efficacy and side effects, which is lacking in amount and consistency within the literature.

In addition, all of the literature supports hormone replacement therapy for women on an individual risk-assessed basis. Should a woman have any contraindications for HRT, alternatives are widely available and can be recommended to manage individual symptoms following a holistic assessment by their specialist healthcare professional.

References

1. Quality in nursing. Excellence in cancer care: the contribution of the clinical nurse specialist. We are Macmillan. Cancer support. https://www.macmillan.org.uk/documents/aboutus/commissioners/excellenceincancercarethecontributionoftheclinicalnursespecialist.pdf
2. Macmillan Cancer Support. The recovery package. https://www.macmillan.org.uk/about-us/health-professionals/programmes-and-services/recovery-package#297633
3. Frumovitz M, Abu-Rustum RN, Ramirez PT (2018) The principles of gynecologic oncology surgery. Elsevier, Philadelphia, PA
4. Guy's and St. Thomas' NHS Foundation Trust. Having a hysterectomy. http://gti/resources/patientinfo/womens/abdominal-hysterectomy-having-a.pdf
5. Wheatley RG, Schug SA, Watson D (2001) Safety and efficiency post-operative epidural anaesthesia. Br J Anaesth 87(1):47–61. https://academic.oup.com/bja/article/87/1/47/304216
6. Principles of monitoring postoperative patients (2013) Nurs Times 109(22):24–26. https://www.nursingtimes.net/Journals/2013/05/31/g/l/a/050613-Principles-of-monitoring-postoperative-patients.pdf
7. Royal College of Obstetricians and Gynaecologists (2013) Enhanced recovery in gynaecology. Paper no. 36. https://www.rcog.org.uk/globalassets/documents/guidelines/scientific-impact-papers/sip_36.pdf
8. Macmillan.org.uk
9. Eveappeal.org.uk
10. GTI/resources/patientinfo/oncology_haematology/radiotherapy_for_gynaecology_cancer.pdf
11. Jostrust.org.uk
12. www.guysandstthomas.nhs.uk/resources/patient-information/vascular/lymphoedema.pdf
13. www.lymphnet.org
14. www.ncbi.nim.n.h.gov/pmc/articles/pmc5526302
15. www.nhs.uk/conditions/lymphoedema
16. www.macmillan.org.uk/info/support/lymphoedema
17. Gynae oncology clinical nurse specialist experience
18. www.macmillan.org.uk/info/psychological-self-help-therapies.html
19. Levine P (1997) Waking the tiger. North Atlantic Books, Berkeley, CA
20. www.guysandstthomas/nhs.uk/resources/patient-information/gynaecology/abdominal-hysterectomy-having-a.pdf
21. National Institute of Health and Care Excellence (2015) Menopause: diagnosis and management: clinical guideline NG23. NICE, London
22. Biliatis I, Thomakos N, Rodolakis A, Akrivos N, Zackarakis D, Antsaklis A (2012) Safety of hormone replacement therapy in gynaecological cancer survivors. J Obstet Gynaecol 32:321–325
23. Harvey RE, Coffman KE, Miller VM (2015) Women-specific factors to consider in risk, diagnosis and treatment of cardiovascular disease. Womens Health 11:239–257
24. Hinds L, Price J (2010) Menopause, hormone replacement and gynaecological cancers. Menopause Int 16:89–93

25. Guidozzi F (2013) Estrogen therapy in gynaecological cancer survivors. Climacteric 16:611–617
26. Hickey M, Szabo R, Hunter M (2017) Non-hormonal treatments for menopausal symptoms. BMJ 359:j5101. https://doi.org/10.1136/bmj.j5101

Suggested Reading

Royal College of Nursing (2014) Menopause: lifestyle and therapeutic approaches. http://www2. rcn.org.uk/_data/assets/pdf_file/0012/596928/Meopause_guidance_Oct2014_WEBFINAL. pdf. Accessed 1 Jul 2018
Royal College of Obstetricians and Gynaecologists (2011) Alternatives to hormone replacement therapy for symptoms of the menopause. http://www.rcog.org.uk/en/patients/patient-leaflets/ alternatives-to-hrt-for-symptoms-of-the-menopause/. Accessed 1 Jul 2019
The British Menopause Society (2018) Ovarian cancer and HRT. http://www.the bms.org.uk/fact-detail.php?id10. Accessed 1 Jul 2019
The British Menopause Society (2018) Premature menopause. https://thebms.org.uk/. Accessed 1 Jul 2018

The Menopause

10

Nikki Noble and Debra Holloway

10.1 Prevalence/Background

Menopause is a natural part of aging and the reproductive cycle. Women's periods stop and they are no longer able to reproduce. It is a physiological process of ovarian failure due to loss of follicular activity. Females are born with all their oocytes: seven million are present at 20 weeks' gestation, diminishing to 600,000 at puberty and the number diminishes over their lifetime, dropping drastically after the age of 35 and continuing to decline until all the follicles have run out [1, 2]. Periods become irregular and eventually stop. This is when the menopause occurs.

The endocrinology of the menopause is complex and can vary between women [3]. Follicle-stimulating hormone (FSH) is controlled by the pulsatile secretion of gonadotrophin-releasing hormone (GnRH), which is moderated by the negative feedback of oestradiol, progesterone and inhibin B. Luteinising hormone (LH) is also controlled by GnRH and surges mid-cycle owing to positive feedback from oestradiol, which triggers ovulation [4]. At this stage, the pituitary gland produces high levels of FSH trying to force the ovaries to release an oocyte. This leads to permanently elevated FSH levels. The average age for the menopause in the UK is 51.

Menopause is defined by the National Institute for Clinical Excellence in Health Care (NICE) [5] as when a woman stops having periods as she reaches the end of her natural reproductive life. It is a gradual process during which women experience peri-menopause before reaching post-menopause.

Women undergoing the menopause are seen across a variety of primary and secondary care settings, and by nurses of various disciplines [6]. It is important that

N. Noble
Aneurin Bevan University Health Board, Caerleon, UK

D. Holloway (✉)
Guys and St Thomas NHS Foundation Trust, London, UK
e-mail: Debra.Holloway@gstt.nhs.uk

© Springer Nature Switzerland AG 2019
D. Holloway (ed.), *Nursing Management of Women's Health*,
https://doi.org/10.1007/978-3-030-16115-6_10

nurses in primary care and women's health have a general awareness and understanding of the menopause to support and signpost women. This should include knowledge of the symptoms, psychosocial implications and the treatments available including hormonal, non-hormonal and alternative therapies in addition to lifestyle advice. Nurses should also have knowledge of the implications of menopause for women's future health and well-being [7].

Surgical menopause occurs when the ovaries are removed, which may be for a variety of reasons such as fibroids, endometriosis, cancer or for risk-reducing surgery when a BRCA gene is present [8]. Symptoms can be more intense than a physiological menopause and there is a risk of long-term health conditions.

Premature ovarian insufficiency occurs when ovarian function ceases before the age of 40. It is discussed in more detail later in the chapter.

10.2   Signs

Many women experience the menopause with relatively minor symptoms; however, some women request advice and help because of the significant impact their symptoms are having on their work and home life. Around 10–20% of women find the symptoms of menopause intolerable and approach a health care professional for help with managing their symptoms [9].

10.3   Symptoms

Menopause symptoms typically last for 4–5 years, but can be present for up to 15 years in some women [10]. Hot flushes and night sweats are the most common menopausal symptoms [11], but symptoms of the menopause are varied and wide-ranging and are described in detail below.

Other symptoms include low mood, anxiety, frequency of micturition, low libido, muscle and joint pain, itching and loss of concentration.

10.3.1   Vasomotor Symptoms

The most common menopausal symptoms are the vasomotor symptoms of flushes and hot sweats. The pathophysiology of hot flushes are still an enigma and not well understood; however, there are several theories of why they occur. One theory is that women who experience hot flushes have a narrower thermoregulatory zone in the hypothalamus than those who do not have symptoms. A slight change to core body temperature can lead to a hot flush [12]. Another theory is that a decrease in oestrogen levels causes reduced endorphins in the hypothalamus, which leads to an increase in the release of the neurotransmitters serotonin and noradrenaline. Serotonin and noradrenaline lower the set point in the thermoregulatory nucleus, triggering inappropriate heat loss [13]. Oestrogens are clearly involved in the aetiology of a hot flush; this is supported by the fact that oestrogen replacement therapy practically eliminates them [12].

A hot flush starts as a spontaneous sensation of warmth, usually on the chest spreading to the neck and face and can be accompanied by anxiety, perspiration and palpitations [13]. They vary in intensity, frequency and duration and last for several minutes. They may be triggered by hot drinks, stress and warm environments [13]. Two thirds of women experience some vasomotor symptoms and a small number of these feel discomfort at a level that significantly diminishes their quality of life [14]. In addition, recent research has suggested that women who have more severe vasomotor symptoms may be at a greater risk of cardiovascular events later on in life [15].

10.3.2 Psychological and Cognitive Symptoms

For some women, the menopause is a positive experience and a positive time in their lives. It can mark the end of painful periods, worries about contraception and conceiving, or pre-menstrual tension.

For other women, the menopause can be a negative experience, as it signals the loss of the ability to reproduce, the start of old age and a perceived loss of femininity. Impaired memory and difficulty in concentrating are common symptoms experienced by women. This may be caused by lack of sleep, stress and low mood [4]. It is not known why psychological symptoms occur during the menopause; they may be unrelated to hormones and may be multifactorial. There may be life stresses present that can contribute to these symptoms [8]. Psychological symptoms can include a loss of confidence, panic attacks, irritability and low mood.

Different cultures have varied perspectives of menopause, some more positive than others. Western society has negative attitudes towards aging, whereas Eastern cultures view older women as wise and they are well respected as part of the community.

10.3.3 Loss of Libido

Loss of libido is multifactorial and relates to the decline of testosterone and oestrogen, but it can depend on bio-psycho-social problems. These factors are outlined in Table 10.1 [16].

Table 10.1 Factors in the loss of libido

Physical factors	Psycho-social factors
Oestrogen and testosterone deficiency	Quality of relationships
Aging	Culture
Physical illness	Lifestyle factors
Menstrual difficulties, i.e. irregular, painful	Education and employment
Surgical menopause	Negative attitude towards the menopause

10.3.4 Genitourinary Symptoms of the Menopause/Vulvo-Vaginal Atrophy

Postmenopausal vaginal dryness is termed vulvo-vaginal atrophy (VVA) or genitourinary syndrome of the menopause (GSM), which is the preferred term [17], because it also encompasses the urinary symptoms that can be experienced due to the lack of oestrogen in the urethra and trigone muscle of the bladder [18].

Vaginal dryness is a very common symptom of menopause [19]. Physiological changes occur in the vagina because of the lack of oestrogen. The vagina becomes thin, with pale dry vaginal walls [20]. The symptoms of GSM include itching, dryness and dyspareunia, increased susceptibility to urinary tract infections and a watery vaginal discharge. These symptoms can have an impact on sexual function, daily activities, quality of life and relationships [19].

The physiological decrease in vaginal oestrogens modifies the characteristics of the vaginal epithelium, which becomes squamous and stratified, whereas it was wet and wrinkled before the menopause [21].

10.4 Diagnosis and Investigations

Diagnosis of the menopause is only truly made in retrospect, as according to the definitions above it is 1 year after the last menstrual period (LMP). However, the diagnosis of peri-menopause can be made clinically and blood tests are not generally needed. There are several tools available to aid a menopause diagnosis: a full medical history should be taken and should include the date of the LMP, current symptoms and the effect the symptoms are having on the woman's quality of life. A baseline assessment of cardiovascular and venous thromboembolic risk should be undertaken because of the potentially increased risks associated with hormone replacement therapy (HRT) [22].

Diagnosing and treating the menopause is easy [2], as it does not require any blood tests (in women over 45) and should be made clinically [5]. By replacing the oestrogen that is deficient in the body, the women's symptoms improve dramatically [20].

10.5 Treatment

There are many treatment options for women who are experiencing menopausal symptoms. Lifestyle changes may be enough, but some women may need pharmacological treatment. HRT is the gold standard, but for women who are unable or unwilling to take HRT, there are other drug treatments available. There are complimentary therapies available that have varying levels of evidence of their effectiveness. All treatments are discussed in detail here.

10.6   Lifestyle Changes

Many women benefit from lifestyle changes to relieve menopausal symptoms. Women should be advised on lifestyle factors such as diet, exercise, smoking and weight. Routine health screenings, such as cervical screening, breast mammography and bowel cancer screening should be undertaken and up to date.

Smoking: cessation should be advised, as it is known that women who smoke over 14 cigarettes per day have an earlier menopause and more severe vasomotor symptoms than women who do not smoke [8]. Smoking can increase the number of hot flushes; therefore, stopping smoking helps with this symptom [23]. The benefits of stopping smoking for people of all ages are well known and should be included in a discussion of lifestyle factors.

Alcohol: government recommendations for alcohol consumption are that women drink no more than 3 units of alcohol daily, with weekly consumption capped at 14 units [24]. Alcohol is known to trigger hot flushes and should be avoided if possible [8]. An increased alcohol intake can increase the risk of breast cancer, heart disease, stroke and hypertension [8].

Diet: Menopausal women should eat a diet that is protein-rich, as muscle mass can decline after the menopause [4]. Spicy foods can trigger hot flushes and should be avoided. Women should aim to eat at least five portions of fruit and vegetables daily, two portions of fish per week, and ensure an adequate calcium intake [6].

Weight: it has been found that women who have a normal body mass and regularly exercise cope better with menopausal symptoms than women who are overweight and do little to no exercise [25].

Exercise: it is also beneficial and studies have shown yoga to be specifically helpful.

Advice given regarding contraception should be up to date and evidence-based. The Faculty of Sexual and Reproductive Health (2017) guideline [26] "Contraception for Women over Aged Over 40 Years" is particularly useful for this.

10.7   Hormone Replacement Therapy

The basis for the use of HRT in the menopause is that by replacing the deficit of oestrogen that is causing the symptoms, an improvement should be seen [27]. Oestrogen was first approved and used as a hormone replacement in the 1940s [13] and is now a commonly used treatment for moderate to severe symptoms of menopause [27].

In general, the benefits of HRT outweigh the risks in symptomatic women aged 50–59, or less than 10 years after the onset of menopause, when there are no contraindications [22].

When prescribing HRT, there are several factors that need to be considered before deciding on what type and preparation of HRT to prescribe. If a woman has had a hysterectomy, she only requires oestrogen for symptom control. This is available orally, transdermally through the skin as a gel or patch or as an implant. If a woman still has a uterus, then the HRT should be a combined preparation that contains oestrogen and progestogen. The oestrogen is for symptom management and progestogen to prevent the endometrium thickening, which can lead to hyperplasia and potentially endometrial cancer. This is termed "opposing" the oestrogen.

If a woman still has a uterus, then the HRT depends on when the woman's LMP was. If over a year ago, then a continuous combined preparation would be the most appropriate. This means that oestrogen and progestogen are given daily and there should not be any bleeding, although bleeding may occur during the first 3–6 months. Continuous combined HRT is available orally or transdermally. If the LMP was less than a year ago, then a sequential combined HRT would be more appropriate. This consists of continuous oestrogen (taken daily) with progestogen taken for 12–14 days of the cycle, this results in a regular monthly bleed. This type of HRT is available orally and transdermally.

The Mirena intra-uterine system (IUS) is also licensed for HRT as the progestogen component and can be used in any women with a uterus regardless of her LMP; this results in a bleed-free HRT. Oestrogen can then be added as a tablet, gel or patch.

There are different types of oestrogen and progestrogen, with differing side-effects profiles.

If the only symptoms are genitourinary, then a topical vaginal oestrogen as a pessary or cream is more appropriate and can effectively treat vaginal dryness [28]. It can be used twice weekly to relieve symptoms and as it is a chronic condition, life-long management is required to prevent a recurrence of symptoms [17]. A summary of the care of women in the menopause is shown in Fig. 10.1.

10.7.1   Testosterone

Testosterone levels steadily decline throughout a woman's 30s and at the time of the menopause, as oestrogen levels drop, there is a change in the oestrogen/testosterone ratio, which can have a negative effect on libido. Research has shown testosterone to be of benefit in women who have a low libido post-menopause as long as they are also utilising oestrogen therapy. The NICE [5] supports the use of testosterone under these circumstances.

10.7.2   Monitoring and Follow-Up

The NICE [5] recommends that women should be reviewed 3 months after starting HRT and then yearly. Women should be advised that vaginal bleeding is a common side-effect within the first 3 months of commencing HRT and it should be reported at the 3-month check. If bleeding occurs after 3 months, it should be reported promptly in line with the NICE guidelines on suspected cancer [5].

Side-effects vary and the different hormones have differing side-effects. Oestrogen can cause bloating, breast tenderness, headache, fluid retention and

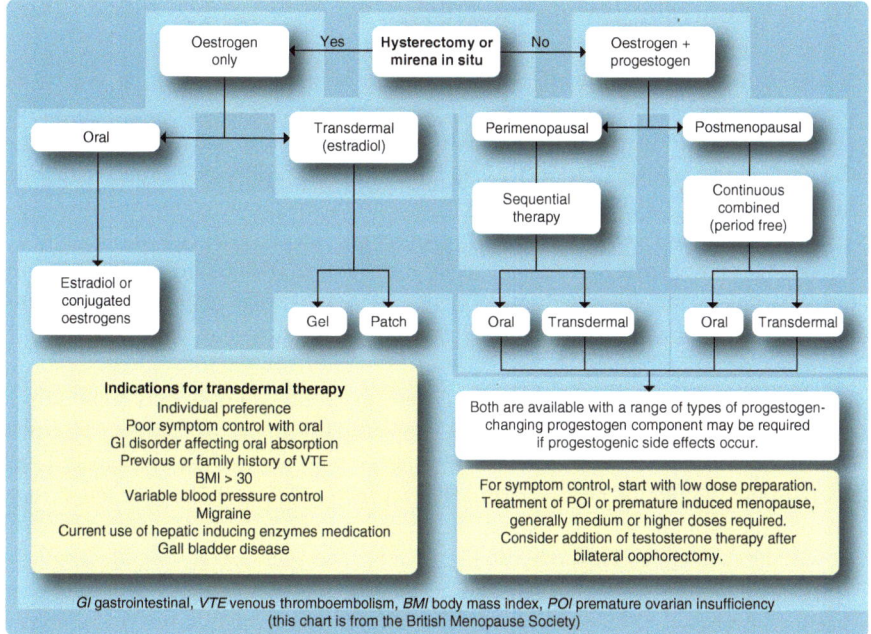

Fig. 10.1   Management of the menopause

nausea. Side-effects of progestogens include premenstrual-like syndrome, fluid retention, mood changes and breast tenderness [29]. Testosterone side-effects include acne, a slight increase in hair growth, thickening and local irritation to the gel [30]. Women using a patch may experience contact sensitisation.

10.7.3   Benefits of HRT

The main benefit of HRT is that it relieves the symptoms of menopause and improves quality of life; however, there are other known benefits.

Women can become prone to osteoporosis post-menopause as a result of bone loss caused by oestrogen deficiency [31]. HRT can prevent bone loss by preserving bone density, thus reducing the risk of a fragility fracture later in life [20]. Oestrogen is known to be beneficial to cardiovascular health in women and premenopausal women are at a lower risk of cardiovascular disease (CVD) compared with age-controlled men [4]. Commencing HRT in the peri-menopause or early menopause may maintain the benefits of oestrogen for the cardiovascular system. There is no increased risk of CVD in women aged between 50 and 59 years when commencing HRT. Several large trials have shown that taking HRT at this age may have beneficial effects on cardiovascular health [32].

10.7.4 Contraindications and Risks

Hormone replacement therapy is contraindicated in women with an oestrogen-dependent cancer (breast and endometrial cancer), undiagnosed vaginal bleeding, pregnancy, active liver disease, uncontrolled hypertension and recent thrombosis. Caution should be exercised in women with migraine, epilepsy, fibroids and endometriosis [20].

Taking oral HRT can increase the risk of stroke. The level of risk varies, depending on other risk factors such as age, body mass index (BMI), smoking, immobility, hypertension and the type and route of HRT used. In women under 60, the absolute risk of stroke is low [28] and low-dose transdermal oestrogen is not associated with an increased risk of stroke [4].

A previous history or the presence of thromboembolism is usually a contraindication to taking oral HRT. The risk of a deep vein thrombosis or pulmonary embolism is increased by twofold to fourfold in women taking oral HRT compared with the baseline population risk [4]. Transdermal rather than oral HRT should be considered for women who are at an increased risk of venous thromboembolism, including those with a BMI over 30 [5].

The relationship between HRT and breast cancer is complex. Evidence suggests that the combined HRT (oestrogen and progestogen) increases the risk of breast cancer when taken for longer than 5 years [20]. For most symptomatic women the use of HRT for 5 years or less is safe and effective [28]. HRT does not affect the risk of dying from breast cancer [33].

10.7.5 Discontinuing Hormone Replacement Therapy

There is no set time limit for how long HRT can be taken and no upper age limit. However, symptoms of the menopause are transient; the average is a few years but can be up to 10 years for some women [23] and there is no indication for treatment once symptoms have stopped [20]. The difficulty is that the woman does not know if her symptoms have gone until she stops HRT. The risks of stopping HRT should be assessed on an individual basis, because they may change as the woman becomes older and depending on the length of time she has been using HRT. The benefits should always outweigh the risks if the woman is to continue to use HRT. There is limited evidence to support either stopping HRT abruptly or tapering the dose and stopping more slowly [34]. This lack of evidence means that the patient and prescriber can reach a collaborative decision regarding the discontinuation of HRT and stop it in the way in which the woman prefers [34].

10.8 Non-hormonal Treatments

There are several non-hormonal medicines available for women in whom HRT is contraindicated or who choose not to take HRT. These drugs are listed in Table 10.2, with a summary of dosage and side-effects:

Table 10.2 Prescribed alternatives to HRT

Drug	Class/type of drug	Indication	Dose	Side-effects	Comments
Clonidine	Anti-hypertension	Vasomotor symptoms	50–75 µg twice daily	Difficulty sleeping, dry mouth, sedation, constipation	Only licensed option
Venlafaxine	SSRIs/SNRIs	Vasomotor symptoms Anti-depressant effect	37.5–150 mg daily	Side-effects include dizziness and sexual dysfunction	Reduces flushes by 37–61%
Paroxetine	SSRIs/SNRIs	Vasomotor symptoms	10–20 mg daily	Nausea, dizziness, sexual dysfunction	Interacts with tamoxifen
Citalopram	SSRIs/SNRIs	Vasomotor symptoms	20 mg daily	Nausea, dizziness, sexual dysfunction	Can be used with tamoxifen
Gabapentin	Gamma amino-butyric acid analogue	Vasomotor symptoms Improved sleep	300–1600 mg	Dizziness, dry mouth, weight gain	
Pregabalin	Anti-epileptic	Vasomotor symptoms Improved sleep Anti-depressant effect	50–300 mg daily in divided doses	Dizziness, dry mouth, weight gain	Better tolerated than gabapentin

SSRIs selective serotonin reuptake inhibitors, *SNRIs* serotonin–norepinephrine reuptake inhibitors

10.8.1 Clonidine

Clonidine is the only non-hormonal drug licensed in the UK for the treatment of hot flushes [35]. It is an antihypertensive alpha-2 adrenergic agonist and the mechanism of action for reducing hot flushes is not fully understood [36]. It has been shown in clinical trials to be more effective than placebo for reducing hot flushes. It is usually prescribed in a dosage of 25 µg twice daily, which is increased to a maximum of 50 µg three times a day. Sleep disturbance is a side-effect in 50% of users. Caution must be used when stopping clonidine, as abrupt withdrawal can cause rebound hypertension [35].

10.8.2 Selective Serotonin Reuptake Inhibitors and Serotonin–Norepinephrine Reuptake Inhibitors

Selective serotonin reuptake inhibitors (SSRIs) and serotonin–norepinephrine reuptake inhibitors (SNRIs) are traditionally used to treat depression and anxiety

[35]. Evidence is emerging that serotonin, noradrenaline and dopamine reactions may be involved in the aetiology of a hot flush [23] and evidence shows that SSRIs and SNRIs can improve mild to moderate vasomotor symptoms. Caution must be taken when prescribing SSRIs and SNRIs as paroxetine and fluoxetine can interfere with the cytochrome P2D6 pathway and disrupt the metabolism of tamoxifen [28].

10.8.3 Gabapentin

Gabapentin is a gamma amino-butyric acid analogue primarily indicated for epilepsy [29]. It can be used to reduce the severity of hot flushes. It may also be beneficial to women with aches and pains. Numerous side-effects include drowsiness, fatigue and weight gain.

10.8.4 Ospemifene

Ospemifene is new drug and belongs to the selective oestrogen receptor modulator (SERM) group of drugs. It is suitable for women with GSM, particularly dyspareunia, who are unable to take hormonal treatments [22]. In the UK, it is marketed under the brand name Senshio and it is available as 60-mg tablets to be taken once daily with food [37]. It is licensed for the treatment of moderate to severe symptomatic VVA in post-menopausal women who are not candidates for local vaginal oestrogen therapy.

The safety of using Senshio concomitantly with oestrogens or other selective oestrogen receptor modulators, such as tamoxifen, bazedoxifene and raloxifene, has not been studied, and its concurrent use is not recommended [37].

Ospemifene may be beneficial to women with a previous history of breast cancer or who currently have breast cancer (but this is off license use), or simply in women who prefer to avoid such treatments as vagainal oestrogens.

10.9   Cognitive Behavioural Therapy

Cognitive behavioural therapy (CBT) is a brief, non-medical therapy that can be helpful for a range of menopausal symptoms including hot flushes and sweats, sleep disturbances and low mood [38]. Paced breathing and relaxation can help during a hot flush to reduce anxiety due to the stress of having a hot flush. CBT may help with sleep disturbances as it is aimed at reducing worrying thoughts and improving relaxation [38].

Research has proved that CBT is beneficial to women with breast cancer who are experiencing vasomotor symptoms [39].

10.10   Lubricants and Moisturisers

Lubricants and moisturisers are effective for women with mild to moderate vaginal dryness to relieve discomfort and pain during sexual intercourse [19]. The difference between lubricants and moisturisers are their intended use.

Lubricants are used before sex to relieve vaginal dryness and associated pain. There are a wide variety of lubricants available and can be water-, oil-, silicone- or plant oil-based [19]. Oil-based lubricants should not be used with condoms.

Moisturisers can be used regularly (every day/alternate days) to relieve symptoms. They work by rehydrating the vaginal mucosa as they are bio-adhesive; this allows the epithelial cells to retain water. They can be used regularly and in the long term [18].

10.11   Complementary Therapies

Evidence for complementary therapies is mixed and there is more evidence for some than for others with regard to effectiveness. The most commonly used therapies are discussed below.

10.11.1   Phytoestrogens

There are two types of phytoestrogens: isoflavones and ligands. They are thought to have a chemical structure similar to oestrogen and are commonly found in soya products. Evidence from the use of phytoestrogens is limited at present.

10.11.2   Black Cohosh

A Cochrane systematic review of black cohosh for relieving menopause symptoms undertaken in 2012 showed that there was insufficient evidence to support its use.

10.11.3   Novogen Red Clover

A commercially available tablet form of isoflavone. There is some evidence from short-term trials for its efficacy [36].

10.11.4   Herbal Preparations

There is no or limited evidence for the following herbal remedies: Omega 3 acids, ginseng, flax seeds, wild yam, dong quai [36].

10.11.5 New Developments

The use of neurokinin 3 receptor antagonists (NK3R) has been prompted by a better understanding of how GnRH is regulated and how NK3R antagonists lead to the reduction of LH [10]. This better understanding of the link between GnRH and LH and a reduction in hot flushes led to a small placebo randomised control trial, which showed a 40% reduction in vasomotor symptoms. Larger trials will be underway soon [35]. Although unlikely to replace HRT as the standard treatment for vasomotor menopausal symptoms NK3R antagonists may prove to be beneficial for women who are unable to take HRT, such as those with active breast cancer [40].

10.12 Contraception and the Menopause

Women who are peri-menopausal have a low fertility rate, but are still at risk of unintended pregnancy at this stage in their reproductive life. Contraceptive choice can be limited by co-morbidities in this older age group [26]. Current advice for stopping non-hormonal contraceptives in women aged 50 years or over is to wait until 1 year of amenorrhoea and women aged under 50 years should wait for 2 years of amenorrhoea before stopping contraception when using a non-hormonal contraceptive. However, for women using a progestogen-only method, such as a progestogen-only pill, implant or IUS, amenorrhoea is not a reliable indicator of menopause. Stopping contraception is an individual choice for the woman, and she should be supported to make an informed choice. Women should be aware that HRT does not act as contraception (see Chap. 13) [41].

10.13 Long-Term Effects of Oestrogen Deficiency

10.13.1 Cardiovascular Disease

Severe hot flushes and sweats have been linked to decreased cardiovascular health [42]. CVD is the leading avoidable cause of death in women and it is important to understand that HRT does not increase the risk of CVD in women when started under the age of 60 [8].

10.13.2 Osteoporosis

Osteoporosis is a disease of structural deterioration of the bone tissue leading to low bone density. This can contribute to an increase in susceptibility to fracture. In fact, over 300,000 patients present with fragility fractures to hospitals in the UK each year [43].

Increased bone loss after the menopause in women combined with age-related bone loss means that the prevalence of osteoporosis increases markedly with age, from 2% at 50 years to more than 25% at 80 years in women [43]. In the UK, 1 in 2 women aged 50 and over will have a fragility fracture due to osteoporosis. Over the age of 50, as oestrogen levels decline, the risk of osteoporosis increases.

10.14 Premature Ovarian Insufficiency

As discussed above, the average age at menopause is 51; however, women can undergo the menopause at any age. This can be natural or surgical or induced by medications such as chemotherapy or radiotherapy. When women have an early menopause or POI, then this does require medical intervention to help with symptoms and to prevent against the long-term health consequences.

The standard agreed definition of POI is women under the age of 40 [44], who have a loss of ovarian function, which is characterised by no or infrequent periods and raised FSH and LH and low oestradiol. Formerly, the terms to describe this used to be premature ovarian failure or premature menopause [44]. They were changed to include insufficiency, as this does not have the negative connotations of failure for women, and the ovarian function is intermittent and there may even be spontaneous pregnancy. This is estimated to affect 1% of women [45], which rises to 7% if surgical and iatrogenic menopause is included, and 0.1% if the age is lowered to 30 [46]. The term premature menopause applies to women over the age of 40 and under 45. These definitions, however, can vary in different countries. There are many guidelines for the management of this special group of women [5, 44], but despite this, women still struggle to gain access to specialist services, and to get the correct diagnosis, as there can be preconceived ideas that women under the age of 50 are too young for the menopause. Many women see three or more clinicians before they get a diagnosis, which can be delayed for 5 years or more [46]. This can lead to women being frustrated and left with multiple symptoms that are not treated, in addition to the long-term impact on cardiovascular and bone health, and increased mortality. There is evidence that bilateral salpingo-oophorectomy before the natural age of menopause is associated with increased mortality, coronary heart disease, dementia, parkinsonism, osteoporosis, mood disorders and sexual dysfunction [45].

A woman who presents with amenorrhea at any age, up to the natural age of menopause, needs to be investigated. There can be many causes for periods stopping, as have be seen summarised in Table 10.3. These need to be excluded before the diagnosis of POI is made.

The investigations that a woman needs if periods have stopped are dependent on her history and presentation symptoms. All women who present with cessation of periods should be asked about symptoms of low oestrogen [46]. Women need to undergo FSH/LH/oestradiol/prolactin measurement as a baseline and then further tests dependent on the results of these [47]. Hormone tests are normally repeated after at least 6 weeks as they can fluctuate in line with changes that can be seen with the menstrual cycle [47]. Some women may have raised levels (and symptoms), but continue to have normal cycles

Table 10.3 Causes of cessation of periods

Cause of no periods	Diagnostics
Pregnancy	History and pregnancy test
Breastfeeding	History
PCOS	History, ultrasound, bloods (raised LH and oestradiol and testosterone)
Hypergonadotropic hypogonadism	History and bloods (low FSH, LH and oestradiol)
Medications	History examples may be IUS, Depo, POP, cocaine
Low BMI/excessive exerciser	Hormone tests normal to low, AMH normal
Hyperthyroidism	Bloods TSH (symptoms can be irregular periods, hot flushes, hair loss and weight loss)
Hypothyroidism	TSH (symptoms HMB, or no periods, fatigue, hair loss, dry skin, weight gain)

PCOS polycystic ovary syndrome, *BMI* body mass index, *LH* luteinising hormone, *FSH* follicle-stimulating hormone, *IUS* intra-uterine system, *POP* progestogen-only pill, *AMH* anti-Müllerian hormone, *TSH* thyroid-stimulating hormone, *HMB* heavy menstrual bleeding

as the peri-menopausal phase can last for a few to many years. A diagnosis of POI can be made on FSH being raised on two occasions and oestradiol being low [44, 46, 47].

Women with POI may present with different menopausal symptoms from those with menopause at a natural age. There seem to be fewer hot flushes and more issues with vaginal dryness, irregular cycles and inability to conceive [46]. However, those who have a sudden menopause because of surgery or in relation to chemotherapy (type, dose and amount and age at time of treatment determine the risk of POI) or radiotherapy often find that they have more severe symptoms and they can be difficult to manage, as in some cases, the use of oestrogens is contraindicated by the cancer, if it is hormone-dependent. This is often compounded in women who have treatments for breast cancer that are anti-oestrogen. Women who have had a hysterectomy with conservation of the ovaries may find that they have an earlier menopause [47]; the diagnosis in this case is guided by symptoms and not the absence of periods, and in some cases hormone profiles can be helpful. In addition, as there are more children who survive childhood cancers, they have a higher risk of developing POI either at the time of treatment or after treatment [46].

The causes of POI are varied, with most women not knowing the reason for it. There is ongoing research to look for genetic causes, and a woman is 10–15% more likely to have POI if she has a first-degree relative with POI [46]. The main known causes of POI are shown in Table 10.4.

Premature ovarian deficiency is a multi-factorial disorder in which in up to 85–90% of women, no cause is currently found [46, 47]. Women are born with a finite number of oocytes and they gradually decline over their lifetime. POI can occur in three main ways:

1. Reduced peak number of follicles.
2. Increased follicle depletion.
3. Follicle dysfunction.

Table 10.4 Causes of premature ovarian insufficiency (POI)

Cause	Comment
Autoimmune component (about 5%) [47]	Normally associated with thyroid, ovarian or adrenal auto-antibodies. Other conditions include diabetes, lupus rheumatoid arthritis
Enzyme deficiencies	
Genetic	Abnormalities on the X chromosome occur in about 14% [47] Most common is Turner syndrome Fragile X carriers more at risk of POI If found in POI, women should be referred for genetic counselling and discussion with the wider family considered Rare inherited syndromes such as blepharophimosis, ptosis, epicanthus inversus syndrome type 1
Infections	Mumps or pelvic TB, malaria, women with HIV may have POI (may be due to HIV or the medication used)
Iatrogenic	1. Chemotherapy. Many chemotherapy regimens cause POI, especially alkylating agents. There is a correlation among age at treatment, dose and POI. In women with combination therapies, there is the highest risk of POI 2. Radiotherapy to abdomen, pelvis or spine 3. Surgery Removal of ovaries, some possibility of earlier menopause if hysterectomy undertaken

Protective factors have been found to include later menarche, irregular menstruation and breastfeeding [48].

Whatever the cause of the POI, women need specialist care to help them manage the symptoms, psychologically cope with the diagnosis and lack of fertility, and manage the longer-term consequences of POI such as osteoporosis, CVD and higher mortality, as recommended by current guidelines. It is recommended that these women are referred to specialist services to be managed [5, 44]. In addition to the physical symptoms, women often struggle with the diagnosis and lack peer support.

10.14.1 Diagnostic Tests

To establish a diagnosis, women need to have at least two hormone profiles (FSH/LH/oestrdiol taken 4–6 weeks apart as well as prolactin and TSH). Once these are complete and no other cause for the cessation of periods has been found, then other investigations include thyroid and adrenal auto-antibodies, genetics for karyotyping and Fragile X testing, and baseline bone density with dual-energy X-ray absorptiometry (DEXA) [47]. If adrenal antibodies are present, then the woman needs to be referred to an endocrinologist and if the thyroid is positive but TSH is normal, then this should be repeated yearly and the patient referred if raised [44]. Previous guidelines had suggested routine screening for diabetes, but this is now not recommended owing to a lack of evidence [44]. Table 10.5 shows a summary of the investigations for women who are diagnosed with POI.

In terms of general health, there is evidence that smokers may tend to have an earlier menopause; thus, women with a strong family history of POI should be

Table 10.5 Investigations into POI

Test	Results
FSH/LH/oestradiol	High/high/low Repeated two times
Prolactin	Normal
TSH	If abnormal refer to the endocrinologist
Karyotyping	
Fragile X	If positive referral for genetics
Thyroid and adrenal auto-antibodies	If thyroid positive but TSH normal, check TSH yearly, with adrenal referral to the endocrinologist
Bone density (DEXA)	Repeat as guidelines

DEXA dual-energy X-ray absorptiometry

encouraged to stop smoking [44]. Despite all these tests, there are many women in whom no cause of POI is identified and are classed as unexplained.

Although there are some family links for POI, there is no current test that identifies whether a woman is going to have POI or to prevent this; therefore, relatives of women with POI should also have discussions on the risks of an earlier menopause and the implications that this may have for their fertility. Anti-Müllerian hormone (AMH) is a good marker for fertility treatments and has some potential in predicting POI; however, it is not currently in use [46].

10.14.2 Surgical Menopause

All women who are going to have procedures or treatment that are likely to mean that they will have a menopause before the age of 51 should have access to counselling because of the impact on their future and long-term health, in addition to fertility status and the implications of this [44, 49].

10.14.3 Fertility and POI

Women with POI often have questions relating to fertility. These can be managed within the specialist clinic with a fertility specialist if available or by referral to a fertility clinic [5]. There is a spontaneous pregnancy rate of 5–10%, which is often quoted to women, even when they have high FSH and low AMH [44]. This is often because they have some ovulation, which is partly why the term has been changed from failure to insufficiency, in addition to the negative connotations for the women of the word failure.

There are currently no treatments that can increase ovarian activity and increase conception rates; therefore, the main fertility option is ovum donation [44]. The other options are surrogacy and adoption. Currently, within the NHS there is limited or no funding for these women who require fertility help.

In contrast, as there is a spontaneous conception rate within this group of women, an assessment should be made of the fertility needs and if a woman does not want to become pregnant then she needs to ensure that she is using adequate contraception and not relying on her diagnosis [44, 47]. This can be any suitable form of contraception taking into consideration her medical history. The IUS (Mirena) is the only licenced progestogen-only contraceptive that can also be used as part of HRT [26]; otherwise contraception would be used in addition to or in place of, for example, the combined oral contraceptive pill.

Women who have a diagnosis of cancer who are likely to become menopausal because of the treatments should discuss this and a referral to a fertility clinic should be made to explore the possibilities before treatment starts [49]. Cancer patients should discuss fertility options before any treatment that may have an impact on future fertility. These options may be egg/sperm freezing or freezing of fertilised gametes (see Chap. 6) [50].

10.14.4 Long-Term Consequences

As women with POI are at risk of a reduced life expectancy [44–46], this is mainly due to cardiovascular disease; therefore, in addition to HRT, women would be advised to reduce these risks by cessation of smoking, regular exercise and maintaining a healthy weight and good diet. HRT is cardio-protective in this group and should be given until the natural age of menopause. Blood pressure, weight and smoking should be monitored annually, with additional tests for women with Turner syndrome. This helps not only the CVD, but bone health as well.

- Bone health—POI is linked to low bone mineral density and this may be related to an increased fracture rate later in life, but there is limited evidence for this currently [45]. Women with POI should be advised on bone health and have a healthy lifestyle, weight-bearing exercises, stop smoking and have a normal BMI. In addition, there should be a balanced diet with calcium and vitamin D, or a supplement if the diet is insufficient [44, 46, 47].
- Hormone replacement therapy is best for maintaining bones and prevention of osteoporosis in this group of women and the combined oral contraceptive pill (COCP) can be used, but it may be less effective. As before, this needs to be balanced with the need and the wishes of the woman [47]. Medications such as bisphosphonates could be given with guidance or under a specialist osteoporosis team. DEXA scans should be a baseline in all women. The need for repeat is dictated by treatment and the baseline value.
- General well-being—women diagnosed with POI have a reduced quality of life and psychological wellbeing and interventions can be used if needed, such as CBT [46].
- Sexual function—it should be standard to ask all women with menopause, and not just POI, questions about sexual function. Women do not often volunteer this information and wait for it to be brought up by a health care provider. The baseline in managing any issues should be adequate oestrogen replacement, both systemic and local. Once this is established, then women may need to use testos-

terone replacement as well, especially in surgical menopause, but this is generally off-licence and the long-term safety effects are not yet known [5, 46, 47]. If the only symptoms is vaginal dryness, then local oestrogen can be used in addition to advice on lubricants [5].
• Cognitive function—there is a detrimental effect of cognition in women with POI and this should be discussed with women before risk-reducing surgery. In women with POI, the risk can be reduced by oestrogen replacement.

10.14.5 Sources of Information

Often, women in this age group may have difficulty accessing accurate information about the use of HRT and need to be reminded. The health care providers that publish the studies do not include this age group; thus, the risks do not apply and as far as is currently known, there is no increased risk of cancer in this group related to HRT until they take it once they reach the age of natural menopause [47]. A good source of information for these women are support groups and charities such as the Daisy Network [51].

10.14.6 Treatment

Women with POI may need to have off-licence dosage of oestrogens to control symptoms and for the maintenance of bones. This may mean that they take 100–150 μg via a patch or 4 mg of an oral preparation [46]. This would be managed by a specialist [5].

Once diagnosed, then treatment should be offered, for symptoms, and for long-term health benefits such as CVD prevention and bone protection. There is an ongoing debate about HRT versus COCP, especially if contraception is not needed. In some small studies, HRT plays a more protective role in bone and CVD than the COCP [47]. However, this normally depends on the woman's choice.

Hormone replacement therapy is indicated for women with POI for symptoms and long-term health benefits. In this age group, no increased risk of breast cancer from HRT before the natural age of menopause has been found. As with all HRT, progestogen should be given if the uterus is in situ and the route and method of administration of HRT should be individual. Once established on HRT, after an initial 3-month review, women should have an annual review, looking at symptoms, compliance and any health changes. No specific tests are required.

Once started on a treatment, or if a woman is not on treatment, she needs to be monitored by DEXA at regular intervals, or if she needs advice on bones, diet (calcium and vitamin D) and exercise, she can obtain this.

Women with POI should be kept under review until the age of at least 51–52, when symptoms, bones and medical history can be assessed in line with the general menopause population and a decision can be made as to how long and if they want to continue on HRT.

Women who cannot take HRT can be managed with lifestyle and diet changes, and sometimes bisphosphonates can be given for bones in addition to the prescribed alternatives outlined in the section above.

Risk-reducing surgery—women with BRCA are increasingly undergoing risk-reducing surgery and this group of women may constitute a large cohort of a menopause clinic. In general, if they have had breast cancer, then HRT is normally contraindicated. If not, and they have had risk-reducing surgery, then they should be encouraged to use HRT, being aware that the uterus is normally left in situ; thus, combined HRT or an IUS is needed.

Women often ask about the role of alternative or complementary medicine in the treatment and management of POI. In general they are not recommended in this group, as treatment is needed for the prevention of the long-term consequences and not just the symptoms; there are no data to support their role in this.

10.15 Nurses and Their Role in Menopause

Nurses are in a prime position to be seeing and advising women during the menopause. Within the NICE guidance, women with specialist conditions [5], such as cancer or previous venous thromboembolism, need to be referred to specialist services. There is, however, no definition of a specialist; therefore, the British Menopause Society (BMS) has published such a definition [52]. There is no distinction between medical and nurse specialist and the RCN have developed guidance for nurses who wish to become specialised nurses in the menopause, which builds on the BMS definition and encompasses the four pillars of advanced practice [6].

In addition to being specialist, any nurse at any level should be able to direct women to appropriate sources of evidence and help. For example, in the UK, women should be directed to the Daisy Network (for POI), the Royal College of Obstetricians and Gynaecologists menopause hub, "Menopause Matters" and "Manage My Menopause", the BMS and "Women's Health Concern". The role of the nurse in relation to menopause care is developing. The Royal College of Nursing (RCN; 2017) document Nurse Specialist in the Menopause [6] has outlined how the role of the nurse can develop within the field of menopause care. It identified that there is a need for the nurse specialist in the menopause to lead and develop specialist menopause services and outlined the educational requirements and clinical skills needed to be able to take on the role [6]. Menopause services are currently ad hoc, with limited availability across the UK. In Wales, there are only two specialist menopause clinics [53] and in England there are currently no commissioned services for women with symptoms of the menopause; however, the specialist service requirements are likely to change this [6]. A nurse specialist in the menopause would be expected to have a range of skills and knowledge, including:

- An expert knowledge of the menopause, including all treatment options.
- At least 100 patients per year, including 50 new referrals.

- Independent consultations, including detailed assessments, ordering appropriate investigations and referring on as necessary.
- Independent prescribing.
- Master's level education, with Master's level problem-solving and critical thinking.

Women should be referred for secondary/specialist menopause care when there is poor symptom control, persistent side-effects, or a complex medical history such as venous thromboembolism or hormone-dependent cancer. Depending upon local agreements, women should be referred for ultrasound assessment and/or gynaecology with the following bleeding problems: if there is an increase in the heaviness or duration of bleeding, or if bleeding is irregular with sequential HRT; if bleeding for longer than 6 months after initially starting HRT or bleeding after a period of amenorrhoea when taking continuous combined HRT.

References

1. Djahanbakhch O, Ezzati M, Zosmer A (2007) Reproductive aging in women. J Pathol 211:219–231
2. Al-Azzawi F, Palacios S (2009) Hormonal changes during menopause. Maturitas 63:135–137
3. O'Neill S, Eden J (2017) The pathophysiology of menopausal symptoms. Obstet Gynaecol Reprod Med 27(10):303–310
4. Hillard T, Abernethy K, Hamoda H, Shaw I, Everett M, Ayres J, Currie H (2017) Management of the menopause, 6th edn. British Menopause Society, London
5. National Institute of Health and Care Excellence (2015) Menopause: diagnosis and management: Clinical guideline NG23. NICE, London
6. Royal College of Nursing (2017) Nurse specialist in menopause. RCN, London
7. Noble N (2018) Symptom management in women undergoing the menopause. Nurs Stand 32(22):53–62
8. Royal College of Nursing (2017) Menopause: RCN guidance for nurses, midwives and health visitors. RCN, London
9. Singer D (2004) Counselling and stress management. In: Rees M, Mander T (eds) Managing the menopause without oestrogen. The Royal Society of Medicine Press Limited, London, pp 91–95
10. Simpson PD, Morris EP (2015) Is it possible to manage the symptoms of the menopause without oestrogen. Womens Health (Lond) 11(4):429–431
11. Avis N, Greendale G (2015) Duration of menopausal vasomotor symptoms over the menopause transition. JAMA Intern Med 175:539–531
12. Freedman RR (2014) Menopausal hot flashes: mechanisms, endocrinology, treatment. J Steroid Biochem Mol Biol 142:115–120
13. Nelson HD (2004) Commonly used types of postmenopausal oestrogen for treatment of hot flashes, scientific review. JAMA 291(13):1610–1620
14. Godfrey JR, Low Dog T (2008) Toward optimal health: menopause as a rite of passage. J Women's Health 17(4):509–514
15. Thurston R (2018) Vasomotor symptoms; natural history, physiology and links with cardiovascular health. Climacteric 21(2):96–100
16. Rani S (2009) The psychosexual implications of menopause. Br J Nurs 18(6):370–373

17. Gandhi J, Che A, Dagur G, Suh Y, Smith N, Cali B, Ali Khan S (2016) Genitourinary syndrome of menopause: an overview of clinical manifestations, pathophysiology, aetiology, evaluation and management. Am J Obstet Gynecol 215(6):704–711
18. Primary Care Women's Health Forum (2017) Guidelines on diagnosis and management of urogenital atrophy or genitourinary syndrome of the menopause (GSM). PCWHF, Letchworth Garden City
19. Edwards D, Panay N (2015) Treating vulvovaginal atrophy/genitourinary syndrome of menopause: how important is lubricant and moisturiser composition? Climacteric 19(2):151–161. https://doi.org/10.3109/13697137.2015.1124259
20. Abernathy K (2015) Making sense of hormone replacement therapy. Nurs Prescrib 13(9):452–456
21. Palacios S, Cancelo MJ (2016) Clinical update on the use of ospemifene in the treatment of severe symptomatic vulvar and vaginal atrophy. Int J Women's Health 8:617–626
22. Stuenkel CA, Santen RJ (2016) An introduction to the Endocrine Society Clinical Practice guideline on treatment of symptoms of the menopause. Post Reprod Health 22(1):6–8
23. Holloway D (2017) Managing women's health in the menopause. Nurs Pract. www.nursingin-practice.com/article/managing-women's-health-menopause. Accessed 2 Dec 2017
24. Department of Health (2016) UK chief medical officers' low risk drinking guidelines. DOH, London
25. Lindh-Astrand L, Nedstrand E, Wyon Y, Hammar M (2004) Vasomotor symptoms and quality of life in previously sedentary women randomised to physical activity or oestrogen therapy. Maturitas 48(2):97–105
26. FSRH (2017) Contraception for women aged over 40 years. FSRH, London
27. Voican A, Francou B, Novac L, Chabbert-Buffet N, Canonico M, Meduri G, Lombes M, Scarabin P, Young J, Guiochon-Mantel A, Bouligand J (2012) Pharmacology of hormone replacement therapy in menopause. In: Gallelli L (ed) Pharmacology. Intech, Rijeka, pp 313–338
28. Hickey M, Elliot J, Davidson SL (2012) Hormone replacement therapy. BMJ 244:763
29. Joint Formulary Committee (2017) British national formulary, 74th edn. British Medical Association and Royal Pharmaceutical Society of Great Britain, London
30. Maclaran K, Panay N (2012) The safety of postmenopausal testosterone therapy. Women's Health 8(3):263–275
31. Hennefer D, Lawson E (2009) The safety of postmenopausal testosterone therapy Kate Maclaran12. Nick Panay1 Women's Health. 8(3):263–275. First Published May 1, 2012
32. Harman S, Vittinghoff E, Brinton E et al (2011) Timing and duration of menopausal hormone treatment may affect cardiovascular outcomes. Am J Med 124(3):199–205
33. Shaw I (2016) Menopause – guidance on management and prescribing HRT for GPs based on NICE guidance 2015. Accessed 28 Jul 2017
34. Files JA, Mayer AP, Sandya P (2012) Anything goes: discontinuation of hormone therapy. J Women's Health 21(5):567–568
35. Woyka J (2017) Consensus statement for non-hormonal-based treatments for menopausal symptoms. Post Reprod Health 23(2):71–75
36. Holloway D (2017) Update on non-hormonal treatment options during the menopause. Nurs Prescrib 15(1):28–32
37. European Medicines Agency (2015) Summary of product characteristics Ospemifene http://www.ema.europa.eu/ema/index.jsp?curl=pages/medicines/human/medicines/002780/human_med_001837.jsp&mid=WC0b01ac058001d124. Accessed 12 July 2018
38. Hunter M, Smith M (2017) Cognitive behaviour therapy (CBT) for menopausal symptom. Post Reprod Health 23(2):77–82
39. Mann E, Smith MJ, Hellier J, Balabanovic JA, Hamed H, Grunfeld EA, Hunter MS (2012) Cognitive behavioural therapy for women who have menopausal symptoms after breast cancer treatment (MENOS): a randomised control trial. Lancet Oncol 13(3):309–318
40. Simpson P, Currie H, Morris E (2018) Neurokinin 3 receptor antagonism – is this the end of HRT? Post Reprod Health 24(2):61–62

41. Bateson D, McNamee K (2017) Perimenopausal contraception: a practice based approach. Aust Fam Physician 46(6):372–377
42. Mikkola TS, Savolainen-Peltonen N, Yikorakal O (2017) New evidence for the cardiac benefit of postmenopausal therapy. Climacteric 20:15–20
43. National Institute of Health and Care Excellence (2012) Osteoporosis: assessing the risk of fragility fracture: clinical Guideline CG146. NICE, London
44. European Society for Human Reproduction and Embryology. https://www.eshre.eu/Guidelines-and-Legal/Guidelines/Management-of-premature-ovarian-insufficiency.aspx. Accessed 1 July 2016
45. Faubion S, Kuble C et al (2015) Long term health consequences of premature or early menopause and considerations for management. Climacteric 18:483–491
46. Maclaran K, Panay N (2015) Current concepts in premature ovarian insufficiency. Womens Health 11(2):169–182
47. Hamoda H (2017) The British Menopause Society and women's health concern recommendations on the management of women with premature ovarian insufficiency. Post Reprod Health 23(1):22–35
48. Chang SH, Kim CS, Lee KS et al (2007) Premenopausal factors influencing premature failure and early menopause. Maturitas 58:19–30
49. National Institute for Health and Care Excellence. https://www.nice.org.uk/guidance/qs143/chapter/Quality-statements
50. https://www.rcn.org.uk/professional-development/publications/pub-005986
51. https://www.daisynetwork.org.uk/
52. https://thebms.org.uk/menopause-specialists/overview/
53. BBC (2018) Menopause: lack of specialist care 'limits treatments'. https://www.bbc.co.uk/news/uk-wales-44860468. Accessed 18 Jul 2018

Suggested Reading

Nurses

Faculty of Reproductive and sexual healthcare www.frsh.org.uk
Royal college of Nursing Women's Health forum www.rcn.org.uk/get-involved/forums/womens-health-forum
The British Menopause Society www.bms.org.uk

Patients

Daisy network
Manage my menopause
Menopause matters
Women's Health Concern www.womens-health-concern.org

Urogynaecology

11

Ellie Stewart

11.1 Introduction

This chapter will detail the role of the urogynaecology nurse. It will detail the importance of their role, the treatments they can offer and useful information to those in or starting in the role.

11.2 The Role of the Clinical Nurse Specialist in Urogynaecology

The clinical nurse specialist (CNS) in urogynaecology provides the mainstay of treatment for women presenting with pelvic floor dysfunction and bladder symptoms. They advise on conservative treatments, fit and change pessaries, teach intermittent catheterisation, perform urodynamic investigations and help to support the medical team. There are no specific urogynaecology courses, but there are continence courses available and some excellent resources to read such as the NICE guidelines [5], Minimum Standards for Continence Care in the UK [1] and the ICI guidelines. Urogynaecology CNSs often form close links with their local urology and colorectal nurse specialists who will be able to provide support and clinical supervision to assist with the continuous development of their skills. Women's health physiotherapists are also a useful resource

E. Stewart (✉)
West Suffolk NHS Foundation Trust, Bury Saint Edmunds, UK
e-mail: Ellie.Stewart@wsh.nhs.uk

© Springer Nature Switzerland AG 2019
D. Holloway (ed.), *Nursing Management of Women's Health*,
https://doi.org/10.1007/978-3-030-16115-6_11

for advice on more complex pelvic floor treatments such as biofeedback and electrical stimulation, although some urogynaecology CNSs may do this too. With multidisciplinary working becoming more important and prevalent, most hospitals will have specialist pelvic floor multidisciplinary teams (MDTs), usually consisting of urogynaecologists, urologists and colorectal surgeons with physiotherapists, clinical scientists and CNSs from each discipline who meet regularly to discuss and plan care for women with more complex pelvic floor dysfunction.

Many more nurses are becoming nurse prescribers. This is an excellent skill to have as a urogynaecology CNS as it allows more advanced practice and prevents having to write to the GP to suggest a new medication or medication change/ review. Medications can be started earlier, which will hopefully help to treat the symptoms that are being experienced, and more holistic care can be provided by the CNS.

11.3 QOL Issues

Female urinary incontinence is a very common problem amongst women of all different ages. Many women don't report their symptoms or seek help because of perceptions that urinary incontinence is an inevitable consequence of ageing [1] and they have low expectations of successful treatment. They also feel embarrassed to admit that they are having symptoms and try to cope with them for as long as possible.

The reported prevalence of urinary incontinence varies between 6% and 69% in women [2]. The EPIC study [3] found that 66.6% of women aged over 40 years suffered with at least one lower urinary tract (LUT) symptom. Seeking help is associated with symptom bother and severity [4], so the more symptoms someone has, the higher the chance of them presenting to the GP with their symptoms.

11.4 Definition of Types of Incontinence

There are a number of different types of incontinence which women presenting in the urogynaecology clinic will be experiencing. Table 11.1 defines these different types according to the ICS-IUGA joint terminology report [6].

It is vital that the correct diagnosis is made during the assessment period to ensure that women receive the most appropriate advice and treatments. To do this effectively, the assessor needs to have a good understanding of all types of female urinary incontinence, conservative treatments available and when to refer to a specialist [7] and also be experienced [8].

Table 11.1 Definitions of types of female urinary incontinence

Stress urinary incontinence	The complaint of involuntary leakage upon effort or exertion or upon sneezing or coughing
Urge urinary incontinence	The complaint of involuntary leakage of urine associated with urgency
Functional incontinence	Urinary incontinence where no organic cause can be found: may be due to cognitive and physical factors
Mixed urinary incontinence	The complaint of involuntary leakage associated with urgency and also with exertion, effort, sneezing or coughing
Overflow incontinence	The involuntary leakage of urine associated with poor bladder emptying
Nocturnal enuresis	The complaint of loss of urine during sleep
Postural urinary incontinence	The complaint of involuntary loss of urine associated with change of body position
Insensible urinary incontinence	The complaint of urinary incontinence where the woman has been unaware of how it occurred
Coital incontinence	The complaint of involuntary loss of urine with coitus; this can be further divided into that occurring with penetration or with orgasm

11.5 Important Things to Discuss When Undertaking a Continence Assessment

11.5.1 Do Their Current Symptoms Affect Quality of Life (QOL)?

Urinary incontinence is often extremely QOL limiting. Patients can easily become depressed, suffer with sexual dysfunction and loss of respect, have low self-esteem and incur extra expenses due to the cost of managing their problem [9] such as buying pads, taking time off work and increased laundry. Women often 'cope' with their symptoms for long periods of time because they are too embarrassed to discuss things with their GPs or are unaware that anything can be done and that incontinence is an 'inevitable outcome of getting older'. When they do present for help, symptoms are often quite severe and difficult to tackle initially, but do respond well when the advice given is taken on board.

11.5.2 How Bothersome Is the Problem?

Different symptoms will bother different people in different ways. One of the most important things to ascertain during the assessment is which problem is the most bothersome for them. For example, it may not be the fact that a woman is going to the toilet every hour in the daytime that bothers her the most, but that she is up five times a night so isn't getting adequate sleep for her to do her job safely. It is essential to find out what the most bothersome problem is because if this can be addressed and realistic goals and expectations set, then she may be more likely to comply with any treatment plans that are suggested for her.

11.5.3 Red Flags

It is essential that the CNS assessing a woman's continence needs is aware of the red flags and knows who to refer to and how to refer onward if any are noted. Onward referral to the appropriate secondary care specialist should be initiated immediately if any of the following red flags are detected during the assessment [1, 5]. Examples of such red flags are in Table 11.2.

11.5.4 Drug History

It is essential to review the patients' current medications during the assessment. Many common medications can exacerbate urinary symptoms. During the assessment it is important to find out whether any such medications are being taken by the patient [10] and refer the patient to their GP or urogynaecologist to consider alternatives or consider stopping them if the CNS isn't a nurse prescriber. Table 11.3 details some of the most common drugs affecting continence.

11.5.5 Obstetric and Gynaecological History

The number of births, type of delivery, tears and whether the deliveries were instrumented all have an impact on the pelvic floor [11] and consequently bladder symptoms. Women often report problems with their bladder following a hysterectomy or a vaginal repair, so it is important to know what gynaecological surgery someone has had.

Table 11.2 Red flags requiring referral to secondary care services

Microscopic haematuria in women over 50 years
Visible haematuria
Previous pelvic cancers or suspected malignancy Persistent bladder or urethral pain
Clinically benign pelvic masses
Voiding difficulties
Suspected urogenital fistula
Recurrent urinary tract infections
Previous continence surgery
Previous pelvic cancer surgery or radiation therapy
Suspected neurological disease
Associated faecal incontinence
Symptomatic urogenital prolapse
Failure of conservative management
Complex symptoms such as a combination of storage and voiding symptoms

Adapted from NICE [5]

Table 11.3 Common drug types affecting continence

Drug name/type	Effect on continence	Examples
Alpha-adrenergic agonists	Contract the bladder neck causing retention and overflow incontinence	Methyldopa
Antipsychotics	Cause stress incontinence	Haloperidol, chlorpromazine
Antidepressants	Retention and overflow incontinence	Amitriptyline, imipramine
Diuretics	Increase urinary frequency, urgency, urge incontinence	Bendroflumethiazide
Calcium channel blockers	Decrease smooth muscle contractility in the bladder causing retention and constipation	Amlodipine, nifedipine, diltiazem
ACE inhibitors	By blocking the angiotensin receptors in the bladder, decreases detrusor contractility and urethral tone which can improve urge incontinence but increase stress incontinence	Enalapril, captopril, lisinopril, ramipril
Opiates	Cause constipation and urinary retention by inhibiting bladder contractions, sedation, faecal impaction and delirium	Codeine, morphine, oxycodone
Anticholinergics	Urinary retention—postvoid dribbling, straining, hesitancy, overflow incontinence	Oxybutynin, tolterodine, solifenacin
Non-steroidal anti-inflammatory	Urinary retention in the elderly	Diclofenac, ibuprofen, naproxen
Laxatives	Faecal incontinence, bloating	Lactulose, senna, bisacodyl, castor oil

11.5.6 Questionnaires

Questionnaires can be used during the assessment phase as they assess how patients view their symptoms [12] and QOL. They can be used to help with feedback and evaluate any progress made as well as to gain lots of information about their current symptoms. Common questionnaires used when assessing female urinary incontinence are the Kings Health Questionnaire, ICIQ-OAB, I-QOL and ICIQ.

11.6   Investigations Following the Verbal Assessment

There are a number of basic tests which should be performed as part of the assessment. These can all be performed during the initial assessment [5].

Urinalysis: This should be performed for all women undergoing a continence assessment. It is a reliable indicator of a urinary tract infection [13]. Urinalysis can also detect any haematuria which is a red flag indication for onward referral. Any infection should be treated and then the assessment repeated [14] to see if symptoms have changed. Overactive bladder (OAB) symptoms are very similar to the symptoms experienced with a urinary tract infection (UTI), so an infection should be excluded prior to treatment for an OAB.

Postvoid residuals show the assessor whether there are any issues or difficulties with voiding. Incomplete voiding can lead to urinary tract infections [13] and can be caused by chronic constipation. A PVR can be performed with an in and out

catheter or bladder scanner. Constipation, large fibroids, pregnancy, vaginal prolapse and previous continence surgery can cause problems with voiding which may
lead to recurrent UTIs, frequency and urgency. A simple technique which can be
taught to help empty the bladder fully is double voiding. This is where a woman is
advised to empty her bladder as normal, but then to tighten and relax her pelvic floor
muscles, rock to and fro, stand up and sit down and try to empty her bladder again.
Often this allows for any extra urine left in the bladder to be passed.

NICE guidance [5] suggests that *bladder diaries* should be completed for 3 days
as part of a thorough continence assessment. They can be a really useful tool for the
assessor. If completed correctly, a bladder diary will provide information about the
types and volumes of fluids ingested and the frequency of micturition [15] and also
the volumes passed which will be an indicator of bladder volume.

Unfortunately, bladder diaries are rarely completed fully or at all. They are difficult to complete and require a good understanding of what needs to be done, so
these may not be suitable for someone with learning difficulties or memory problems. If they are completed, then it shows that the woman is motivated and keen to
improve her symptoms and provides excellent feedback, enabling the CNS to give
pointers and suggestions on where and how to improve or reduce their oral intake.

Vaginal and rectal examination: The vagina should be observed for prolapse—
both anterior and posterior wall prolapse and uterine prolapse. The condition of
the skin in and around the vagina and perineum should be assessed. Many women
presenting with incontinence have incontinence-associated dermatitis or a sore
perineum due to wearing pads and continuous incontinence. Postmenopausal
women may also have atrophic vaginal tissues and complain of a dry, uncomfortable vagina and pain during sex. A cough test should be performed to test for
incontinence. This is done by asking the patient to cough whilst lying down to see
if there is any leakage of urine [16]. A digital examination can also be performed to
assess pelvic floor function and strength if the practitioner has been appropriately
trained.

The CNS should observe the anal area for skin tags, rectal prolapse and skin
condition [15]. Digital rectal examination will diagnose faecal loading or impaction
and also squeeze pressure.

11.7   Skills Needed by the Urogynaecology CNS for High-Quality Assessment

Good communication skills are paramount to obtain all of the important, most
relevant information required to provide the most appropriate treatments [1]. It is
essential that language which is easily understood is used and that technical, medical language is avoided. Try to think about the terms you use and avoid words such
as 'nocturia' or 'urge incontinence' when questioning the patient. Instead try and
use words or phrases which are easily understood such as 'how many times do you

get up to go to the toilet at night?' or 'do you leak on the way to the toilet if you don't make it in time?'. Try to use 'open-ended' questions to encourage the patient to provide useful information [6], instead of closed questions which are easy to answer but don't provide much useful information. You may also need to tailor the way you ask the questions and the language you use depending upon the age or understanding of the patient being assessed. For example, diagrams can be useful to help to explain what type of prolapse they have or what sort of pessaries can be used. Printed information should be given out for them to read once they are at home. This will remind them of what they need to do and will reinforce what you have said during the consultation.

It is important to remember that this may be the first time that the patient being assessed has opened up and discussed their problem at all, or in such detail, with anyone. They may be feeling worried or embarrassed, so it is the CNS's job to put them at ease and enable them to talk about things openly. In the same respect, it is important for the assessor to have an eye out for concerning body language—verbal or non-verbal—and an understanding of when to question further, when to stop questioning or when to be concerned about safeguarding issues. The body language of the assessor is just as important as the observation of the body language of the patient. A smile encourages people to feel relaxed, as does an open posture, nodding and positive response to comments that are made. The assessor needs to be empathetic and sensitive. Excellent interpersonal skills will enable a trusting relationship to be developed between the patient, carer and professional [17] which will increase compliance and hopefully symptom improvement.

11.8 Treatments

Conservative treatments are available for all bladder problems and can be instigated easily by the CNS. Table 11.4 details treatments suggested for each bladder diagnosis. Each will be discussed in more detail below.

Table 11.4 Conservative management of bladder problems

Problem	Conservative treatment
Stress incontinence	Pelvic floor exercises, vaginal cones, Squeezy app, electrical stimulation, Elvie trainer, intravaginal supports
Overactive bladder	Bladder retraining, pelvic floor exercises, fluid advice, medications
Voiding difficulties	Intermittent self-catheterisation, double voiding, constipation prevention advice
Functional incontinence	OT referral for commodes or aids to help with toileting, clothes with elasticated waists or Velcro
Mixed incontinence	Pelvic floor exercises, bladder retraining, fluid advice, constipation management, medications

11.8.1 Treatments for Stress Incontinence

Pelvic floor exercises (pfe): NICE [5] recommends that supervised pelvic floor exercises should be undertaken for at least 3 months. Pelvic floor exercises are an effective way of strengthening the pelvic floor muscle and improving bladder symptoms. NICE [5] suggests that women should perform at least eight contractions three times a day to notice an improvement in symptoms. Women whose symptoms don't improve following a course of pfe should be referred back to the urogynaecologist for further management options [14].

Vaginal cones can be used instead of, or to augment, pelvic floor exercises; however, there is no difference demonstrated in the current literature, in the success rates the literature in the success rates between the use of vaginal cones and pfe alone [18]. 'Squeezy' (squeezyapp.com) is an app designed to motivate and remind women to do their pfe regularly. It is downloaded on to an android phone and programmed to remind women when to do their exercises each day. Whitehouse et al. [19] suggest that women who are motivated and get regular feedback are more likely to continue with their exercise programme and notice an improvement in their symptoms and a reduction in incontinence episodes.

Elvie (Fig. 11.1) is a device which can be synched to a mobile phone. It is inserted into the vagina, and when it is squeezed, a biofeedback mechanism is activated so that women can see how hard they are squeezing their muscles and how long for.

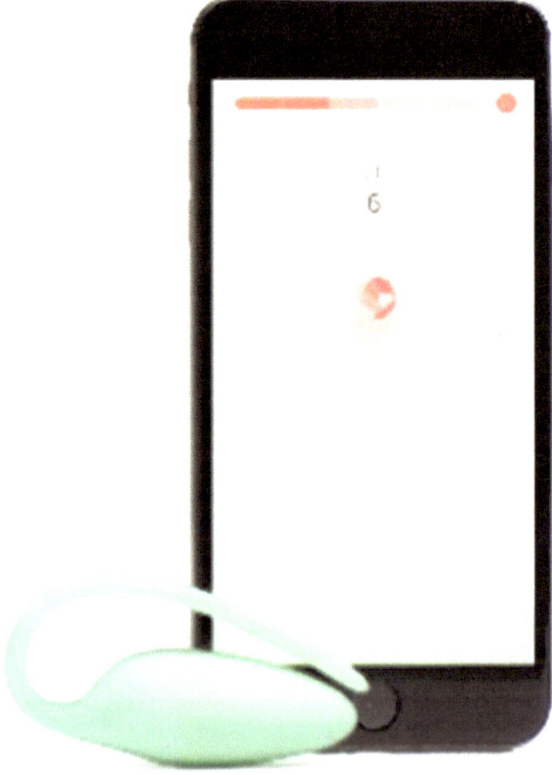

Fig. 11.1 Elvie pelvic floor trainer (I have permission to use this image from the company)

There are programmes and 'workouts' which can be followed to encourage regular use and exercising of the muscle. This helps to motivate women which encourages compliance and a want to do the exercises more regularly to improve. This device will be available on the NHS from August 2018.

Intravaginal devices to support the bladder neck have become more popular since the suspension of mesh surgery as a way of treating those with stress incontinence. There are a number of new devices on the market. They are inserted into the vagina and support the bladder neck, reducing the leakage. See Fig. 11.2 for some available in the UK. They can be a useful adjunct for those who are working on their exercises and strengthening their pelvic floor muscle or those who don't want to consider surgical management at that time. Unfortunately, they aren't always available on the NHS so women often need to buy them if they want to use them.

Electrical stimulation can be used in women with little or no pelvic floor contraction to help to 'teach' them to recognise how a correct pelvic floor muscle contraction feels. Some women are unable to contract their pelvic floor muscles, so this is a good way to help motivate them. Often if women are unable to feel a contraction, they lose motivation quickly as they don't notice any improvement in their symptoms. Electrical stimulation machines can be bought by the patient. In some departments they are loaned to the patient for a specific amount of time so that they can use them at home. Other departments provide the machine for the patient to use in the hospital.

Weight loss: Obesity is a significant adjustable and reversible risk factor for stress incontinence [20]. Subak et al. [21] suggest that moderate weight loss may

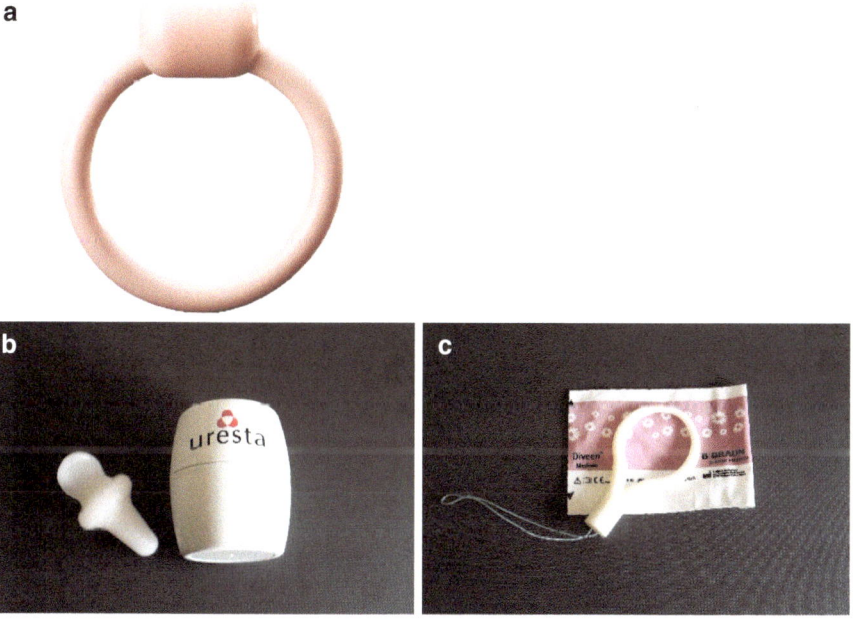

Fig. 11.2 Newer support devices. (**a**) Mediplus Incontinence Ring Courtesy of Mediplus LTD. (**b**) Uresta intravaginal device iMEDicare. (**c**) Diveen intravaginal device B Braun

decrease episodes of urinary incontinence. Women should be supported in their attempt to lose weight and need to understand the general health benefits as well as the potential reduction in their incontinence episodes.

Urodynamics are performed if conservative treatments don't improve a patient's symptoms sufficiently and they want to consider surgical management of their problem.

11.8.2 Overactive Bladder Treatments

Bladder retraining aims to increase the time in between trips to the toilet by getting the patient to 'hold on' when they need to go, whether this be for 30 s or 10 min. This will enable the person to take control of their bladder [16]. In time, this will also help to reduce any symptoms of frequency, urgency and nocturia.

Fluid advice: NICE [22] and Syan and Brucker [23] recommend a reduction in caffeine to improve overactive bladder symptoms. Citrus drinks, fizzy drinks and alcohol are also known bladder irritants [24]. These should be avoided or reduced to see if symptoms improve. Modification of a high or low oral intake should also be considered when looking at improving bladder symptoms [14]. If a patient suffers with nocturia, they should be advised to fluid restrict from earlier in the evening—such as 9 p.m.—to try and reduce these episodes.

Medications: These can be used if lifestyle changes are not effective. Anticholinergics are the most commonly used medications to help treat OAB symptoms of urgency, frequency, urge incontinence and nocturia. NICE suggests [22] that patients are offered the anticholinergic medication with the lowest acquisition cost to treat OAB symptoms or mixed UI in women, see table below.

Darifenacin
Fesoterodine
Oxybutynin (immediate release, extended release, transdermal, topical gel)
Propiverine (immediate release, extended release)
Solifenacin
Tolterodine (immediate release, extended release)
Trospium (immediate release, extended release) with a link to the current guideline

The most common side effects of antimuscarinics are constipation, blurred vision and dry mouth [25]. These potential side effects should be borne in mind when selecting the correct medication.

Pelvic floor exercises: A stronger pelvic floor will help to reduce the urinary frequency and urgency, so regular pelvic floor exercises will also help to improve OAB symptoms.

Suppression techniques: Encourage the patient to squeeze their pelvic floor muscle when they get the urge to go to the toilet. As the muscle strengthens, this will help to reduce the urgency and increase their control. Perineal pressure can also reduce the need to go to the toilet, so crossing their legs or pushing on their perineum (e.g. sitting on their heel, or a hard surface) can help reduce the urge. Also trying to distract themselves when they feel the need to go to the toilet can help to improve the urgency and frequency.

For those failing two or more medications and other conservative treatments listed above, urodynamic investigations should be performed. The treatments to be discussed following this would be botulinum toxin, sacral nerve stimulation (SNS) or percutaneous tibial nerve stimulation (PTNS).

Botulinum toxin (Botox) injections are available for those who have failed two antimuscarinics and conservative treatments and have urodynamically proven detrusor overactivity. Women are often taught intermittent self-catheterisation prior to having the injections as there is a risk of retention or incomplete voiding post-operatively. This will be taught by the nurse specialist. Some women find that they suffer with more frequent UTIs following botulinum toxin injections. The ICIq-OAB is a simple four-questioned questionnaire which can be used to assess the improvement to symptoms following the injections. Each unit will devise its own protocol for following up women post Botox, but they should have a urinalysis and postvoid residual assessment performed when they return to clinic.

Percutaneous tibial nerve stimulation and *sacral nerve stimulation* can also be offered for those failing conservative treatments for their OAB symptoms [22]. Patients requiring these more complex treatments will be discussed in multidisciplinary meetings following their urodynamic investigations, with urologists and clinicians with an interest in pelvic floor dysfunction as per NICE guidance [5]. They may need to be referred to specialist urogynaecology or urology units as not all departments offer these treatments.

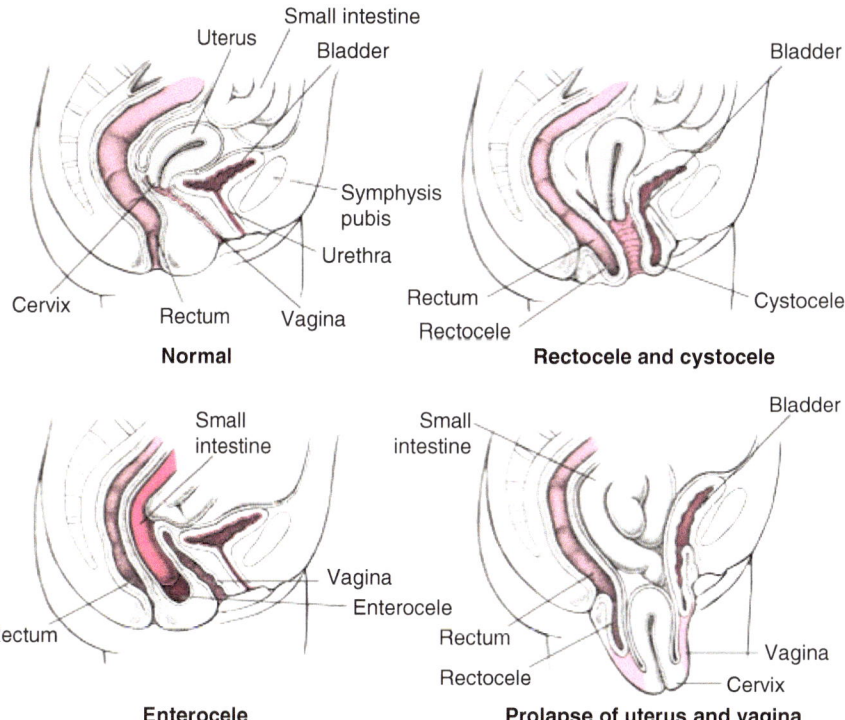

Fig. 11.3 Different types of pelvic organ prolapse

11.8.3 Vaginal Prolapse

There are five main types of pelvic organ prolapse (POP): cystocele, rectocele, uterine prolapse, vaginal vault prolapse and enterocele (see Fig. 11.3).

Pelvic organ prolapse is one of the most common medical disorders with one in two parous women suffering with urogenital prolapse. Thirty per cent of women who have had prolapse surgery will re-prolapse at some point following the repair so surgery should not necessarily be seen as a permenant solution to their problem and womens should be informed of the re-prolpse risk and rate. The only universally accepted risk factor for developing pelvic organ prolapse is age, with the risk of prolapse doubling with each completed decade. Straining to open bowels, obesity, childbirth (especially forceps deliveries), congenital collagen vascular disease such as Ehlers-Danlos, a chronic untreated cough and women whose mothers or sisters report a prolapse are at increased risk of developing a vaginal prolapse. Prolapse prevention advice should be given to women. Low-impact exercise should be advised; women should be advised on the importance of weight loss and the need to avoid heavy lifting if at all possible. They should be taught the correct position to sit on the toilet to avoid unnecessary straining when opening their bowels as this can worsen symptoms of POP. This can be seen in Fig. 11.4.

There are three main treatments for pelvic organ prolapse:

1. Pelvic floor exercises.
2. Vaginal pessary with pelvic floor exercises.
3. Surgery.

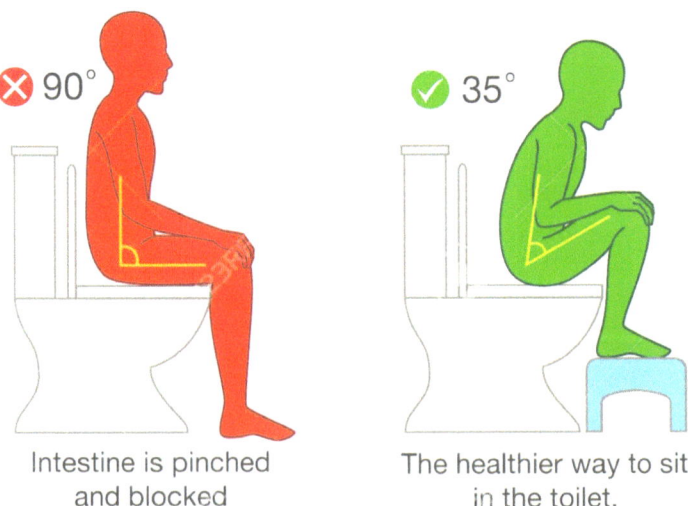

❌ 90°   ✓ 35°

Intestine is pinched   The healthier way to sit
and blocked   in the toilet.

Fig. 11.4 Correct toilet position

Pessaries can be used for those women awaiting surgery, those who are pregnant or who haven't finished their family or those who are unable to or chose not to have surgery. There are a number of different types of vaginal pessaries available to support vaginal prolapse (Fig. 11.5). They are used to support the prolapse and take away the feeling of heaviness which is often a main symptom in those presenting with a prolapse. Anantawat et al. [26] have shown that the use of a vaginal pessary for 6 months improves vaginal symptoms, quality of life and satisfaction in women with pelvic organ prolapse. Ring pessaries are the most commonly used pessaries. They are inserted into the vagina and should be changed every 4–6 months.

Pessaries can be inserted and managed by nurses in primary and secondary care. Training can be gained from the urogynaecology team in secondary care, and pessary-specific study days are available to attend. Companies producing pessaries often run study days to teach nurses about selecting, inserting and removing pessaries and how to manage complications. Figure 11.6 details the types of pessaries available and what they can be used for.

Vaginal pessaries should be changed every 4–6 months. Vaginal tissue quality and evidence of ulceration and bleeding should be checked using a speculum once the pessary has been removed. Nurses managing women with vaginal pessaries need to be aware to observe for or ask about vaginal bleeding. If this occurs in postmenopausal women, then they should be referred, on the cancer pathway, to the oncology team for assessment of the endometrial thickness and possible endometrial cancer.

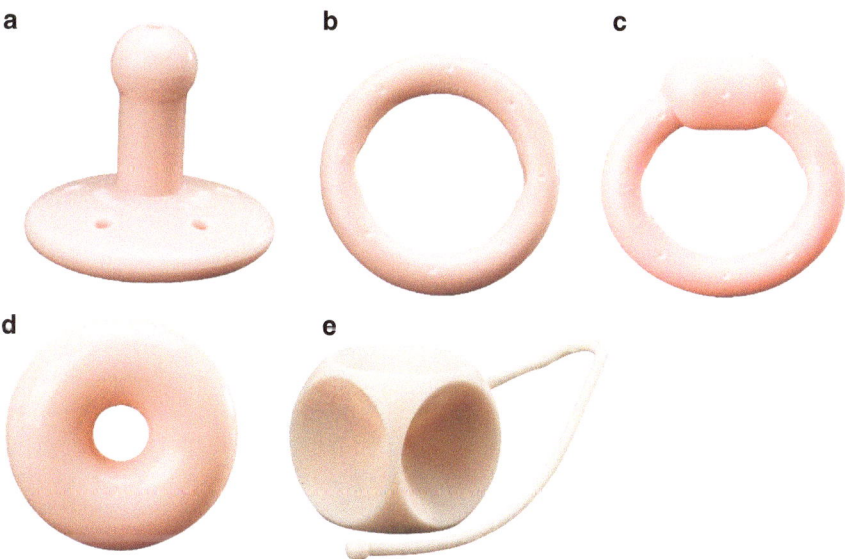

Fig. 11.5 Images of pessaries above courtesy of Mediplus LTD. (**a**) Mediplus Gellhorn pessary. (**b**) Mediplus ring pessary. (**c**) Mediplus ring with knob. (**d**) Mediplus donut pessary. (**e**) Mediplus cube pessary

PROLAPSE									
1-2nd Degree Uterine	2-3rd Degree Uterine	Sexually Active	Vaginal Vault	Stress Urinary Incontinence	Cystocele	Rectocele	Cervical Weakness	Retro Displacement	Most Commonly Used
									MEDIPLUS
	✓								POPY™
	✓								POPY™ SHORT STEM
									MILEX
✓		✓			✓				RING
✓		✓		MILD ✓					RING WITH SUPPORT
✓		✓	✓	MILD ✓	✓				SHAATZ
✓		✓		✓	✓				INCONTINENCE DISH
✓ ✓				MILD ✓					DISH WITH SUPPORT / HODGE WITH SUPPORT
	✓ ✓		✓ ✓	MILD ✓	✓				DONUT / GELLHORN (FLEX 95% RIGID)
	✓	✓		MILD ✓	MILD ✓				INFLATOBALL
	✓	✓	✓	✓	✓	MILD ✓			CUBE, TANDEM CUBE
✓	✓			✓	✓	MILD ✓			GEHRUNG
	✓			✓	✓	MILD ✓			GEHRUNG WITH KNOB
		✓ ✓		✓ ✓					INCONTINENCE RING / RING WITH KNOB
				✓ ✓					HODGE & HODGE WITH KNOB / HODGE WITH SUPPORT & KNOB
	✓	✓		✓	MILD ✓		✓	✓	SMITH, HODGE, RISSER
✓	✓	✓		✓	MILD ✓				RING WITH SUPPORT & KNOB

Fig. 11.6 Types of pessary and indications for use Courtesy of Mediplus LTD

The most common cause of vaginal bleeding for those with a vaginal pessary, in postmenopausal women, is atrophic vaginitis. This is when the tissues in the vagina lack oestrogen and as a result can become dry and thin and may bleed [27]. The movement of a pessary in the vagina, if the tissues are atrophic, may cause ulceration and bleeding. To prevent this or reduce the risk, women with a vaginal pessary are often started on a low-dose, topical vaginal oestrogen in the form of a vaginal tablet or cream [28]. If vaginal bleeding occurs and there is no suspicion of a thickened endometrium, i.e. they are still having periods or have had a hysterectomy, then the pessary should be left out and topical vaginal oestrogen used to help to heal the tissues. Ulceration in the vagina won't heal unless the pessary is left out for at least a month; this allows for the tissues to heal without the continuous rubbing of the tissues from the pessary.

Silicone pessaries, which are very easy to insert and remove and last for 5 years, can be used for self management by younger premenopausal women who don't need the condition of their vagina checking for ulceration and bleeding every 6 months. They can be shown how to insert and remove their pessaries as and when they want to. They should be advised that this should be at least once every 6 months, to clean them. Some women remove them to have sex; others use them for extra support and symptom relief if they know they will be spending a day on their feet or doing anything strenuous. Some women use them and don't remove them in between their routine removal and wash of the pessary. Some women don't find them as supportive as the plastic ones because they are slightly thinner. Premenopausal women don't need to attend for a face-to-face clinic follow-up but can manage their pessaries independently with a telephone follow-up every 6 months with the agreed understanding that they contact their health care professional if they do experience any abnormal bleeding, or have any problems or concerns.

11.9   Atrophic Vaginitis and Vaginal Oestrogens

Atrophic vaginitis is a common condition experienced by postmenopausal women [29]. These women frequently complain that their vagina feels dry, sore and uncomfortable. If questioned, postmenopausal women will regularly complain of inadequate lubrication during sex in spite of being turned on, and as a result they find sex uncomfortable or painful [27]. They then start to avoid it, which can put a strain on their relationship. It is essential for those being assessed to be questioned about their sex lives, especially if they are postmenopausal, as incontinence and atrophic vaginitis can both have a significant impact. Rantell [30] agrees with this saying that a third of women will not initiate discussion about their sexual issues with their doctor. Almost half of the women questioned for the REVIVE survey [31] stated that they had not discussed their vaginal symptoms with their healthcare professional and that 40% expected their assessor to initiate a conversation about menopausal symptoms.

Atrophy of the vaginal tissues can also lead to decreased strength in pelvic floor muscles and urge incontinence [7]. Oestrogen helps to maintain normal structure and function of the urogenital tissue. NICE [22] however suggests that topical vaginal oestrogens aren't used as a first-line treatment for urinary incontinence but can be considered in postmenopausal women with OAB and vaginal atrophy.

Topical vaginal oestrogens can be given in the form or tablets (e.g. Vagifem) and cream (e.g. Ovestin) to re-oestrogenise the vaginal tissues. The tablets are less messy than the creams so are often preferred and should be used as a maintenance dose twice weekly. They can also be used together, for example, Vagifem can be inserted inside the vagina and a topical oestrogen cream used around the vulva if the vulval tissues are also dry, sticky and sore.

For those who don't want to use or can't use topical vaginal oestrogen (caution should be taken in women who have previously had breast cancer—advice should be sought from their oncologist), moisturisers and lubricants can be used. There are many moisturisers available on the market such as Yes, Hyalofemme and Sylk. They don't treat the atrophic tissues but can be inserted into the vagina to ease the dry and uncomfortable symptoms. Vaginal moisturisers are bio-adhesive so attach to mucin and epithelial cells on the vaginal wall to retain water. They can help balance vaginal pH and can be used on a long-term basis. Water- and oil-based moisturisers are available. They can be used frequently depending upon the severity of the dryness and should also be used regularly, rather than just with sex [32]. A selection should be given to patients for them to try at home.

11.9.1 Functional Incontinence

Functional incontinence is where someone is aware of the need to urinate, but for one or more physical or mental reasons, they are unable to get to a bathroom before being incontinent. This may be because they have arthritis or had a stroke or have many layers to remove or take down before they can sit on the toilet. Often an OT referral needs to be made to assess for suitability of aids which may make getting to the toilet easier, for example, a commode near the bed at night or a walking frame or something as simple as using Velcro or an elasticated waist instead of buttons or a zip.

Women with dementia may struggle to recognise the need to go to the toilet or may not remember where the toilet is or how to remove their clothes to enable them to go without being incontinent. *Timed voiding or prompted voiding* can be instigated for patients with dementia or Alzheimer's. They may benefit from regular verbal reminders to try and establish a routine which could help them to recognise the signs of needing to go to the toilet [33]. Morgan et al. [34] suggest that a personalised toileting programme (timed voiding) works well in pre-empting the need to go to the toilet. However, this type of intervention can be very labour-intensive. When prompted voiding is used, women should be reminded to go to the toilet, before an episode of incontinence occurs. Simple, recognisable signs can be put up to remind someone where the toilet is, or they can be taken to make sure that they get there without getting lost or hopefully without leaking. It is important to get carers and family involved when this type of management is suggested to ensure that everyone is working together to help to reduce incontinence episodes.

11.9.2 Voiding Difficulties

Some women find it difficult to empty their bladder properly. There are a number of causes for voiding difficulties including constipation, urinary tract infections (UTI), fibroids, pelvic organ prolapse, multiple sclerosis and pregnancy. Prior to investigation, assess for and treat any constipation and UTIs, and see if the voiding issues resolve. A postvoid residual should be obtained if improvement isn't noted to assess the volume being retained. This can be done with a bladder scanner or an in and out catheter.

It is advisable to teach the patient how to 'double void' to make sure that they are emptying their bladder as fully as they can. This involves asking them to empty their bladder normally, then to stand up, sit back down, rock forward and backward, squeeze their pelvic floor muscle and try to go again. It is important that they don't strain to push the urine out as this can worsen any prolapse.

Women who are unable to empty their bladder properly will be advised of the need to learn intermittent self-catheterisation (ISC) to ensure that any residual is removed. This will help to reduce urinary tract infections and may also improve other symptoms, such as frequency and nocturia, as the bladder is emptied fully. The frequency of the ISC will depend upon the residual volume. Video urodynamic investigations can be performed to check for any other causes of the voiding issues.

11.10 Links with Maternity Colleagues

Close links with the maternity teams and midwives should be established to try and ensure that women who are labouring or those who are post-partum are looked after with regard to their bladder function. The risk of urinary retention intra- or

Table 11.5 Signs and symptoms of retention to warn post-natal women about or following catheter removal

Signs and symptoms of urinary retention
Frequency
Urgency
Incomplete voiding
Inability to pass urine at all
Pain in the bladder

post-partum increases with primiparity, instrumented delivery, epidural analgesia, prolonged labour and perineal trauma [35]. Women should be encouraged to go to the toilet regularly during labour and the volume documented in the notes. They should pass urine within 4–6 h of delivery [35].

A local guideline should be written to ensure that bladders are being managed consistently by doctors and midwives. There are no national guidelines for this, so one needs to be written locally. There is a distinct lack of evidence about best practice for bladder management intra- and post-partum.

In most units, women are sent home for the bladder to rest for around a week if they go into retention of over a litre. Ideally to prevent this happening, women should have been given information explaining the importance of going to the toilet to empty their bladder postdelivery and what to do if they feel they aren't able to empty properly (see Table 11.5). Any bladder symptoms and the inability to empty fully should be assessed regularly during and after labour to prevent episodes of acute urinary retention and subsequent bladder damage. It is important to note that acute retention in the post-partum period can be painless, especially following epidural anaesthesia. There are many local guidelines on the Internet to compare when writing your own.

11.11 Specialist Investigations

11.11.1 Urodynamics

Urodynamic investigations are recommended to diagnose the type of incontinence [22, 36] if conservative management or previous surgical management has failed and surgical management is an option [23]. These are often performed independently by the urogynaecology CNS or in conjunction with members of the medical team.

There are three main types of urodynamics—simple urodynamics, video urodynamics (where X-rays are used to check bladder outline and reflux to the kidneys) and ambulatory urodynamics (where the patient is catheterised and asked to walk around and carry on their normal activities for 3–4 h to assess bladder function).

Catheters are inserted into the bladder and vagina/rectum which measure pressures in the bladder and abdomen as the bladder fills. The pressures are observed as the bladder fills. Detrusor overactivity and low compliance can be seen during this phase, the bladder capacity can be assessed and the sensations experienced as the bladder fills are noted. The woman is then asked to stand or sit and cough with a full bladder, to assess whether there is any stress incontinence. The aim of the test is to replicate their current bladder symptoms so that further treatments can be discussed.

It is essential that the nurse performing the urodynamic tests has attended a certified urodynamic course. There are courses available which last 3 days. They are held in Bristol, Manchester, London and Newcastle. Information on these courses can be found at www.ics.org and www.baus.org.uk.

Nurses often run urodynamic clinics independently or with support from medical colleagues.

11.12 Other Resources Useful to the Urogynaecology CNS

11.12.1 BSUG Accreditation

Most urogynaecology units are striving for accreditation or have already been accredited by the British Society of Urogynaecologists (BSUG). Details of the standards and objectives needed to achieve accreditation can be found on the BSUG website www.bsug.org.uk.

The BSUG website also has patient information leaflets for all urogynaecology surgery. The leaflets are endorsed by the society and are useful to hand out to those considering urogynaecological surgery.

11.12.2 Useful Websites and Relevant Associations

The International Urogynaecological Association (IUGA) is a good association to become a member of. They hold annual conferences and are in the process of developing a working stream for nurses and physiotherapists and other allied health professionals working within urogynaecology (www.iuga.org).

www.yourpelvicfloor.org is an excellent website which provides support and information for patients and healthcare professionals. Leaflets are available for download, there are videos to watch and it provides information on resources available—for example, pelvic floor apps to download to help with pelvic floor exercise compliance.

The Association for Continence Advice (ACA) is another group of nurses who have an interest in continence promotion. They run study days and conferences. It is a good resource to use for networking with colleagues working in incontinence and continence promotion. www.aca.uk.com, www.bladderhealthuk.org and www.bladderandbowel.org are other sites which provide useful information to professionals and patients on bladder issues. There is also a telephone helpline available for patients/professionals to ring for advice.

The British Association of Urological Nurses (BAUN) is designed for urology nurses, but as a lot of the urogynaecology CNS role links very closely with urology, this may be another society to be aware of/join. They have many guidelines relevant to the procedures and treatments which the CNS deals with too (www.baun.co.uk).

References

1. Rantell A, Dolan L, Bonner L, Knight S et al (2016a) Minimum standards for continence care in the UK. Neurourol Urodyn 35:400–406
2. Hunskaar S, Burgio K, Clark A, Lapitan MC, Nelson R, Sillen U, Thom D (2005) Epidemiology of urinary incontinence (UI) and faecal incontinence (FI) and pelvic organ prolapsed (POP). In: 3rd international consultation on incontinence. Basics and evaluation, vol 1. Health Publication Ltd, Plymouth, pp 255–312
3. Coyne K, Sexton C, Thompson C, Milsom I et al (2009) The prevalence of lower urinary tract symptoms (LUTS) in the USA, the UK and Sweden: results from the Epidemiology of LUTs (EpiLUTS) study. Br J Urol Int 104:352–360
4. Irwin D, Abrams P, Mislom I, Kopp Z et al (2008) Understanding the elements of overactive bladder: questions raised by the EPIC study. BJU Int 101:1381–1387
5. National Institute for Health and Care Excellence (2019) Urinary incontinence and pelvic organ prolapse in women: management. NICE guideline [NG123]. NICE, London
6. Haylen B, De Ridder D, Freeman R, Swift S et al (2010) An International Urogynaecological Association (IUGA)/International Continence Society (ICS) joint report on the terminology for female pelvic floor dysfunction. Int Urogynaecol J 21:5–26
7. Bardsley A (2016) An overview of urinary incontinence. Pract Nurs 8(11):537–545
8. Mc Clurg D, Jamieson K, Hagen S et al (2013) Improving continence education for nurses. Nurs Times 109(4):16–18
9. Yates A (2017) Incontinence and associated complications: is it avoidable? Nurs Prescrib 15(6):288–295
10. Harris A (2007) Assessing urinary incontinence in women. Nurs Times 103(26):50–53
11. Herbert J (2009) Pregnancy and childbirth: the effect on pelvic floor muscles. Nurs Times 105(7):38–41
12. Robinson D et al (2007) Outcome measures in urogynaecology: the clinicians' perspective. Int Urogynecol J 18:273–279
13. Davis C, Rantell A (2017) Lower urinary tract infections in women. Br J Nurs. https://doi.org/10.12968/bjon.2017.26.9.S12
14. Ostle Z (2016) Assessment, diagnosis and treatment of urinary incontinence in women. Br J Nurs 25(2):84–91
15. Nazarko L (2015) Person centred care of women with urinary incontinence. Nurs Prescrib 13(6):288–293
16. Rantell A (2017) Assessment and diagnosis of overactive bladder in women. Nurs Stand 27(52):35–40
17. Rantell A (2013) Assessment and diagnosis of overactive bladder in women. Nurs Stand 27(52):35–40
18. Haslam J (2008) Vaginal cones in stress incontinence treatment. Nurs Times 104(5):44–45
19. Whitehouse T (2012) Patient motivation in managing stress urinary incontinence. Nurs Times 108:18–20
20. Faiena I, Patel N, Parihar JS et al (2015) Conservative management of urinary incontinence in women. Rev Urol 17(3):129–139
21. Subak LL, Wing R, Smith West DS et al (2009) Weight loss to treat urinary incontinence in overweight and obese women. N Engl J Med 360(5):481–490
22. National Institute for Health and Care Excellence (2017) Urinary incontinence in women: management clinical guideline. nice.org.uk/guidance/cg171
23. Syan R, Brucker B (2016) Guidelines of guidelines: urinary incontinence. Br J Urol Int 117:20–33
24. Stewart E (2011) Prescribing antimuscarinics for women with an overactive bladder. Nurs Prescrib 9(2):82 87
25. Robinson D, Cardozo L (2012) Antimuscarinic drugs to treat overactive bladder. BMJ 344:e2130. https://doi.org/10.1136/bmj.e2130

26. Anantawat T, Manonai J, Wattanayingcharoenchai R et al (2016) Impact of a vaginal pessary on the quality of life in women with pelvic organ prolapse. Asian Biomed 10:249–252
27. Domoney C (2014) Treatment of vaginal atrophy. Womens Health 10(2):191–200
28. Bulchandani S, Tooz-Hobson P, Verghese T et al (2015) Does vaginal estrogen treatment with support pessaries in vaginal prolapse reduce complications? Post Reprod Health 21(4):141–145
29. MacBride M, Rhodes D, Shuster L (2010) Vulvovaginal atrophy. Mayo Clin Proc 85(1):87–94
30. Rantell A, Cardozo L, Khullar V (2017) Personal goals and expectations of OAB patients in the UK. Neurourol Urodyn 36:1194–1200
31. Wysocki S, Kingsberg S, Krychman M (2014) Management of vaginal atrophy: implications from the REVIVE study. Clin Med Insights Reprod Health 8:23–30. https://doi.org/10.4137/CMRH.S14498
32. Primary Care Womens Health Forum (2017) Guidance on diagnosis and management of genitourinary syndrome of the menopause (GSM). Primary Care Womens Health Forum, Hertfordshire
33. Price H (2011) Incontinence in patients with dementia. Br J Nurs 20(12):721–725
34. Morgan et al. 2008 cited by Price H (2011) Incontinence in patients with dementia. Br J Nurs 20(12):721–725
35. Kearney R, Cutner A (2008) Review: postpartum voiding dysfunction. Obstet Gynaecol 10:71–74
36. Thuuroff J, Abrams P, Andersson K, Artibani W et al (2011) 2011 EAU guidelines on urinary incontinence. Eur Assoc Urol 59(2011):387–400

Hannah Gamlen

Medical techniques and technological advances mean a growing number of gynaecological procedures historically performed under general anaesthetic in theatre are now done in an outpatient setting. One such example of this is outpatient hysteroscopy, which has been performed in the UK for some years now [1]. Development of flexible and rigid hysteroscopes with smaller diameters, and simplification of the procedure, means that it is best practice for hysteroscopy to be performed as an outpatient [2]. This is reflected in guidance from the RCOG [1] and in the best practice tariff set by Monitor [3]. Operative hysteroscopy is also becoming increasingly common, with new scopes and devices (bipolar electrodes and morcellators) enabling removal of polyps and fibroids and radiofrequency technology enabling endometrial ablation. In addition to appropriate training as can be seen from previous chapters, these outpatient developments put nurses in a prime position to see and manage the care of women within the outpatient setting.

12.1 Advantages for Patients

There are many advantages to procedures being performed in outpatients rather than in theatre under anaesthetic. For the patient, it can be more convenient as they can have their procedure done quickly, often in a 'one-stop' clinic model requiring just one appointment. This means less time spent in hospital and negates the requirement for an escort home and time off work for recovery that would be required after an anaesthetic [4]. To prepare for a general anaesthetic, most patients require an additional appointment for preoperative assessment to identify and manage risks for anaesthesia [5]. Some patients have comorbidities that greatly increase the risk

H. Gamlen (✉)
Guys and St Thomas NHS Foundation Trust, London, UK
e-mail: Hannah.Gamlen@gstt.nhs.uk

© Springer Nature Switzerland AG 2019
D. Holloway (ed.), *Nursing Management of Women's Health*,
https://doi.org/10.1007/978-3-030-16115-6_12

235

posed by a general anaesthetic, such as morbid obesity. For these patients, guidance states general anaesthesia should be avoided if possible [6]. Therefore, if it is possible to perform the procedure without a general anaesthetic, with the patient's consent, this should be attempted first.

12.2   Advantage for Service Providers

Procedures in outpatients are more time- and cost-efficient for a combination of reasons. Administering anaesthesia requires the presence of an anaesthetist and multiple trained support staff, as well as the surgeon [7]. Procedure duration is shorter in outpatients, and less resources and staff are required, therefore less costs incurred [8]. The benefit of performing procedures in outpatients is increased by the fact that the tariff (payment received) for the procedure is the same, or higher, for those performed in outpatients as in theatre. This is despite costs to the hospital being higher for procedures in theatre. For example, the tariff for a hysteroscopy and biopsy in outpatients is £465, whereas for a day case, it is £420 [9]. This is to provide an incentive for best practice [10].

12.3   Outpatient Hysteroscopy

Clear guidance for outpatient hysteroscopy clinics is provided with the RCOG's Green-top Guideline [1]. This was reviewed in 2014 and no changes made and therefore remains effective. The guideline gives an overview of clinic set-up, types of hysteroscopes, pain relief, distension media and staffing but does not go into detail. It recommends that practitioners are assisted/chaperoned by up to three staff, including at least one registered nurse. One registered nurse is adequate for diagnostic and simple operative procedures, provided the set-up of the clinic is such that they can assist the clinician whilst also talking to the patient and acting as a 'vocal local' [11].

The RCOG guideline [1] leaves the choice of hysteroscope to the practitioner, as there are advantages and disadvantages to different methods. Flexible hysteroscopes with a 3 mm diameter can be used for diagnostic hysteroscopy. These are single channel and therefore cannot be used for any operative work. Whilst the small diameter and flexibility mean that cervical dilatation is rarely required, flexible hysteroscopes make it more difficult to do procedures vaginoscopically, and this can reduce the amount of discomfort experienced by the patient during the procedures. However, if pathology were found, it would not be possible to take a targeted biopsy or attempt removal. A semi-rigid hysteroscope used with disposable sheath and operative channel can also be used, which can mean increased success of using a vaginoscopic approach and the ability for a 'see and treat' if pathology is found. However, these have a larger diameter and can therefore be more uncomfortable for the patient.

Saline is an effective and simple to administer distention medium. Carbon dioxide is also effective but cannot be used for operative hysteroscopies using bipolar electrodes as saline is required for conduction. The RCOG guidance [11] found that carbon dioxide was more likely to induce a vasovagal reaction. Saline can be administered using an IV giving set, either with a manual pressure cuff or pump system. The manual pressure cuff is cheaper and simpler to set up but requires the assisting nurse to continually monitor and adjust the pressure as required, throughout the procedure [12]. There is not a definite consensus on the optimum intrauterine pressure, but pressures of 40–100 mmHg have been shown to be effective [13–15] without causing prohibitive pain. Pressure should be slowly increased just to the level required to achieve and maintain a good view. Increased pressure has been linked to higher pain scores; therefore the lowest possible pressure should be used to minimise patient discomfort [14, 15].

12.4 Suggested Equipment for Diagnostic Hysteroscopy Clinic

- Stack consisting of light source, processor, good quality monitor, printer, facility for picture storage if needed, camera head.
- Procedure chair with electric controls to allow for correct patient positioning and manoeuvrability during the procedure, with tray for instruments.
- Appropriate seat for practitioner to ensure correct posture and manual handling during the procedure, e.g. height-adjustable saddle stool.
- Gynaecological examination light.
- Small diameter hysteroscope with light lead, as per RCOG guidance this can be flexible or rigid/semi-rigid depending on practitioner preference and procedure requirements.
- Drip stand with multiple hanging points (suggested minimum of two).
- Pressure infusers for saline, 250–1000 ml bags, pressure range of at least 0–150 mmHg.
- Trolley with large top surface, smooth to allow for thorough cleaning, with drawers for equipment.
- Sterile pack prepared by sterile service department or purchased as a single-use set. To enable this to be used for all procedures (diagnostic, operative and IUD insertion/removal), suggested items are gallipot for iodine/antiseptic for cervixes, cotton wool balls, tenaculum (small enough to be tolerated without anaesthetic), sponge holder, Spencer Wells forceps, two double-ended dilators sizes 3–4 and 5–6, uterine sound and curved scissors. The instruments need to have the longer handles for access to the cervix via the speculum.
- Suggested supplementary items available: dental syringe (disposable or re-usable, disposable syringes may not have a long enough barrel to be used with longer speculums), cervical polyp forceps.
- Suggested single-use items/consumables: saline bags of 250 ml and giving sets, OS finders in various sizes, endometrial sampler curettes, antiseptic solution, sample pots for histopathology and cytology, cervical cytology brushes, charcoal and chlamydia swabs.
- Suggested medications available: anaesthetic antiseptic lubricant with appropriate instillation device; anaesthetic for cervical block, e.g. citanest with octapres-

sin; pain relief for pre- or post-procedure, such as paracetamol, mefenamic acid and diclofenac; and silver nitrate in case of incidental finding of cervical ectropian or cautery after cervical polyp removal.

- Appropriate monitoring and resuscitation equipment, medications and support to manage complications such as anaphylaxis, seizures and vasovagal reactions.

12.5   Operative Hysteroscopy

The main types of operative hysteroscopy performed in outpatients are removal of endometrial polyps and fibroids. There are two different ways of removing polyps hysteroscopically in outpatients. These are with a bipolar electrode or with a morcellator. Both require the use of a hysteroscope with an operating channel as well as the fluid input channel. For larger polyps and fibroids, morcellators are required, as with resection pathology would need to be removed with forceps or similar through the cervical canal. Although possible it would usually necessitate taking the hysteroscopy and forceps in and out repeatedly to remove sections of poly/fibroid. This is technically difficult but also can take longer and be more painful and with greater risk of perforation and trauma to the cervix. It also means intrauterine pressure cannot be maintained; bleeding is likely to occur and therefore loss of view. Using a morcellator allows bigger pathologies to be removed, without needing to remove scope of forceps, allowing greater control over intrauterine pressure and therefore maintaining a better view in the cavity. This does, however, require a larger diameter scope, and therefore for small polyps possible to remove in one manoeuvre, bipolar electrode resection may be preferable if a small diameter hysteroscope, such as an AlphaScope with disposable sheath, can be used or on some occasions simply a pair of forceps.

For removal of fibroids, a morcellator and fluid management system are required. Hysteroscopic morcellation in outpatients has been found to be safe and tolerated well, giving improvement in quality of life scores in women with heavy menstrual bleeding [16, 17].

For more complex procedures such as morcellation, involving mid-procedure set-up, there will be the need for an additional circulating person. The nature of these procedures mean that the set-up can be complex and requires understanding of the procedure and aseptic technique. They are likely to be more anxiety provoking for the patient and more painful than diagnostic hysteroscopy as local anaesthetic and cervical dilatation are more frequently required, along with more fluid at a higher pressure to maintain distension and view, and the length of the procedures is greater. The 'vocal local' aspect of these procedures is therefore even more important. There is also a greater possibility of the patients having a reaction (vasovagal or pain) for the same reasons [1]; therefore it may be pertinent to have two registered nurses assisting the practitioner for these cases, dependent on skill mix and personnel.

Other types of operative hysteroscopy performed in an outpatient setting include division of intrauterine adhesions, removal of intrauterine devices (IUDs), targeted endometrial biopsy and removal of retained products of conception. For these procedures a semi-rigid scope with sheath and operating channel would be required, along with semi-rigid hysteroscopic instruments such as scissors (blunt or sharp tipped), graspers, IUD removers and biopsy cup forceps [12].

12.6   Additional Equipment for Operative Hysteroscopy

- Rigid hysteroscope + operative sheath and light lead.
- Equipment required for specific procedure, e.g. bipolar electrode and generator, morcellator and fluid management system or suction tubing and wall/portable suction, saline (500–3000 ml bags depending on procedure), tissue collection device for connection to suction, or hysteroscopic forceps for manual removal, fluid management system.
- Hysteroscopic instruments; biopsy cup forceps, IUD remover, scissors, graspers (usually 3 or 5 Fr).
- Vulsellum.

12.7   Other Outpatient Procedures

Alongside hysteroscopy there are a number of other procedures that can be performed in an ambulatory setting. Insertion (and removal) of IUS or IUDs can be performed, using the same set of instruments in the pack described above for outpatient hysteroscopy.

Small cervical polyps can also be removed in outpatients. This will depend on the size, shape (broad based or not) and vascularity and on access to cautery. Small polyps can be removed with cervical polyp forceps and silver nitrate used for cautery. Larger polyps or those with a broad base can sometimes be removed in colposcopy with the use of the loop diathermy, if the original can be clearly visualised and they are definitely cervical rather than endometrial.

Vulval cysts and skin tags can be removed with a disposable suture pack and local anaesthetic. Again, this will depend on size, location and vascularity.

Cervical ectropians can be quickly and easily treated with silver nitrate and, for more persistent ones, if appropriate, using cold coagulation.

12.8   Patient Comfort

Pain and anxiety are associated with outpatient procedures, even when regarded as minor, and this in turn affects patient experience and success rates of procedures [2, 18]. Minimising these is therefore extremely important.

Local anaesthetic for outpatient hysteroscopy is not recommended for routine diagnostic hysteroscopy unless there is cervcial dilatation. In fact, at the time of writing, there is no strong enough evidence to support the routine use of any specific analgesia although women should be advised to have analgesia before the procedure. A recent Cochrane review found only a limited number of studies in this area which were not of good quality and therefore could not make any recommendations [19]. In procedures for which cervical dilatation is required, such as for patients with cervical stenosis (most common in postmenopausal women), and operative procedures, evidence does support local anaesthetic injection into the cervix [1, 19]. The RCOG guidance [1] also recommends topical anaesthetic to the cervix if a tenaculum is required.

Aside from pharmacological methods, several other interventions, such as distraction and music, have demonstrated reduction in patient pain and anxiety during outpatient procedures. One study has demonstrated that transcutaneous nerve stimulation (TENS) can decrease pain and increase patient satisfaction during outpatient hysteroscopy [20]. A Cochrane review from 2006 (not yet updated) [21] looked at acute, chronic and cancer pain and found that music reduced opioid requirements, but the effect was small and not necessarily clinically significant. One more recent study found that music played during the procedure decreased both pain and anxiety scores [22]. Having someone to talk to the patient during the procedure to act as a distraction, sometimes known as 'vocal local', has been shown to be effective in reducing pain [11].

12.9   Staff Training

The RCOG recommends a registered nurse who assists with hysteroscopic procedures. It is important that staff setting up for and assisting with the procedures have a good understanding of the procedure, aseptic technique, the instruments commonly used and other items that may be required, as well as the drugs given, signs and symptoms of potential reactions (to the procedure itself as well as any medications) and how to manage these. It is also important that they can troubleshoot any equipment problems. Communication is a key skill, not only to provide the vocal local but also required to liaise with other departments and services, such as equipment providers and sterilisation departments. It may be useful to use a set of local competencies for staff assistant with ambulatory procedures in outpatients, an example of which is provided in Tables 12.1 and 12.2. It may also be useful to have a document clearly outlining the responsibilities of those assisting with the procedures, including a set-up guide for those most commonly performed. An example of this is provided in Fig. 12.1. Figure 12.1 shows the standard contents for an IUCD pack. Both will assist in training new starters and giving clear instructions on expectations and requirements when assisting with procedures.

Ensuring all equipment is sterile and items that are in direct contact with the patient are tracked is a legal requirement. Tracking specimens to ensure they are all labelled correctly and sent to the lab after each procedure is the

Table 12.1 Responsibilities

Nurse responsibilities in the minor procedure room
Complete hysteroscope checklist—if equipment missing check and ring CSSD to chase missing equipment
Set up room in readiness for the first patient—dressing trolley (stocked), fluids primed and in pressure bag, etc.; bring scopes and fiddle boxes around from the clean room
Put patient stickers in the record folder, have one ready for labelling samples and put on the scope packaging and computer if applicable
Call patient from waiting room and prepare them for the procedure
Ensure the patient provides a urine sample for pregnancy test if required (any hysteroscopic procedure, IUCD insertion/removal)—do test and leave on sink for clinician to see or have an agreed protocol with clinicians
Provide patient support during procedure—chatting helps!
Act as patient advocate—if you feel the patient is experiencing too much discomfort, make the practitioner aware
Once finished ensure all specimens have patient labels on, pictures are printed and clinician takes notes, specimens and pictures with them on leaving
Offer patient tissues and a sanitary towel before they leave the room
Complete patient record—pregnancy test
Procedure undertaken—CSSD tracking
No. of specimens taken
Clean the couch, trolley, light and clinician's seat and any other contaminated areas between patients
Ensure all contaminated items are disposed of or stored correctly until the end of clinic
Cover the bin with a paper towel between patients
Clean and flush hysteroscope, repackage ensuring patient's hospital no. and barcode are stuck to the packaging for tracking
Clean hysteroscope camera head and stack keyboard and remote control
At the end of the clinic
Pack used IUCD packs into the box to be sent back to CSSD, fill out the CSSD form and put in with the packs. Put into fiddle box, close using yellow cable tie and put in sluice for collection
Ensure all used scopes are put in sluice for collection and unused scopes are returned to clean room (unless there is another clinic)
Ensure no remaining specimens are left in the room
Primed fluids can only be kept for 48 h, discard after this
Ensure the room is adequately stocked for the next clinic
Empty the bin, tie up laundry back and take to sluice
Ensure the room is clean and tidy—sign cleaning record
Turn off equipment (stack, chair, light, etc.) at the wall
Hysteroscopic procedures
All premenopausal and perimenopausal patients should have a pregnancy test performed prior to the procedure. Write result in the folder
Input patient details into the monitor
Input patient details into the folder and record any specimens taken
Check if scope packaging is not damaged and vacuum seal is maintained
Ensure scope number is written in the folder

(continued)

Table 12.1 (continued)

Patient sticker to be placed in hysteroscopy box with used hysteroscope for tracking purposes at the end of the procedure

Have the scope ready to go but vacuum pack should not be opened

During the procedure wait for the clinician to give the OK, get the scope out and connect it to the stack without contaminating it and then attach the camera head and fluid to the scope

White balance should be done on the first use of the stack

Capture and print pictures on clinician's request

Table 12.2 Equipment set up for procedures

Diagnostic hysteroscopy

Equipment required:
- Hysteroscope
- 250 ml saline through a giving set/pressure bag ~80 mmHg
- IUCD sterile pack
- Antiseptic—Videne (or chlorhexidine if allergic)
- Speculum
- Gel
- Sterile gloves

Hysteroscopic removal of IUS/IUCD

Equipment required:
- Operative hysteroscope (Storz, Versascope or AlphaScope)
- Sheath
- Hysteroscopic forceps or IUD remover
- 250 ml saline through a giving set/pressure bag
- IUCD sterile pack
- Antiseptic—iodine (or chlorhexidine)
- Speculum
- Gel
- Sterile gloves

Hysteroscopic resection of polyp

Equipment required:
- Operative hysteroscope
- Hysteroscopic forceps
- 500 ml bag of saline in pressure bag
- Resector or morcellator
- Under buttock drape
- IUCD sterile pack
- Dental syringe + Citanest with octapressin ×2 vials
- Antiseptic—Videne or chlorhexidine
- Speculum
- Gel
- Sterile gloves

Insertion of IUS

Equipment required:
- IUCD sterile pack
- Mirena IUS (or copper IUD if requested)

Table 12.2   (continued)

• Antiseptic—Videne (or chlorhexidine if allergy)
• Speculum
• Gel
• Sterile gloves
• Pipelle
• Have local anaesthetic on standby

Removal of cervical polyp

Equipment required:

• IUCD sterile pack
• Polyp forceps
• Antiseptic—Videne (or chlorhexidine)
• Speculum
• Gel
• Have silver nitrate on standby

Removal of vulval skin tag

Equipment required:

• Suture pack
• Antiseptic
• Suture (3-0 Vicryl Rapide or check with clinician)
• Small disposable syringe (5 ml) + orange subcut needle
• Local anaesthetic
• Scalpel
• Sterile gloves

Removal of vulval cyst

Equipment required:

• Suture pack
• Antiseptic
• Small disposable syringe (5 ml) + orange subcut needle
• Local anaesthetic
• Scalpel
• Sterile gloves

Vulval biopsy

Equipment required:

• Suture pack
• Antiseptic
• Small disposable syringe (5 ml) + orange needle
• Lignocaine
• Eppendorfer ⟶ or Punch biopsy (various sizes)

Colposcopy

Equipment required:

• Colposcope positioned correctly
• Wound pack
• Extra gallipot

(continued)

Table 12.2 (continued)

• Ascetic acid
• 2 large cotton buds
• 4 small cotton buds
• Eppendorfer ━━━━━ (ready but not opened)
• Lugol's iodine ready but not poured
• Sachet of saline on standby, some clinicians use this
Cold coagulation of the cervix
Equipment required:
• IUCD sterile pack
• Antiseptic—Videne or chlorhexidine
• Speculum
• Gel
• Dental syringe + Citanest with octapressin × 2 vials
• Cold coagulator + probes (attach probe cover *before* turning on the machine). Treatment time is 30 s
• Timer/fob watch with second hand

Fig. 12.1 IUCD pack set-up

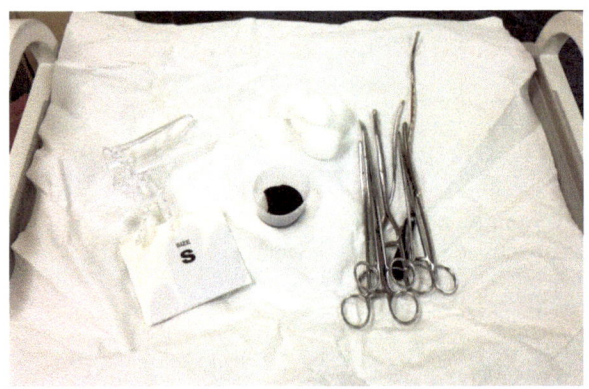

joint responsibility of the assistant and practitioner performing the procedure. Although patients are awake, it is important to ensure that consent is documented [1] and that the correct procedure is carried out with the necessary safety checks (pregnancy status, allergies, site if applicable, type of IUD being inserted, etc.). A safety checklist completed at the beginning and end of the procedure can be useful in the regard, and one can be developed using the World Health Organization checklist as a basis [23]. A log book of the procedures performed, equipment serial numbers used (if applicable), specimens taken and safety checks completed and the name of the clinician performing the procedure and the assistant, in addition to the record in the patients notes, are important and quickly accessible if there are any queries.

References

1. Royal College of Obstetricians and Gynaecologist/BSGE (2011) Best practice in outpatient hysteroscopy (Green Top guideline no. 59). https://www.rcog.org.uk/en/guidelines-research-services/guidelines/gtg59/. Accessed 7 Jul 2018
2. Gambadauro P, Navaratnarajah R, Carli V (2015) Anxiety at outpatient hysteroscopy. Gynecol Surg 12(3):189–196. https://doi.org/10.1007/s10397-015-0895-3
3. Benavent-Caballer V, Biviá-Roig G, Marín-Buck A (2015) 2016/17 national tariff payment system. NHS England, London. Publication code: IRG10/16 NHS England Publications Gateway Reference: 04953 NHS
4. Shah J (2016) Assessment of activity and outcome from a one-stop clinic for men with suspected prostate cancer: five years' experience. J Clin Urol 9(1):5–10
5. Solca M (2006) Evidence-based preoperative evaluation. Best Pract Res Clin Anaesthesiol 20(2):231–236. https://doi.org/10.1016/j.bpa.2005.10.003.7
6. Association of Anaesthetists of Great Britain and Ireland (2015) Peri-operative management of the obese surgical patient. Anaesthesia 70:859–876
7. Association of Anaesthetists of Great Britain and Ireland (2010) The anaesthetic team. Association of Anaesthetists of Great Britain and Ireland, London. http://www.aagbi.org/sites/default/files/anaesthesia_team_2010_0.pdf. Accessed 27 Aug 2017
8. Penketh R, Bruen E, White J, Griffiths A, Patwardhan A, Lindsay P, Hill S, Carolan-Rees G (2014) Feasibility of resectoscopic operative hysteroscopy in a UK outpatient clinic using local anesthetic and traditional reusable equipment, with patient experiences and comparative cost analysis. J Minim Invasive Gynecol 21(5):830–836
9. NHS Improvement (2017) Annexe A: the national prices and tariffs workbook. NHS Improvement, London. https://improvement.nhs.uk/uploads/documents/Copy_of_Annex_A_National_tariff_workbook.xlsx. Accessed 30 Jun 2017
10. Department of Health (2012) Payment by results guidance for 2012–13 (gateway reference: 17250). https://www.gov.uk/government/uploads/system/uploads/attachment_data/file/216212/dh_133585.pdf. Accessed 18 February 2017
11. Keogh SC, Fry K, Mbugua E, Ayallo M, Quinn H, Otieno G, Ngo TD (2014) Vocal local versus pharmacological treatments for pain management in tubal ligation procedures in rural Kenya: a non-inferiority trial. BMC Womens Health 14:21
12. Wong M, Miller V (2017) Why you should be performing office hysteroscopy…now. Contemporary OB/GYN 62(10):24, 26, 28, 30-31, 52 and 54
13. Haggag H, Hassan A, Wahba A, Joukhadar R (2017) A randomized double-blind controlled trial of different filling pressures in operative outpatient hysteroscopy. Int J Gynecol Obstet 139(1):55–60
14. Karaman K, Kolusari A, Çetin O, Çim N, Alkış İ, Karaman Y, Güler S (2017) What should the optimal intrauterine pressure be during outpatient diagnostic hysteroscopy? A randomized comparative study. J Obstet Gynaecol Res 43(5):902–908
15. Haggag H, Hassan A (2016) The impact of altering filling pressures in diagnostic outpatient hysteroscopy on the procedure completion rates and associated pain: a randomised double-blind controlled trial. Aust N Z J Obstet Gynaecol 56:97–101
16. Rajesh SK, Guyer C (2015) Myosure hysteroscopic morcellation for the management of submucous fibroids in an outpatient hysteroscopy setting. J Minim Invasive Gynaecol 22(S1-S2):53
17. Rubino RJ, Lukes AS (2015) Twelve month outcomes for patients undergoing hysteroscopy morcellation of uterine polyps and myomas in an office or ambulatory surgical center. J Minim Invasive Gynaecol 22(2):285–29020
18. Doyle C, Lennox L, Bell D (2013) A systematic review of evidence on the links between patient experience and clinical safety and effectiveness. BMJ Open 3:e001570. https://doi.org/10.1136/bmjopen-2012-001570

19. Ahmad G, Saluja S, O'Flynn H, Sorrentino A, Leach D, Watson A (2017) Pain relief for out-patient hysteroscopy (review). Cochrane Database Syst Rev 2017(10):CD007710

20. Lisón J, Amer-Cuenca J, Piquer-Martí S (2017) Transcutaneous nerve stimulation for pain relief during office hysteroscopy: a randomized controlled trial. Obstet Gynecol 129(2):363–370

21. Cepeda MS, Carr DB, Lau J, Alvarez H (2006) Music for pain relief. Cochrane Database Syst Rev 2006(2):CD004843. https://doi.org/10.1002/14651858.CD004843.pub2

22. Bettocchi S, Bramante S, Bifulco G, Spinelli M, Ceci O, Fascilla FD, Sardo A (2016) Challenging the cervix: strategies to overcome the anatomic impediments to hysteroscopy: analysis of 31,052 office hysteroscopies. Fertil Steril 105(5):e16–e17. https://doi.org/10.1016/j.fertnstert.2016.01.030

23. World Health Organisation (2009) Surgical safety checklist. WHO, Geneva. http://www.who.int/patientsafety/safesurgery/checklist/en/. Accessed 23 Jul 2018

Ruth Bailey

13.1 Integrated Sexual Health

Consensual, enjoyable, negotiated sex can nurture intimacy and enrich relationships. It can increase confidence, feed self-worth and add joy to life. Good sexual health, where people have gratifying sex lives, exercise control over fertility and are free from physical and mental ill-health, can be life enhancing. Conversely, people with poor sexual health can suffer misery. The status of a person's sexual health can be a meaningful barometer of their general wellbeing.

The current UK strategic action plan for sexual and reproductive health (SRH) identifies sexual health as a key public health concern. It traces the links between poor SRH and population morbidity and mortality and wider societal wellbeing and highlights inequities in sexual health within marginalised and vulnerable groups. Improving sexual health has the potential to improve general health and wellbeing and is highly cost-effective [1].

The current SRH priorities are identified as:

- Reduce sexually transmitted infections (STIs).
- Reduce unintended pregnancies.
- Reduce teenage conceptions.
- Reduce onward ward HIV transmission acquisition and avoidable deaths.

The delivery of SRH is complex, within the UK, and takes place in a wide range of settings including primary care, schools and colleges, maternity services, community clinics, abortion providers, the voluntary sector and specialist services. Services are delivered at one of three specified levels, with a move towards providing a specialised integrated service at level 3. This aims to ensure that patients

R. Bailey (✉)
Sexual Health and Contraception, Brighton and Sussex University Hospitals Trust,
Brighton, UK

© Springer Nature Switzerland AG 2019
D. Holloway (ed.), *Nursing Management of Women's Health*,
https://doi.org/10.1007/978-3-030-16115-6_13

receive an accessible, responsive service that meets all their sexual and reproductive needs and onwards referral in a "one-stop" shop [2].

13.2 The Nurse's Role

Nurses have a huge contribution to make to this area of care, which requires a highly specialised skill set, regardless of setting or level of service level [1]. They need to be able to create a confidential safe space where patients feel able to explore sensitive subjects safely, in an environment where they do not feel judged. Nurses need to be confident to ask difficult questions and to support patients through disclosure of trauma. They need skills in explaining information, health promotion and in negotiating person-centred care. Enabling patients to attain control over their sexual health can have a great impact on their general wellbeing, and it can be enormously rewarding.

The current direction in service development is to provide an integrated service so that increasingly nurses are required to be "dual trained," that is, to have developed expertise in both sexual health and contraception [2]. This chapter reflects this by outlining step by step the basis of an integrated consultation, highlighting the basics of assessment and management of common issues.

13.3 Confidentiality

It is key that the consultation starts by outlining the parameters of confidentiality. Under the NMC code of professional conduct, nurses and midwives are required to protect the patients' right to privacy and confidentiality and operate under the Caldicott principles to keep patient's data secure [3, 4]. In sexual health, it is essential that patients trust the clinician to keep their information private and understand how information will be held and under what circumstances it is shared. If samples are sent under a clinic number, rather than the patient's name, this should also be explained.

It is helpful to prepare the patient for the consultation by explaining that they will be asked very personal questions about their private life, so that their individual needs can be fully met.

Patients may ask to bring a friend or partner into the consultation, and this request needs to be considered carefully. The patient may not appreciate the level of intimacy of the questions which they will be asked, and for that reason, it may be better to undertake the history-taking with the patient alone, giving the patient the option to invite their friend or partner in at the stage of examination or care planning if they wish.

13.4 Taking a Sexual History

The basis of any consultation should begin with taking a comprehensive sexual history so that assessment and diagnosis can take place. This requires skilled communication so that the patient is put at ease and able to describe their request or concerns [5].

It is important to use the name that the patient asks to be called by and to use the pronoun of their choice, recognising that patients may not identify with the gender they were assigned at birth or may be gender-fluid [6].

The purpose of the history-taking should be explained clearly to the patient, ensuring that they understand and consent to being asked intimate questions. The rationale for such questions should also be explained.

For some patients, it may be the first time they have had to discuss the intimate details of their sex lives. The consultation may touch on areas that are difficult for patients to discuss and it may unearth painful memories, so the nurse taking the history must be able to support the patient through this process and be equipped to take any appropriate action.

Care should be taken to use terminology that is acceptable to the patient. The use of sexually explicit language can be alarming to patients, and it is helpful to use the words that they use themselves.

The patient may have specific communication requirements. If English is not their first language, an independent translator should be used. It is rarely appropriate to use a family member or friend to act as an interpreter.

Similarly, patients should be offered support with communication if they have visual or hearing impairments. Vulnerable patients may need to be supported with a key worker or independent advocate [5].

13.5 Recording Signs and Symptoms

The sexual history-taking should start by asking an open question to elicit the patient's key concern [5]. Questions such as 'What has brought you here today?' and 'What can I do for you?' give the patient opportunity to describe their worry in their own words. This opens the conversation so that the nurse can explore the nature of the symptoms and onset to start to plan appropriate investigations.

Patients should be asked about their experience of any other symptoms that they may not have recognised as significant. Table 13.1 outlines a guide for history-taking:

Table 13.1 Guide for history-taking

A change in normal vaginal discharge	Colour, volume, smell, irritation
Unexpected bleeding	Breakthrough bleeding, post-coital bleeding, change in volume and colour
Dyspareunia (pain during sex)	Onset, superficial or deep, sexual activity that aggravates pain
Abdominal pain	Onset, location, crampy, sharp, dull, constant, intermittent, what aggravates or relives it
Pain/stinging passing urine	Onset, relief
Lumps/bumps/itching/sores	Onset, location

13.6   History of Sexual Contact

The patient should then be asked about the sexual activity that they have had in the last 3 months, as this covers the window period of incubation for sexually transmitted infection. They should be asked about type of sex they have had which may be oral, vaginal or anal, masturbation and use of sex toys and whether a condom was used or not, as these help assess risk of infection and direct from where appropriate samples to be taken [5].

It is important to establish who they have had sex with (male, female, gender-fluid, group sex); if it was with a regular or casual partner, known friend or sex worker; or if they were a victim of sexual assault, as these will help assess the risk for sexually transmitted infection.

13.7   Medical History

The history should include an assessment of any relevant pre-existing physical and mental health conditions; for example, a history of cardiovascular disease, stroke, venous thromboembolism, migraine with aura and underlying chronic disease are important to uncover, as they will impact on the suitability of contraceptive choices.

Patients accessing contraception should also be asked about the medical history of first-degree relatives, as a family history of venous thromboembolism, stroke, cardiovascular disease, osteoporosis and breast cancer can affect contraceptive choice [7].

The patient should be asked about any allergies and prescribed drugs they are currently taking, including the use of over-the-counter medication and herbal remedies, as they may affect the choice of contraception or prescription.

Gynaecological history should record the date of the last menstrual period (LMP), cycle length and any menstrual problems such as heavy periods, dysmenorrhoea, irregular cycle and premenstrual syndrome.

Details of any pregnancies including terminations, miscarriages and ectopic pregnancies should be recorded. Patients aged 25 and over should be asked about their attendance of cervical screening and treatment of any abnormalities as these will impact on the examination. There is growing recognition that attendance at screening appointments is falling, so engagement with the national cervical screening programme should be encouraged at every consultation [8].

It is a mandatory requirement to ask all patients, regardless of their age or ethnicity, if they have ever experienced cutting on their vaginal area, to screen for the incidence of female genital mutilation (FGM). This has been illegal in the UK since 1985 and should be reported to the police as a safeguarding issue in patients under 18 [9]. Patients over 18 should be supported to discuss any ongoing health issues and referred to appropriate services for advice and support. The risk of FGM within the family unit should also be assessed [9].

If the patient is accessing contraception, the assessment will need to include recording of height, weight and body mass index and a recording of blood pressure, as these factors will affect contraceptive choice and are required for baseline measurement.

13.8   Assessment of Risk of Blood-Borne Virus (BBV)

Sexually transmitted blood-borne viruses (BBV) are human immunodeficiency virus (HIV); hepatitis A, B and C; and syphilis. Anyone who has unprotected sex is potentially at risk from acquiring a BBV, and a risk assessment and appropriate testing should be carried out [10]. HIV is now a completely treatable medical condition with most patients remaining fit and well if fully engaged in medical treatment. Patients with an undetectable viral load are unable to pass the infection on [11], and the consultation is a good opportunity to share this information, which can contribute to the de-stigmatisation of HIV.

Late diagnosis is the most important factor in HIV-related morbidity and mortality [10], and so testing is paramount to initiate early treatment and to stop the infection being passed on.

13.8.1 Assay Tests

BHIVA recommend the use of a fourth-generation assay blood test which will detect the majority of HIV, 4 weeks following exposure. Retesting at 4 weeks should be offered to people at high risk to completely clear the window of exposure, and those with ongoing risk should be advised to test at regular intervals [10].

13.8.2 Point-of-Care Tests (POCT)

These tests have the advantage of giving a result within a few minutes from a mouth swab or blood from a finger prick. They have less specificity and sensitivity and should be followed up with a confirmatory venous blood sample.

All patients should be offered appropriate retesting after appropriate window periods. Full details on current STI testing guidelines can be found at www.bash. org.

Nursing management of patients with HIV is beyond the scope of this chapter, but further information may be found on the British HIV Association website, www. bhiva.org.

A risk assessment should include asking if the patient or their partners are from one of the following groups:

- HIV positive.
- Bisexual.
- Intravenous drugs user.
- Commercial sex worker.
- From a geographical area of high risk.
- Recent exposure to bodily fluids.

Patients should be asked about their history of vaccination for hepatitis A and B, and if born after 1995, about their history of human papilloma virus (HPV) vaccination, so that appropriate vaccination can be arranged if required [5].

Vaccination for hepatitis B may be indicated in patients who have sustained a needlestick injury or sexual assault or who have had unprotected sex with a partner from an identifiable high-risk group [12].

Nurses administering vaccines should be fully equipped to advise on the immunisation programme, including the risks and benefits of immunisation and managing side-effects. They should also have completed an accredited theoretical study and competency assessment [13, 14].

13.9   Social History

A holistic assessment should explore social history that may impact on sexual health and wellbeing. The patient should be asked about the quality of their relationship, to ensure that they feel safe and happy and able to negotiate sex. They should be asked directly if they have ever experienced sexual assault or domestic abuse, as this is an opportunity for patients to access professional help to address issues that may be either current or historical [15].

History-taking should include asking the patient about any experiences of sexual exploitation or assault. Some examples of useful open-ended questions are:

- 'Do you feel safe and happy in your relationship?'
- 'Have you ever been made to do something sexually that you didn't want to do?'
- 'Have you ever been made to feel afraid at home?'

Patients should also be asked about the use of smoking, recreational drugs and alcohol, as this may impact upon their sexual risk-taking. NICE [16] specifically recommends screening for alcohol use with an evidence-based tool in patients who attend GU clinics or who repeatedly access emergency contraception. It is a good opportunity to offer brief interventions and support to make healthy changes if the patient is ready [17]. Smoking history affects contraceptive choice, as combined hormonal methods are contraindicated in smokers aged 35 and over [7].

13.10 Assessing the Needs of Young People Under the Age of 18

There is compelling evidence that young people under the age of 25 have dispro-portionately poorer sexual health with higher rates of common sexually transmit-ted infection and unintended pregnancy. Although rates of teenage pregnancy have halved in the last 10 years, the UK has the highest rates in Western Europe [18]. Under 18 years are particularly vulnerable, and great care should be taken to ensure that this group have a positive experience in the consultation, so that their needs are comprehensively assessed, and they are fully engaged in their care.

Under UK law [19], the age of consent to have a sexual relationship is 16; how-ever consensual sex under the age of 16 is unlikely to lead to prosecution if there is no evidence of coercion or exploitation.

Patients under the age of 16 may consent to receive contraception without parental consent if they are assessed to be competent using Fraser guidelines [20]. This guidance enables a clinician to assess the young person's capacity to make an informed decision and the risk of harm to them, if they continue sexual activity without access to contraception. The assessment should be undertaken and docu-mented every visit.

The consultation should begin by explaining the limits of confidentiality and the requirement to share the patient's information if they are assessed to be at risk of harm or harm to others.

Clinicians working with young people need to be fully conversant with the national child safeguarding framework [21] so that they are alert to signs of abuse and able to take appropriate action working within the multi-professional safeguard-ing team. This should include an assessment of risk of child sexual exploitation, which can occur when an individual or group takes advantage of the child to coerce or manipulate them into any form of sexual activity (see Chap. 4) [22].

13.11 Modern Slavery

NHS England estimates that approximately 13,000 adults and children are victims of trafficking for exploitation in the UK, 55% of victims are female, and 35% are trafficked for sexual exploitation [23]. One in five victims reports meeting a health-care professional, so it is vital that nurses working in sexual health are alert to the signs of physical and emotional harm and confident to take appropriate action to protect and support victims.

Victims of slavery may present with symptoms of sexually transmitted infection, unplanned pregnancy or requests for contraception. They may be accompanied by someone who appears controlling and who may insist on being present during the consultation. It is imperative that the patient is seen on their own at some point, and an independent interpreter should be used if the patient has limited English.

Concerns should be shared with safeguarding leads; clear and accurate records should be documented, and immediate action should be taken to protect those in immediate danger [24].

Advice can be accessed from the national Modern Slavery Helpline *08000121 700*.

13.12 Sexual Assault

Anyone can be a victim of sexual assault. It is defined as the perpetration of any sexual activity that takes place without consent. The Sexual Offences Act 2003 in England, Wales and Northern Ireland defines rape as the non-consensual penile penetration of the mouth, vagina or anus [19]. In law, children under the age of 13 cannot consent to sexual intercourse, so it is recognised as statutory rape and should always be reported to the police.

Victims of sexual assault need the support of the specialist multidisciplinary team to ensure that their immediate needs are met and to prevent the long-term sequelae of infection, unwanted pregnancy, psychological trauma, mental health issues, increased use of substances and damage to relationships [25].

Victims should be given a safe space to tell their story, supported through disclosure by attentive listening. The details of the assault should be meticulously documented. If this is the 'first disclosure', the nurse may be called as a witness in court proceedings.

Victims reporting sexual assault that has taken place in the last 7 days should be referred to a Sexual Assault Referral Centre (SARC) if one is available locally, for medical care, forensic examination, psychological care and victim support.

The following issues should be addressed:

- Emergency contraception.
- Full STI screening.
- Consider post-exposure prophylaxis after sexual exposure (PEPSE).
- Consider antibiotic prophylaxis.
- Vaccination against hepatitis B.
- Forensic sampling (undertaken at specialist centres).
- Psychological support and counselling.
- Follow-up.

13.13 Examination

A full sexual health screen for patients who are asymptomatic requires a self-taken vulvovaginal swab to test for chlamydia and gonorrhoea and a venous blood test to test for HIV and syphilis [10, 18].

A full examination and collection of samples may be indicated if the patient has symptoms and the cause is unknown. The purpose and nature of the examination should be fully explained for the patient to give informed consent. The patient should always be offered a chaperone for support, regardless of the setting or staffing levels [26].

Examination should only be undertaken by a nurse fully competent in the procedure or a learner under direct supervision with patient consent. Examination can be uncomfortable and distressing and may bring back buried memories of childbirth, trauma or assault. The privacy, dignity and comfort of the patient are paramount, and the patient should be advised that they are always in control and may stop the procedure at any time they wish.

The procedure will require the nurse to gently examine the inguinal lymph nodes, external and internal genitalia, taking appropriate samples from any lesions or sores, the vaginal walls, the posterior fornix and the endocervix. Specialist level 3 centres may provide a microscopy service so that samples may be analysed under the microscope while the patient is in the department, assisting immediate diagnosis and treatment.

13.14 Diagnosis and Management

The diagnosis, whether confirmed or a working diagnosis, should be reported back to the patient as soon as possible, to help minimise anxiety.

An overarching principle of care is that management should be person-centred, so treatment options should be offered and a plan negotiated with the patient. The nurse should explain the treatment regimens and discuss the management of side-effects and follow-up in a way that meets their specific information needs. This should be supported by evidence-based written information [27].

13.15 Partner Notification

Partner notification is the process of contacting the sexual contacts of a person who has a sexually transmitted infection (the index patient) and advising them that they have been exposed to infection. This gives them the opportunity to receive screening and appropriate treatment and support and is an important factor in contributing to public health by breaking the chain of infection [28].

Treating partners of the index patient reduces the risk of long-term complications from untreated infection and reduces the risk of reinfection.

Partner notification is best carried out by the index patient, though to do that, they will need to be fully aware of the infection that they have and understand how it is transmitted. They may find it difficult to have this conversation, and they should be supported to plan how and what they will say. If they are unable to do it themselves, a healthcare professional may need to assist, ensuring that they confidentiality of the index patient is not compromised.

13.16 Diagnosis and Management of Common Sexually Transmitted Infections

13.16.1 Chlamydia (CT)

Chlamydia is the most common bacterial STI in the UK, accounting for 48% of all new STI diagnoses. It can occur in the vagina, rectum or eyes and can be passed by non-penetrative sex and through vaginal delivery.

It is particularly prevalent in young people, and the National Chlamydia Screening Programme provides opportunistic screening for young people between the ages of 15 and 24, enabling the disease to be identified and treated. In 2017, 126,828 chlamydia diagnoses were made in this age group, equivalent to a detection rate of 1882 per 100,000 population. It is recommended that sexually active young people are tested annually or when they change partners if untreated can have a significant impact on pelvic pain, fertility and rises the risk of ectopic pregnancies.

The incubation period for chlamydia is 2 weeks, so repeat screening may be necessary to ensure that the window period is covered. Table 13.2 shows the signs and symptoms and treatment for chlamydia.

Table 13.2 Signs and symptoms and treatment for chlamydia

Symptoms	Most frequently asymptomatic. It can cause increased or changes to vaginal discharge, changes to bleeding pattern or bleeding after sex, lower abdominal pain, dyspareunia and dysuria
Investigations	Nucleic amplification test (NAAT) from a self-taken vulvovaginal swab Rectal and throat swabs may be indicated by sexual health history A full symptomatic screen should be undertaken if symptoms are present Exclude pregnancy
Treatment	Uncomplicated chlamydia is usually treated with broad-spectrum antibiotics, currently doxycycline or azithromycin, according to current BASH guidelines Partner notification and treatment of all sexual contacts in the last 3 months Abstain from sex for 1 week Provide written and verbal patient information Encourage condom use
Follow-up	Follow-up is not required in uncomplicated chlamydia Retesting in 3 months should be encouraged

Table 13.3 Management of gonorrhoea

Symptoms	Asymptomatic in up to 50% of women It can cause changes to the volume and colour of vaginal discharge, changes to bleeding pattern or bleeding after sex, lower abdominal pain, dyspareunia and dysuria
Investigations	Nucleic amplification test (NAAT) from a self-taken vulvovaginal swab Rectal and throat swabs may be indicated from the sexual history A full symptomatic screen should be undertaken if symptoms are present An endocervical swab taken if microscopy is available Microscopy on Gram-stained slide allows detection of Gram-negative diplococci inside polymorphonuclear leucocytes An endocervical sample should be used to inoculate a culture plate Exclude pregnancy
Treatment	Intramuscular injection of a cephalosporin +/− broad-spectrum antibiotics, in line with current BASH guidelines Partner notification and treatment of all sexual contacts in the last 3 months Abstain from sex for 2 weeks Patients should be advised to re-refer if symptoms exacerbate Provide written and verbal patient information Encourage condom use
Follow-up	Follow-up is for a test of cure (TOC) Repeat STI testing in 3 months

13.16.2 Gonorrhoea (GC)

The bacterium *Neisseria gonorrhoea* causes infection of the vagina, anus, throat or eyes. There was an overall 22% increase in new diagnoses in 2017, and with growing concern over antibiotic resistance, it presents a public health challenge.

Table 13.3 shows the signs, symptoms and management of gonorrhoea.

13.16.3 Trichomonas Vaginalis (TV)

Trichomonas vaginalis (TV) is an infection with a flagellate protozoan, passed via vaginal sex or the use of sex toys. It is not transmitted via anal sex. It is uncommon, with a prevalence estimated at about 0.3% and a higher risk in non-Caucasians. There is increasing recognition that TV increases the likelihood of HIV transmission, and all symptomatic patients should be tested [29]. Table 13.4 shows its investigations and management.

13.16.4 Anogenital Warts

Genital warts are the most common viral sexually transmitted infection. Table 13.5 shows its presentation and management. Ninety percent are caused by the human

Table 13.4 Management of TV

Symptoms	70% of patients have a change in discharge. Classic frothy yellow discharge which may have an unpleasant smell Cervix may have classic strawberry-like cervicitis Pain or burning passing urine
Investigations	Nucleic amplification test (NAAT) from a self-taken vulvovaginal swab Visualise the cervix and look for cervicitis Take a sample of discharge from the posterior fornix and mount on a wet slide Viewing under microscope allows visualisation of protozoa Test the pH of vaginal discharge on litmus paper Exclude pregnancy Ensure full STI testing
Treatment	Treatment is with metronidazole, according to current BASH guidelines Partner notification and treatment of all sexual contacts in the last 3 months Abstain from sex for 1 week Provide written and verbal patient information Advise the patient to avoid alcohol during the treatment and for a further 2 days Encourage condom use
Follow-up	Vaginal sample for TOC after 1 week Retesting in 3 months should be encouraged

Table 13.5 Management of warts

Symptoms	Soft cauliflower-like growths of varying size; flat, plaque-like or pigmented May be soft and non-keratinised; those on dry and hairy skin, firm and keratinised Lesions may be broad based, flat or pedunculated Usually painless but may cause itching or inflammation
Investigations	Examination of the anogenital region Diagnosis may be aided by the application of liquid nitrogen; wart tissue will hold the spray and appear as white Full STI screening
Treatment	Treatment is optional, as warts will resolve spontaneously within a year Encourage self-care with good nutrition and reduction of smoking to support the immune response Application of creams or ablation with liquid nitrogen Surgical removal may be indicated for very large or obstructive warts Treatment of partners indicated only if they are symptomatic Provide written and verbal information Encourage safer sex with condoms
Follow-up	Follow-up is not required after symptoms resolve

papilloma virus (HPV) types 6 + 11. They are transmitted by penetrative vaginal and anal sex and close skin-to-skin contact. Warts are unsightly and may cause distress; however, most will clear within a year, so treatment is optional [30]. HPV is preventable by HPV quadrivalent immunisation, and the introduction of immunisation to school-age girls has seen a relative reduction of 90% of new diagnoses with the programme soon to be extended to include boys.

Table 13.6 Care of women with PID

Symptoms	Lower abdominal pain Deep pain during sex (dyspareunia) Abnormal vaginal bleeding Abnormal vaginal discharge Fever or feeling generally unwell May be asymptomatic
Investigations	Full sexual health screen including tests for *Mycoplasma genitalium* and blood-borne viruses Bimanual examination to determine cervical motion pain and adnexal tenderness Urine test to exclude pregnancy and urinary tract infection Recording of temperature
Treatment	Two-week course of antibiotics, along with analgesics as required, and rest Abstain from any sexual contact for 2 weeks Partner notification and treatment Patient information, psychological support, encourage safer sex Follow-up in 2–4 weeks May need admission for further investigations and treatment with intravenous antibiotics if the patient is acutely unwell or pregnant Sexual partners of the last 3 months will need to be treated as contacts Patients should abstain from sex for 2 weeks until all partners complete treatment Verbal and written patient information
Follow-up	Two-week follow-up to review progress TOC if symptoms have not resolved

13.16.5 Pelvic Inflammatory Disease (PID)

PID is inflammation of the reproductive organs. It is usually caused by a bacterial infection with a sexually transmitted infection responsible in 25% of affected women, most commonly chlamydia, gonorrhoea or *Mycoplasma genitalium*. Table 13.6 shows the management, signs and care of women with PID. Left untreated, it can lead to pelvic scarring, pelvic abscess, risk of ectopic pregnancies and infertility [31].

13.16.6 Herpes Simplex Virus (HSV)

Herpes simplex is a common viral sexually transmitted infection. There are two types that cause this condition, HSV-1 and HSV-2, which are very similar. HSV-1 is the usual cause of orogenital herpes and the most common overall. HSV-2 is the most likely to cause recurrence of symptoms. The management is the same. Incubation occurs between 2 days and 2 weeks; Table 13.7 shows its management. After primary infection, the virus lies latent in the sensory ganglia and can reactivate to cause recurrence, often after a viral illness or when the patient is run-down and stressed. Careful management is required if a first occurrence occurs in the third trimester of pregnancy due to the risk of vertical transmission in vaginal delivery [32].

Table 13.7 Care and management of women with HSV

Symptoms	Wide spectrum of presentation
	Presence of small fluid-filled blisters anywhere in the anogenital area or the tops of thighs and buttocks, leaving sore painful lesions when they burst
	Feeling unwell with flu-like symptoms
	Fifty per cent patients will not have a recurrence
Investigations	Examination of lesions
	Sampling fluid of lesion taken with a green virology swab
	Exclude pregnancy, the virus can be transmitted via vaginal birth and needs careful management in pregnancy
	Full sexual health screening
Treatment	Self-care, rest and recuperation
	Control of pain and fever with analgesics and topical lidocaine
	Treatment with acyclovir
	Long-term suppression treatment may be indicated if the patient has had six or more recurrences per year
Follow-up	Follow-up is not usually required
	Patients are advised to initiate treatment when they recognise early signs of herpes 'tingling' sensation known as the prodrome

13.16.7 Syphilis

Syphilis is a blood-borne viral infection with the bacterium *Treponema pallidum* which is transmitted through direct contact with secretions from an infective lesion or transplacental passage of bacteria in pregnancy. It is a complicated infection and can manifest in three stages: early (primary and secondary), latent and late (tertiary) [33]. These are shown in Table 13.8. Incubation for primary syphilis is between 3 weeks and 3 months. The UK has seen a 20% increase in the incidence of syphilis in 2017; the burden is largely carried by men who have sex with men.

13.17 Managing Common Non-sexually Transmitted Infection

Many patients will attend the clinic worried about symptoms which arise as the result of common vaginal infections or skin disorders which are not sexually transmitted. Symptoms such as increased discharge or vulval itching can cause great distress and hamper enjoyment of everyday life.

13.17.1 Bacterial Vaginosis (BV)

This is the most common cause of abnormal vaginal discharge caused by an overgrowth of normal vaginal anaerobic bacteria and a decrease in lactobacilli and a rise in vaginal pH to 4.5 or over. It is not sexually transmitted, but it is associated with

Table 13.8 Symptoms and management of syphilis

Symptoms	*Primary syphilis* may present with painless lesions known as chancres, found on the penis, vulva and cervix or in the mouth *Secondary syphilis* may appear 4–10 weeks after chancres have appeared. Symptoms include a non-itchy erythematous rash all over the body, including the palms and the soles of the feet, patchy hair loss, white patches on the tongue or the roof of the mouth, flu-like symptoms and widespread lymphoedema *Latent syphilis* may be asymptomatic but still infectious *Tertiary syphilis* presents with a wide range of complicated multisystem manifestations including gummous lesions affecting the skin and bone and cardiovascular and neurological involvement including progressive dementia
Investigations	Blood test for serology Viewing fluid from lesion to detect *T. pallidum* under dark ground microscopy, if available
Treatment	Intramuscular injection of penicillin, as per BASH guidance Treatment may vary according to the different stages of the disease and associated symptoms Associated symptom control, rest, recuperation and self-care Sexual partners within the last 3 months should be treated as contacts
Follow-up	Follow-up is required

Table 13.9 Management of BV

Symptoms	Watery thin white or yellow discharge Fishy odour Fifty per cent are asymptomatic
Investigations	Vaginal examination Microscopy of vaginal discharge using Hay/Ison criteria to grade vaginal flora Test ph of vaginal discharge on litmus paper
Treatment	Oral/intra-vaginal Metronidazole gel Avoid fragranced shower gels/douching Avoid over-washing Verbal and written advice on treatment
Follow-up	Not usually required

sexual activity and is common in women who have sex with women [34]. The signs, symptoms and treatments are seen in Table 13.9.

13.17.2 Vulvovaginal Candida (Thrush)

This is a very common fungal condition experienced by up to 40% of people in their reproductive lives. Eighty per cent of candida is caused by *Candida albicans*, which results in local irritation of the vaginal area. It is not sexually transmitted but can occur or be aggravated by sexual activity [35]. The signs, symptoms and treatments are seen in Table 13.10.

Table 13.10 Management of Candida

Symptoms	Vulval itching
	Vulval soreness
	Thick creamy discharge
	Superficial dyspareunia
	Stinging passing urine
Investigations	Examination of external genitalia speculum examination of vaginal walls
	Test pH of vaginal discharge using litmus paper
	Swab from left lateral wall, mounted on a dry slide for microscopy
	Bacterial swab for microscopy and culture
	Direct plating on a sabourand solid fungal mediaplate (sabs plate)
	Urine test to exclude, urine infection, pregnancy and diabetes
	Consider investigating immunosuppression
	Investigation for speciation may be required if four or more episodes per year are experienced
Treatment	Replace soap with moisturisers
	Avoid perfumed products
	Avoid tight-fitting synthetic clothing
	Eighty per cent of candida clears with oral and or topical azoles, use regimes according to local guidelines
	Treatment of sexual partners is not usually required
	Verbal/written treatment advice
Follow-up	Not usually required

13.17.3 Vulvodynia

A complex condition of chronic vulval pain, usually described as a burning sensation in the absence of infection and skin disorders. It can occur at any age, is often long standing and often causes huge distress and psychosexual dysfunction (BASH 2014). The are many symptoms, and the main management would depend on the cause. Table 13.11 shows these.

13.17.4 Vulval Skin Conditions

A plethora of vulval skin conditions exist, and the diagnosis and management are beyond the scope of this chapter. These include vulval eczema, vulval psoriasis, lichen planus, lichen sclerosis and vulval tumours. Typically, vulval conditions may be present for many years before they are accurately diagnosed and treated, and often symptoms are dismissed or mistaken for candida and not treated effectively, resulting in unnecessary pain and distress, psychosexual problems and damage to relationships. It is important to exclude common infections and STIs so that an accurate diagnosis can be made. This may involve a

Table 13.11 Vulval pain

Symptoms	A long history of vulval pain Painful, difficult or impossible penetration Unable to use tampons Dry skin
Investigations	Vaginal examination—may not be able to tolerate examination with speculum Exclude STIs and local infection Gentle application of cotton bud to the introitus and clitoris to identify local tenderness Biopsy to exclude dermatosis may be indicated
Treatment	Avoid irritants and encourage use of emollients Daily perineal massage Topical lidocaine prior to sex Consider use of pain modifiers Cognitive behaviour therapy and psychosexual counselling Verbal and written advice Signpost to Vulval Pain Society

skin biopsy and input from dermatologists. Skin disorders can be successfully managed with the application of emollients and topical steroids and psychological support [36].

13.18 Providing Contraceptive Choices

It is estimated that over half of all pregnancies in the UK are currently unplanned. Although not necessarily unwanted, unplanned pregnancies are associated with poor maternal and infant health. The provision of acceptable contraception gives freedom over fertility, so that pregnancy is a planned choice and health outcomes can be maximised [1]. Contraception will be used by people who identify as non-binary or gender-fluid and those in same-sex relationships for cycle control. There is wide recognition that the use of contraception over the lifespan is extensive and the provision of reliable contraception is cost-effective and a public health priority [1, 2, 27].

13.19 The Nurse's Role in the Provision of Contraception

The nurse's role in providing contraception is to carry out a comprehensive assessment and offer appropriate contraceptive choices. They must be able to explain the methods in a way that the patient understands, answer questions, manage uncertainty and support the patient in their choice. They should work with the patient to plan appropriate follow-up to review the method and manage any associated side-effects. Helping the patient to use a method that is right for them can be enormously rewarding.

Nurses may carry out autonomous episodes of care issuing medication using patient group directions (PGDs) or prescribing if they are independent non-medical prescribers (INP).

13.20 Offering Safe Contraceptive Choices

13.20.1 UK Medical Eligibility Criteria (UK MEC)

The UK MEC is a guidance published by the Faculty of Sexual and Reproductive Health (FSRH) that helps clinicians decide what contraceptives they can safely recommend based on the medical conditions of their patients. The integrated assessment outlined earlier in the chapter will indicate appropriate safe options guided by the UK MEC [7]. These are shown in Table 13.12.

Patients should be asked about their lifestyle, specific requirements and any experiences of using contraception in the past as this will influence their choice. They are less likely to discontinue their method if they are positively engaged in selecting it [37].

The FPA current choices chart is a useful tool to guide the discussion of options available and their benefits and risks, and discussion can be enhanced with the use of demonstration models for the patient to handle.

A brief summary of the choices is outlined below: full clinical guidance on each method may be found on the FSRH website: www.FSRH.org.

Table 13.12 UKMEC definitions

UKMEC	Definition of category
Category 1	A condition for which there is no restriction for the use of the method
Category 2	A condition where the advantages of using the method generally outweigh the theoretical or proven risks
Category 3	A condition where the theoretical or proven risks usually outweigh the advantages of using the method. The provision of a method requires expert clinical judgement and/or referral to a specialist contraceptive provider, since use of the method is not usually recommended unless other more appropriate methods are not available or not acceptable
Category 4	A condition which represents an unacceptable health risk if the method is used

Reproduced under licence from FSRH. Copyright © Faculty of Sexual and Reproductive Healthcare. UK Medical Eligibility Criteria for Contraceptive Use 2016. Full guideline available from https://www.fsrh.org/ukmec/

Contraceptive methods that don't depend on you remembering to take or use them.

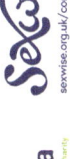

sexwise
sexwise.org.uk/contraception

fpa
the sexual health charity

	Contraceptive implant	Intrauterine device (IUD)	Intrauterine system (IUS)	Contraceptive injection	Sterilisation
What is it?	A small, flexible rod put under the skin of the upper arm releases progestogen.	A small plastic and copper device is put into the uterus (womb).	A small, T-shaped, progestogen-releasing, plastic device is put into the uterus (womb).	An injection of progestogen.	The fallopian tubes in women or the tubes carrying sperm in men (vas deferens) are cut, sealed or blocked.
Effectiveness	Perfect use: over 99%. Typical use: over 99%.	Perfect use: over 99%. Typical use: over 99%.	Perfect use: over 99%. Typical use: over 99%.	Perfect use: over 99%. Typical use: around 94%.	Overall failure rate is about 1 in 200 for females and 1 in 2,000 for males.
Advantage	Works for 3 years but can be taken out sooner.	Works for 5 or 10 years depending on type but can be taken out sooner.	Works for 3, 4 or 5 years but can be taken out sooner. Periods often become lighter, shorter and less painful.	Works for 8 or 13 weeks – you don't have to think about contraception during this time.	Sterilisation is permanent with no long or short-term serious side effects.
Disadvantage	It requires a small procedure to fit and remove it.	Periods may be heavier, longer or more painful.	Irregular bleeding or spotting is common in the first 6 months.	Can't be removed from the body so side effects may continue while it works and for some time afterwards.	Shouldn't be chosen if in any doubt about having children in the future.

Contraceptive methods that you have to use and think about regularly or each time you have sex.

PERFECT USE MEANS USING THE METHOD CORRECTLY EVERY TIME. TYPICAL USE IS WHEN YOU DON'T ALWAYS USE THE METHOD CORRECTLY.

	Contraceptive patch	Contraceptive vaginal ring	Combined pill (COC)	Progestogen-only pill (POP)	External condom	Internal condom	Diaphragm/cap with spermicide	Fertility awareness methods
What is it?	A small patch stuck to the skin releases estrogen and progestogen.	A small, flexible, plastic ring put into the vagina releases estrogen and progestogen.	A pill containing estrogen and progestogen, taken orally.	A pill containing progestogen, taken orally.	A very thin latex (rubber) polyurethane (plastic) or synthetic sheath, put over the erect penis.	Soft, thin polyurethane sheath that loosely lines the vagina and covers the area just outside.	A flexible latex (rubber) or silicone device, used with spermicide, is put into the vagina to cover the cervix.	Fertile and infertile times of the menstrual cycle are identified by noting different fertility indicators.
Effectiveness	Perfect use: over 99%. Typical use: around 91%.	Perfect use: over 99%. Typical use: around 91%.	Perfect use: over 99%. Typical use: around 91%.	Perfect use: over 99%. Typical use: around 91%.	Perfect use: 98%. Typical use: around 82%.	Perfect use: 95%. Typical use: around 79%.	Perfect use: 92–96%. Typical use: 71–88%.	Perfect use: up to 99%. Typical use: around 76%.
Advantage	Can make bleeds regular, lighter and less painful.	One ring stays in for 3 weeks – you don't have to think about contraception every day.	Often reduces bleeding and period pain, and may help with premenstrual symptoms.	Can be used if you smoke and are over 35.	Condoms are the best way to help protect yourself from sexually transmitted infections.	Condoms are the best way to help protect yourself from sexually transmitted infections.	Can be put in any time before sex.	No physical side effects, and can be used to plan as well as prevent pregnancy.
Disadvantage	May be seen and can cause skin irritation.	You must be comfortable with inserting and removing it.	Missing pills, vomiting or severe diarrhoea can make it less effective.	Late pills, vomiting or severe diarrhoea can make it less effective.	May slip off or split if not used correctly or if wrong size or shape.	Not as widely available as male condoms.	You need to use the right size. If you have sex again extra spermicide is needed.	Need to avoid sex or use a condom at fertile times of the cycle.

Last updated April 2018 | Copyright FPA | sexwise.org.uk/contraception

Reproduced with kind permission of the Family Planning Association

13.20.2 Long-Acting Reversible Contraceptives (LARCs)

LARCs, sometimes called 'fit and forget', are methods which are administered less than once per cycle and are not dependent upon the user. They are cost-effective and convenient with a high efficacy, and it is recommended that every patient is offered advice and written information about LARCs [38].

13.20.3 Contraceptive Implant

The progestogen-only implant is a single rod containing 68 mg of etonogestrel and barium. The implant is fitted subdermally in the upper arm, by an appropriately trained clinician. It is over 99% effective, and it may last up to 3 years. Its primary action is to supress ovulation. If it is fitted between days 1 and 5 of the cycle, it will work immediately. If the clinician is reasonably certain that the patient is not pregnant, the implant may be 'quick-started' at any time of the cycle if the patient is able to abstain from sex or use extra precautions for 7 days [39].

Patients should be fully counselled about the method and the risk of side-effects, which include irregular bleeding, mood swings, nausea and bloating, most of which settle in the first 3 months. The most common side-effect is change to bleeding pattern, which is often a factor for discontinuation. Patients should also be advised of the risks of bruising and infection during fitting and removal procedures and the rare risk of device migration.

13.20.4 Intrauterine Contraception

There are two types of intrauterine contraception (IUC) which are the hormonal levonorgestrel intrauterine system (LNG-IUS) and the non-hormonal copper-bearing intrauterine device (Cu-IUD) [40].

Both methods are over 99% effective but differ in the way they work, associated side-effects and duration of use. There are very few absolute contraindications, and they include patients with untreated pelvic infection, septic abortion and active pelvic cancer. The method can be used successfully by people who have never been pregnant.

The selection of the appropriate choice depends largely on the patient's preference, and the nurse has an important part to play in helping the patient choose their device and preparing them for and supporting them through the fitting procedure.

An assessment of the risk of sexually transmitted infection should take place, and any screening indicated should be carried out before the fit.

The patient should be fully versed on the risks of the procedure which include discomfort, cervical shock and infection. However, these risks can be minimised with careful planning and supportive nursing care.

13.20.5 Copper-Bearing Intrauterine Device (Cu-IUD)

The Cu-IUD contains 380 mg of copper that is toxic to sperm and so prevents fertilisation to take place. It has an inflammatory effect on the lining of the womb, making it a hostile environment for implantation. There are various types of Cu-IUD that are effective for between 5 and 10 years depending on the type. It may be safely fitted at any time during the cycle if there is no risk of pregnancy (unless fitted as emergency contraception), and it will provide immediate contraceptive cover [40].

Patients should be advised that the impact on the womb lining means that they are likely to experience longer and heavier periods, and it may not be suitable for those who are already experiencing these.

13.20.6 Levonorgestrel Intrauterine System (LNG-IUS)

There are currently four types of IUS (Jaydess, Kyleena, Mirena, Levosert) available in the UK which last between 3 and 5 years, depending on the type. The primary action of the IUS is to thicken the cervical mucus to hamper sperm so that fertilisation cannot take place. It also thins the lining of the womb so that implantation cannot be sustained.

The impact of the progesterone on the endometrium reduces blood loss and may result in amenorrhoea, and patients should be counselled about changes to their bleeding pattern. Side-effects include acne, bloating, headaches and back pain, but most side-effects settle within 3–6 months.

The Mirena and Levosert is also licensed to treat heavy menstrual bleeding. The Mirena can also be fitted to provide endometrial protection for women using oestrogen as part of hormone replacement therapy and treatment of hyperplasia. If the Mirena is fitted to provide contraception in women over the age of 45, it may be used for up to 7 years if not being used as part of HRT.

The IUS will work immediately if fitted on days 1–5 of the cycle. It may be 'quick-started' and fitted on any day of the cycle if the clinician is reasonably certain the patient is not pregnant, and the patient uses extra precaution for 7 days.

13.20.7 Contraceptive Injections

There are currently two progesterone-only injections available. The primary action of both is to supress ovulation, and they are over 99% effective if used correctly. The risks and side-effect profile are identical, and although the licence for administration differs slightly, they may be used interchangeably. Both injections will be immediately effective if administered during days 1–5 of the menstrual cycle. They can both be 'quick-started' if no unprotected sex has taken place since the last menstrual cycle [41].

Depo-Provera® containing 150 mg medroxyprogesterone acetate in 1 ml is an intramuscular injection administered to the upper outer quadrant of the buttock. It is licensed to be administered every 12 weeks, although it may be administered safely out of specific product characteristics up to 14 weeks.

Sayana Press® is a subcutaneous injection containing 104 mg of medroxypro-gesterone acetate in 0.65 ml and is administered to the patient's abdomen or upper thigh. It is licensed to be administered every 13 weeks, although it can be given safely out of specific product characteristics up to 14 weeks. Patients can be taught to self-administer Sayana Press®, giving them control over their contraception and freeing them from dependency upon clinic appointments.

Patients should be advised that they are likely to experience a change of bleeding pattern using the contraceptive injection. Other side-effects include mood swings, headaches and local reaction at the injection site. It is associated with approximately 2 kg weight gain as it may increase appetite. It is also associated with lowering bone density and so may not be first choice for patients under 18. Patients should also be advised that there may be a delay in the return of fertility up to a year after stopping the method.

13.20.8 Combined Hormonal Methods

The primary action of combined hormonal methods action are to supress ovulation and if used perfectly are more than 99% effective. These are available as an oral pill, a transdermal patch or a vaginal ring. Patches and vaginal rings are useful for people who struggle to swallow pills or who have conditions that limit digestive absorption or who find it difficult to remember to take a pill. The combined oral contraceptive pill (coc) is licensed to be taken once a day every 21 days, followed by a break of 4 or 7 days. This is known as the hormonal-free interval (HFI). The contraceptive transdermal patch is changed once a week for three weeks followed by a 4 or 7 HFI. The contraceptive vaginal ring is inserted into the vagina for three weeks and replaced after a 4 or 7 day HFI. The FSRH has updated its guidance in 2019 in relation to the use of combined hormonal contraception and recommends that all patients are advised that there is no medical benefit of the HFI. All patients should be given information about using extended or tailored regimens, which are effective in avoiding unwanted period-like symptoms of the HFI and may reduce the risk of contraceptive failure. These regimens are unlicensed but supported by the FSRH. Full details may be found in this guidance [42].

Use of oestrogen is associated with increased risk of venous thromboembolism (VTE), and so some restrictions apply. Combined hormonal methods are unsuit-able for people who have a history of venous thrombosis, stroke or cardiovascular disease, a body mass index of over 35, hypertension and migraine with aura or who are smokers over the age of 35. Continued use is associated with a small increase in cervical cancer and breast cancer in users over the age of 35; however, its use is also protective against endometrial, ovarian and bowel cancer. It is important to discuss the risks as well as the benefits with potential users so that their decision to use the method is fully informed.

Combined hormonal methods have the advantage of offering cycle control. Bleeding is predictable and can be eliminated by missing the hormone-free interval (HFI). The effect of the hormone on the endometrial lining means that bleeding in the hormone-free interval is likely to be lighter and less painful, making it a popular choice. The risks, benefits and side-effects profile are the same for all the combined hormonal methods, and so the assessment is identical. All choices may be started with immediate effect on day 1 of the cycle or 'quick-started' at any time of the cycle with extra precautions used for 7 days. An oral pill should be taken once every 24 hours, and more than one missed pill per packet may leave the patient unprotected.

The regimes for use are different, so it is important that the patient is taught how to follow the regime and to know what to do if they miss a pill or forget to change patch, or ring. These are known as the 'pill rules'.

Patients should be advised that side-effects are common when starting combined methods and are likely to settle in the first 3 months. Commonly reported side-effects include breakthrough bleeding, mood swings, headaches, breast tenderness and changes in libido. Patients using combined hormonal contraception should receive annual follow-up to ensure that the method is still suitable. This should include a review of medical history, assessment of body mass index and blood pressure and a discussion about concordance and the experience of any side effects [42].

13.20.9 Progesterone-Only Pill

Progesterone only pills (POPs) are suitable for patients who are unable to use oestrogen and if taken correctly are over 99% effective. Traditional POPs work primarily by creating a cervical mucus plug which is impenetrable to sperm. To maintain efficacy, they must be taken every day within a 3-hour window [43].

POPs containing desogestrel have the additional benefit of suppressing ovulation and have a wider 12-hour window. The pills are taken continuously, and if a patient misses a dose, they won't be protected from pregnancy if they have sex without a condom.

The POP will be immediately effective if it is started on day 1–5 of the cycle, without requiring additional precautions. It can be 'quick-started' at any other time of the cycle if additional precautions are used for 48 hours.

Patients should be advised that changes to their bleeding pattern are likely. Common side-effects include mood changes, acne, headaches and a change to libido. Most side-effects settle after the first 3 months of use.

13.20.10 Male Condoms and Female Condoms

Condoms are widely available hormone-free barrier methods which prevent the delivery of semen into the vagina so that fertilisation cannot take place. They have the advantage of reducing the risk of sexually transmitted infection [44].

Male condoms are 98% effective with perfect use, although typical use has lower efficacy. Patients who elect to use condoms should be offered a demonstration on how to use them and how to avoid common problems. They should be warned that many oil-based products (baby lotion, aromatherapy oils, sunscreen) can weaken condoms, and they should be avoided during sex.

Female condoms are 96% effective when used perfectly. The condom is fitted inside the vagina before sex and held in place over the labia. Female condoms are popular with commercial sex workers, who appreciate the control that the method provides. It is also a useful method for women who have partners who have difficultly achieving or sustaining an erection.

13.20.11 Caps and Diaphragms

Caps and diaphragms are barrier methods of contraception that are placed over the cervix, creating a physical barrier to the sperm. They have lower efficacy rate of between 92% and 96% when used perfectly. They are used in conjunction with spermicide which provides additional protection. Both devices are placed over the cervix prior to sex and left in place for at least 6 hours afterwards [44].

Patients need to be confident to touch their vagina and identify their own cervix in order to use caps or diaphragms successfully, and some contraindications for use apply.

Diaphragms are circular domes made of thin, soft latex (rubber) or silicone with a flexible rim. Patients are usually be measured by a clinician so that an appropriate size can be fitted comfortably. The clinician should teach the patient to place the diaphragm and ensure that they are confident to place and remove it before relying on the method.

A modern version of the diaphragm called Caya (Caya.co.uk) is available for patients to access on the Internet. It is suitable for the 80% of patients that fit between 65 and 85 mm, and it does not require a clinician to measure or fit.

Cervical caps are smaller and are made of latex or silicone. Cervical caps come in three sizes depending on the patient's history of pregnancy and do not need specific measurement.

13.20.12 Natural Fertility Methods

Fertility awareness methods (FAM) give people the ability to identify fertile times of their cycle and avoid unprotected sexual intercourse (UPSI) during this time. Although there is limited data on efficacy, the advantage is that they don't interfere with the cycle or the enjoyment of sex and they offer some control over fertility. Methods include lactational amenorrhoea method (LAM) and combination indicator methods, which require specialist supervision and training [45].

13.20.13 Male and Female Sterilisation

People wishing to access male or female sterilisation should be advised that both methods involve a small surgical procedure and should be regarded as irreversible. Careful counselling should be undertaken that includes a full explanation of the procedure, the risk of complications and success outcomes and the possibility of regret. Inclusion criteria apply, and patients should be signposted to their GP for referral [46].

13.20.14 Emergency Contraception

Emergency contraception is available in the event of contraceptive failure up to 120 hours after unprotected sex has taken place.

The most effective method is fitting a copper bearing intrauterine device (Cu-IUD). If fitted in the first 120 hours after UPSI or within 5 days after expected ovulation, the risk of pregnancy is negligible, and the patient has the extra benefit of continuation with an effective method of contraception. If this is not acceptable or unavailable, the patient has the choice of taking oral emergency contraception, although there is limited evidence of its efficacy post-ovulation [47].

Ulipristal acetate (UPA) is a progesterone antagonist that works to delay ovulation. It is effective up to the 120 hours after unprotected sex. Its efficacy is diminished if hormones have been taken in the 7 days before UPSI. Patients wishing to start a hormonal method will need to delay starting this for a further 5 days.

Patients may be offered levonorgestrel (LNG) if they have had UPSI within the last 72 hours. It is not as effective as UPA, and there is no evidence of efficacy after the start of the luteinsing hormone (LH) surge prior to ovulation. However LNG does not impact on ongoing hormonal methods, so it can be useful if patients want to quickstart a hormonal method immediately or if UPA is contraindicated. There is some evidence that LNG may be less effective in people with a BMI over 26 or who weigh 70 kg or more and so it is recommended that these people are offered a double dose.

13.21 Excluding Pregnancy

Pregnancy should be excluded before initiating contraceptive choices. The date of the last menstrual period (LMP) should be recorded, and the patient should be asked if they have had any unprotected sexual intercourse (UPSI) including withdrawal, since then. If there has been UPSI, it may be appropriate to carry out a pregnancy test, although this may need to be repeated if UPSI has taken place within the last 21 days.

If UPSI has taken place within the last 5 days, emergency contraception should be considered, but may not be indicated [47].

13.21.1 Initiating Contraceptive Choice

When the method of choice has been selected, the nurse needs to work with the patient to ensure that they fully understand how the method works, what the risks and benefits are, what side-effects they may experience and how and when they start the method.

If the method is started on days 1–5 of the menstrual cycle, it will provide contraceptive cover immediately. It may be in the patient's best interests to 'quick-start' a method, which means starting a method mid-cycle, using extra precautions until the method is effective. This is done to start the method as soon as possible to reduce the risk of pregnancy and should only be undertaken if the clinician is reasonably certain that the patient is not pregnant. Although this approach is outside the specific product criteria (SPC), it is recommended as safe by the FSRH.

If the patient is 'quick-starting' a method, condoms should be offered, and a plan for pregnancy testing should be made.

Patients should be issued with clear verbal and written advice about to use their method and have a clear follow-up plan as well as advice on to how to access help if it is needed.

13.21.2 Follow-Up and Managing Problems

Follow-up may be necessary to support ongoing concordance with the method of choice. If the patient is happy with the method and it is suiting them, they can enjoy sex, free from the worry of an unexpected pregnancy.

If the patient is not able to maintain the method or suffering from side-effects, the nurse has a role to play in exploring any difficulties and suggesting ways to manage side-effects. If side-effects are unacceptable, an alternative method may need to be started. Patients will need support and advice in switching to an alternative method safely.

Unscheduled bleeding on hormonal methods is a common side-effect but always requires investigation. This includes testing for infection, excluding pregnancy, examining the cervix if necessary and may require referral for gynaecological investigation [48].

13.22 Education and Training

The RCN has published new comprehensive guidance on education, training and career development in sexual health. This is available at: https://www.rcn.org.uk/professional-development/publications/007-502.

Full details of all courses available for nurses, midwives, nursing associates and unregistered support staff may be found online at https://www.rcn.org.uk/sexualhealtheducationdirectory.

Further information on careers in sexual health may be found at https://www.rcn.org.uk/clinical-topics/public-health/sexual-health.

13.22.1 e-Learning Resources

13.22.1.1 e-Learning for Sexual and Reproductive Healthcare

These free courses have been developed by the Faculty of Sexual and Reproductive Healthcare (FSRH) in partnership with Health Education England e-Learning for Healthcare (e-LfH). It comprises 18 modules covering a wide range of topics in contraception and sexual health including the theoretical component of additional training in gaining letter of competence in LARC fitting.

Courses can be accessed via ttps://portal.e-lfh.org.uk.

13.22.1.2 e-Learning for Sexual Health and HIV

The eHIV-STI has been developed by the British Association for Sexual Health and HIV (BASHH) and the Federation of Royal Colleges of Physicians in partnership with Health Education England e-Learning for Healthcare. It comprises 19 modules covering aspects of STI testing and management and includes the foundation STIF course. Courses can be accessed via ttps://portal.e-lfh.org.uk.

13.22.1.3 Sexually Transmitted Infection Foundation (STIF) Programme

The STIF Intermediate Competency Programme is a nationally recognised training and assessment qualification in sexual and reproductive health for the multidisciplinary team working in any healthcare setting. It was developed and is now administered by the British Association of Sexual health and HIV (BASHH). The STIF Intermediate Competency Programme involves clinical attachments during which time a trainee is observed working with patients, receives training and is assessed in practice. Further information can be accessed via www.stif.org.uk.

13.22.1.4 Microscopy Skills

The British Association for Sexual Health and HIV (BASHH) Special Interest Group BSIG in microscopy provides a 1-day training course to provide training for nurses and healthcare assistants in the practical skills of microscopy. The course gives an overview of the theory and provides experience in using a microscope, reading slides and avoiding common problems. Candidates then need to practise reading slides and undertake competency assessment in their own clinical areas. Details may be found on the following website:https://www.bashh.org/events/training-courses-and-meetings

13.22.1.5   Higher Education Institutes (HEIs)

Modules at level 6 and 7 are provided at several HEIs across the UK. Courses vary in the theoretical and clinical component and credits that are offered.

Details may be accessed on the RCN website:https://www.rcn. org.uk/clinical-topics/public-health/specialist-areas/sexual-health/ sexual-health-education-and-training

13.22.2   The Faculty of Sexual and Reproductive Health (FSRH)

Provides a variety of training programmes.

13.22.2.1   Sexual Reproductive Health (SRH) Essentials

This is a 1-day course aimed at equipping General Practice Nurses with the skills to discuss contraception and sexual health in their consultations. It equips nurses with the practical skills to reissue oral contraception and contraceptive injections and undertake sexual health screening. It is provided at various locations around the country. Details of courses may be found at: https://www.fsrh.org/ education-and-training/srh-essentials/

13.22.2.2   Faculty of Sexual Reproductive Health (FSRH) Diploma

This is a blended learning package aimed to equip nurses and doctors working in contraception and sexual health with the underpinning theoretical knowledge and skill. The preparation for the FSRH is currently being updated and will be launched in 2020 full details are found at https://www.fsrh.org/education-and-training/ diploma%2D%2Dnurse-diploma/.

13.22.2.3   Letters of Competence in LARC Fitting

Nurses wishing to train as LARC fitters need to have completed either the FSRH e-KA or have a recognised Contraception Sexual Health (CASH) module. They will need to complete the appropriate theoretical e- learning SRH modules before undertaking practical training with a faculty registered trainer (FRT). An administration fee is charged, and nurses will be required to pay a fee to become associate members of the faculty to maintain their letter of competence. Recertification of letters of competence is required every 5 years.

Full details may be found at https://www.fsrh.org/recertification/ recertification-requirements-for-letters-of-competence-loc-iut/.

13.22.2.4   Faculty Registered Trainer

Faculty-registered trainers (FRTs) support the delivery of local training in sexual and reproductive health, by facilitating FRSH training programmes such as the course of five and SRH essentials and by teaching and assessing LARC fitting skills necessary to achieve letters of competence.https://www.fsrh.org/education-and-training/ become-a-fsrh-registered-trainer/.

References

1. GOV.UK (2015) Sexual and reproductive health and HIV: strategic action plan. https://www.gov.uk/government/publications/sexual-and-reproductive-health-and-hiv-strategic-action-plan. Accessed 3 Aug 2018
2. Assets.publishing.service.gov.uk (2018) Integrated sexual health services: a suggested national service specification. https://assets.publishing.service.gov.uk/government/uploads/system/uploads/attachment_data/file/731140/integrated-sexual-health-services-specification.pdf. Accessed 3 Aug 2018
3. Read the Code online (2015). Nmc.org.uk. https://www.nmc.org.uk/standards/code/read-the-code-online/#first. Accessed 3 Aug 2018
4. Caldicott2 Principles (2013). Igt.hscic.gov.uk https://www.igt.hscic.gov.uk/Caldicott2Principles.aspx. Accessed 3 Aug 2018
5. Bashhguidelines.org (2013) 2013 UK national guideline for consultations requiring sexual history taking. https://www.bashhguidelines.org/media/1078/sexual-history-taking-guideline-2013-2.pdf. Accessed 3 Aug 2018
6. The Royal College of Nursing (2016) Fair care for trans peoplehttps://www.rcn.org.uk/professional-development/publications/pub-005575. Accessed 3 Aug 2018
7. FSRH UK MEC – Faculty of Sexual and Reproductive Healthcare (2016) Fsrh.org. https://www.fsrh.org/ukmec/. Accessed 3 Aug 2018
8. The Royal College of Nursing (2018) HPV, cervical screening and cervical cancer. https://www.rcn.org.uk/professional-development/publications/pdf-006903. Accessed 3 Aug 2018
9. The Royal College of Nursing (2013) Tackling FGM in the UK: intercollegiate recommendations for identifying, recording and reporting. https://www.rcn.org.uk/professional-development/publications/pub-004531. Accessed 4 Aug 2018
10. BHIVA (2008) BHIVA – UK national guidelines for HIV testing 2008. Bhiva.org. http://www.bhiva.org/HIV-testing-guidelines.aspx. Accessed 3 Aug 2018
11. Terrence Higgins Trust (2018) Viral load and being undetectable. Tht.org.uk. https://www.tht.org.uk/hiv-and-sexual-health/about-hiv/viral-load-and-being-undetectable. Accessed 3 Aug 2018
12. Assets.publishing.service.gov.uk (2017) Hepatitis B immunisation information for public health professionals. https://assets.publishing.service.gov.uk/government/uploads/system/uploads/attachment_data/file/628602/Greenbook_chapter__18.pdf. Accessed 4 Aug 2018
13. ASSETS (2018). National minimum standards and core curriculum for immunisation training for registered healthcare practitioners. Assets.publishing.service.gov.uk. https://assets.publishing.service.gov.uk/government/uploads/system/uploads/attachment_data/file/679824/Training_standards_and_core_curriculum_immunisation.pdf. Accessed 4 Aug 2018
14. Sps.nhs.uk (2018) Immunisation knowledge and skills competence assessment tool. https://www.sps.nhs.uk/wp-content/uploads/2018/01/RCN-Imms-Tool.pdf. Accessed 4 Aug 2018
15. The Royal College of Nursing (2017) Domestic abuse pocket guide. https://www.rcn.org.uk/professional-development/publications/pub-005985. Accessed 4 Aug 2018
16. NICE (2010) Alcohol-use disorders: prevention. Guidance and guidelines. Nice.org.uk. https://www.nice.org.uk/guidance/PH24. Accessed 4 Aug 2018
17. Cks.nice.org.uk (2010) Smoking cessation – NICE CKS. https://cks.nice.org.uk/smoking-cessation. Accessed 4 Aug 2018
18. Assets.publishing.service.gov.uk (2018) Sexually transmitted infections and screening for chlamydia in England, 2017. https://assets.publishing.service.gov.uk/government/uploads/system/uploads/attachment_data/file/713944/hpr2018_AA-STIs_v5.pdf. Accessed 4 Aug 2018
19. Sexual Offences Act 2003 (2003). Legislation.gov.uk. http://www.legislation.gov.uk/ukpga/2003/42/contents. Accessed 4 Aug 2018
20. FSRH (2010) FSRH clinical guidance: contraceptive choices for young people (March 2010) – Faculty of Sexual and Reproductive Healthcare. Fsrh.org. https://www.fsrh.org/standards-and-guidance/documents/cec-ceu-guidance-young-people-mar-2010/. Accessed 4 Aug 2018

21. GOV.UK (2018) Working together to safeguard children. https://www.gov.uk/government/publications/working-together-to-safeguard-children%2D%2D2. Accessed 4 Aug 2018
22. GOV.UK (2017) Child sexual exploitation: definition and guide for practitioners. https://www.gov.uk/government/publications/child-sexual-exploitation-definition-and-guide-for-practitioners. Accessed 4 Aug 2018
23. NHS England (2016) Modern slavery. England.nhs.uk. https://www.england.nhs.uk/ourwork/safeguarding/our-work/modern-slavery/. Accessed 4 Aug 2018
24. The Royal College of Nursing (2017) Modern slavery pocket guide. https://scadmin.rcn.org.uk/professional-development/publications/pub-005984. Accessed 4 Aug 2018
25. Bashhguidelines.org (2011) UK national guidelines on the management of adult and adolescent complainants of sexual assault 2011. https://www.bashhguidelines.org/media/1079/4450.pdf. Accessed 4 Aug 2018
26. The Royal College of Nursing (2016) Genital examination in women: a resource for skills development and assessment. https://www.rcn.org.uk/professional-development/publications/pub-005480. Accessed 4 Aug 2018
27. GOV.UK (2013) A framework for sexual health improvement in England. https://www.gov.uk/government/publications/a-framework-for-sexual-health-improvement-in-england. Accessed 4 Aug 2018
28. Bashh.org (2012) BASHH statement on partner notification for sexually transmissible infections page. https://www.bashh.org/documents/4445.pdf. Accessed 4 Aug 2018
29. Bashhguidelines.org (2014) United Kingdom national guideline on the management of Trichomonas vaginalis 2014. https://www.bashhguidelines.org/media/1042/tv_2014-ijstda.pdf. Accessed 4 Aug 2018
30. Bashhguidelines.org (2015) UK national guidelines on the management of anogenital warts 2015. https://www.bashhguidelines.org/media/1075/uk-national-guideline-on-warts-2015-final.pdf. Accessed 4 Aug 2018
31. Bashhguidelines.org (2018) 2018 United Kingdom national guideline for the management of pelvic inflammatory disease. https://www.bashhguidelines.org/media/1170/pid-2018.pdf. Accessed 4 Aug 2018
32. Bashhguidelines.org (2014) 2014 UK national guideline for the management of anogenital herpes. https://www.bashhguidelines.org/media/1019/hsv_2014-ijstda.pdf. Accessed 4 Aug 2018
33. Bashhguidelines.org (2015) UK national guidelines on the management of syphilis 2015. https://www.bashhguidelines.org/media/1148/uk-syphilis-guidelines-2015.pdf. Accessed 4 Aug 2018
34. Bashhguidelines.org (2012) UK national guideline for the management of bacterial vaginosis 2012. https://www.bashhguidelines.org/media/1041/bv-2012.pdf. Accessed 4 Aug 2018
35. Bashhguidelines.org (2007) United Kingdom national guideline on the management of vulvovaginal candidiasis 2007. https://www.bashhguidelines.org/media/1155/united-kingdom-national-guideline-on-the-management-. Accessed 4 Aug 2018
36. Bashhguidelines.org (2014) 2014 UK national guideline on the management of vulval conditions. https://www.bashhguidelines.org/media/1056/vulval-conditions_2014-ijstda.pdf. Accessed 4 Aug 2018
37. Firman N, Palmer M, Timæus I, Wellings K (2018) Contraceptive method use among women and its association with age, relationship status and duration: findings from the third British National Survey of Sexual Attitudes and Lifestyles (Natsal-3). BMJ Sex Reprod Health 44:bmjsrh-2017-200037
38. NICE (2014) Long-acting reversible contraception. Guidance and guidelines. Nice.org.uk. https://www.nice.org.uk/guidance/cg30/chapter/1-Recommendations#contraception-and-principles-of-care. Accessed 4 Aug 2018
39. FSRH (2014) FSRH clinical guidance: progestogen-only implants – February 2014 – Faculty of Sexual and Reproductive Healthcare. Fsrh.org. https://www.fsrh.org/standards-and-guidance/documents/cec-ceu-guidance-implants-feb-2014/. Accessed 4 Aug 2018

40. FSRH (2015) FSRH clinical guidance: intrauterine contraception – October 2015 – Faculty of Sexual and Reproductive Healthcare. Fsrh.org. https://www.fsrh.org/standards-and-guidance/documents/ceuguidanceintrauterinecontraception/. Accessed 4 Aug 2018
41. FSRH (2014) FSRH clinical guidance: progestogen-only injectable contraception – December 2014 – Faculty of Sexual and Reproductive Healthcare. Fsrh.org. https://www.fsrh.org/standards-and-guidance/documents/cec-ceu-guidance-injectables-dec-2014/. Accessed 4 Aug 2018
42. FSRH (2019) FSRH Clinical Guidance: Combined Hormonal Contraception. Faculty Sexual and Reproductive Health. https://www.fsrh.org/standards-and-guidance/documents/combined-hormonal-contraception/. Accessed May 2019
43. (2015) FSRH Clinical Guidance: Progestogen-only Pills - March 2015 - Faculty of Sexual and Reproductive Healthcare. Fsrh.org. https://www.fsrh.org/standards-and-guidance/documents/cec-ceu-guidance-pop-mar-2015/. Accessed 4 Aug 2018
44. FSRH (2012) FSRH clinical guidance: barrier methods contraception and STI prevention – August 2012 – Faculty of Sexual and Reproductive Healthcare. Fsrh.org. https://www.fsrh.org/standards-and-guidance/documents/ceuguidancebarriermethodscontraceptionsdi/. Accessed 4 Aug 2018
45. FSRH (2015) FSRH clinical guidance: fertility awareness methods – June 2015 – Faculty of Sexual and Reproductive Healthcare. Fsrh.org. https://www.fsrh.org/standards-and-guidance/documents/ceuguidancefertilityawarenessmethods/. Accessed 4 Aug 2018
46. FSRH (2014) FSRH clinical guidance: male and female sterilisation summary of recommendations – September 2014 – Faculty of Sexual and Reproductive Healthcare. Fsrh.org. https://www.fsrh.org/standards-and-guidance/documents/cec-ceu-guidance-sterilisation-summary-sep-2014/. Accessed 4 Aug 2018
47. FSRH (2017) FSRH CEU clinical guidance: emergency contraception - December 2017 – Faculty of Sexual and Reproductive Healthcare. Fsrh.org. https://www.fsrh.org/standards-and-guidance/documents/ceu-clinical-guidance-emergency-contraception-march-2017/. Accessed 4 Aug 2018
48. FSRH (2015) FSRH clinical guidance: problematic bleeding with hormonal contraception – July 2015 – Faculty of Sexual and Reproductive Healthcare. Fsrh.org. https://www.fsrh.org/standards-and-guidance/documents/ceuguidanceproblematicbleedinghormonalcontraception/. Accessed 4 Aug 2018

Suggested Reading

Association for Lichen sclerosis and vulval health. www.lichensclerosus.org
British Society for the study of vulval disease. www.bssvd.org
Caya contoured diaphragm. https://caya.co.uk/
Family Planning Association. https://www.fpa.org.uk/, https://www.contraceptionchoices.org/
Female Sterilisation. https://www.nhs.uk/conditions/contraception/female-sterilisation/
Fertility UK. www.fertilityuk.org
Herpes Viruses Association. https://herpes.org.uk/
Patient UK. https://patient.info/
Terrence Higgins Trust. https://www.tht.org.uk/
Vulval Pain Society. www.vulvalpainsociety.org

Debra Holloway

The development of advanced or specialist roles within the UK has been driven by nurses and also changes within health services and the NHS. The Advanced Practice Framework [1] sets out a path for advanced practice that is not reliant on nursing qualifications and can be followed by all advanced practitioners. This is to upskill professionals owing to multiple challenges within the UK and the NHS:

- Increased demand
- Increased pressures of workload
- Decreased recruitment
- Decreased retention
- Decreased number of nurses qualifying

This new pathway needs to be managed and balanced with decreased finance, increasing quality and by ensuring safety. It does allow nurses to practice to their full potential and ensure a high level of contribution to the care of patients in many different service settings. Key components as are discussed in the education setting are Master's level education and practising within the code. The advantages of these roles include a direct decrease in costs by saving admissions and replacing others in interactions with patients, which frees up other staff, such as medics, to see a different case load of patients. Advanced nursing practice (ANP) and clinical nurse specialist (CNS) also deal with both the medical and nursing aspects of the patients, which leads to holistic care, and brings these together. The workforce is autonomous but also flexible and supports other health care professionals [2]. The rise in advanced roles for nurses and the development of advanced practice in 2004 with the European working time directives led to shortages and gaps in the NHS workforce [3].

D. Holloway (✉)
Guys and St Thomas NHS Foundation Trust, London, UK
e-mail: Debra.Holloway@gstt.nhs.uk

© Springer Nature Switzerland AG 2019
D. Holloway (ed.), *Nursing Management of Women's Health*,
https://doi.org/10.1007/978-3-030-16115-6_14

14.1 Insurance

Within the UK in the NHS, insurance is generally provided by the employer. However, there are a few rules that relate to this. In 2014, the UK government [4] introduced new rules on indemnity insurance. This required all nurses to be aware and ensure that they had indemnity insurance in place.

For a nurse to be covered by this, it generally means that he/she is working within an NHS setting and that the job description that he/she has reflects the work that he/she is doing. For example, if he/she is employed as a hysteroscopist, then this area of practice is covered, but if she were not expected to do this within his/her role and set up this service and there was an issue, the Trust or employer may not cover her. Therefore, a good practice point is to ensure that the job description that you are working to reflects your practice, especially when looking at advanced practice, the extended role and non-medical prescribing. This may have evolved over time, so it is worth reviewing this in line with performance reviews to ensure that it is up to date and reflects daily practice. One aspect that normally needs to be added is non-medical prescribing to ensure that the nurse is covered for this. Many employers/Trusts have a standard appendix to add in, found within the non-medical prescribers' policy.

The level of appropriate cover is determined by the job that you undertake and where this is undertaken, the level of care and the amount of risk involved.

Within primary care, the situation with insurance is different. Some nurses may be covered by the practice and employer and some will need to obtain their own insurance or indemnity.

The Nursing and Midwifery Council (NMC) states [5]:

- Nurses need to have in place an indemnity arrangement, which is a mandatory requirement of the Code. This needs to be declared when registering or renewing during revalidation.
- Each nurse is responsible for making sure that they have the appropriate cover for their role and scope of practice. The cover that they have in place should be relevant to the risks involved in their practice, so that it is sufficient if a claim is successfully made against them.
- While the arrangement does not need to be individually held by the nurse, it is their responsibility to ensure that appropriate cover is in place.
- If it is discovered that a nurse is practising without an appropriate indemnity arrangement in place, they will be removed from the register.
- Nurses in the NHS already have an appropriate indemnity arrangement. The NHS insures its employees for work carried out on its behalf. This means that nurses are covered if a claim is made against them in an NHS role.
- For nurses in private healthcare (for example, a nursing home or general practice), it is likely that the employer will have an appropriate indemnity arrangement, but the nurse needs to check this. This provides appropriate cover for all the relevant risks related to his/her job.
- Nurses who are self-employed, work as a consultant or through an agency are required to have their own indemnity arrangement in place. This can be via a professional body or their own cover directly through a commercial provider.

14.2   Autonomy and Accountability

Nurses have autonomy in many situations, which is normally linked to advanced practice and forms one of the definitions of advanced practice, the freedom to make autonomous decisions around care. Although they have autonomy, they are still accountable for the care that they deliver.

When working as an autonomous practitioner, nurses still have accountability to a line manager and normally someone else who is clinical but may be of a different discipline. In addition to this, nurses should have a clinical supervisor or mentor that they are able to see to discuss clinical questions or work through scenarios that may involve clinical or ethical issues and may not have a correct answer.

Nurses working in advanced roles, either as an ANP or a CNS, need to ensure that the work that they undertake is visible, recorded and generates the income that it should do [6]; they need to ensure that they disseminate the work undertaken to others, including line managers, whether it is requested or not. This needs to include: numbers of patients seen, number of telephone and email consultations, interventions that have led to patients being kept out of hospital or decreased their length of stay, or decreased multiple appointments. Guidelines, teaching sessions, talks and publications and responses to complaints and the number of compliments should all be highlighted within a 6-monthly report to show the visibility of the role and ensure ongoing management support.

Accountability, autonomy and clinical governance sit side by side. Accountability can be blurred, as roles become blurred and care can be delegated to others.

Accountability is taking responsibility for actions and this can be difficult to describe in nursing, especially in advanced practice [7]. The functions of accountability are to protect, deter, regulate and educate. It is hoped that accountability leads to the prevention of negligence and higher quality care.

Nurses working in any role are accountable to:

1. The employer—the employees are accountable and measured in terms of performance goals, outcomes and working within organisational guidelines.
2. The NMC as a professional body [5]—a nurse is responsible for his/her actions, including delegation. This is normally defined by using knowledge from courses and applying this knowledge to the care. To ensure accountability, nurses need to be trained and competent.

    The governance of a new and advanced role must be in place beforehand to protect the employee, the patients and the employer. A portfolio should be available that shows the domains of advanced practice, which can then be aligned with revalidation for either the NMC or in some cases the awarding body of the advanced skill, such as hysteroscopy or colposcopy, as well. In addition to looking at the here and now, there needs to be a plan to reassess and audit the service to ensure that the goals are achieved and that the impact is captured.

14.3 Training

Behind all the education and training in advanced practice is accountability, the governance needed behind the role, and the maintenance and development of professional standards. The governance is related to the professional body, the organisation and the role. Each country that has developed advanced practice have devised their own educational programmes. As discussed before, the key to all of them is Master's qualifications, and this is also highlighted by the International Council of Nurses and the Department of Health [1, 8]

Within this education it is paramount to gain the knowledge, experience and skills needed to function as an ANP, but, as with any role, the learning is lifelong and can take many forms, such as journal reading, courses, webinars, online and distance learning and reflection for revalidation or formal reflection with peers. In addition, some ANPs can develop by undertaking roles in national bodies such as the National Institute for Health and Care Excellence, the Royal College of Obstetricians and Gynaecologists and the Faculty of Sexual and Reproductive Healthcare.

Within the UK, there is no overall governance of the roles and therefore of the educational standard of courses. In the USA, the ANP is a graduate, with an MSc and a licensed examination within their speciality, leading to the title nurse practitioner [9].

The roles that specialist nurses develop and take on within women's health are vast and, in some cases, unique. For many, there would not have been a course that they could undertake to obtain all the skills that would be needed. They may have undertaken different courses and finalised the learning with a Master's, normally in advanced practice. Many nurses may have developed their roles before non-medical prescribing or advanced practice masters and so may have these as additional qualifications. As can be seen throughout the chapters, some areas have specific qualifications such as hysteroscopy, colposcopy, scanning and to some extent the menopause, whereas others such as endometriosis do not. The Royal College of Nursing has developed guides rather than competencies for many specialist roles within women's health [10]. The roles and training also vary by the setting that they are in. As was seen in Chap. 1, there is no regulation of advanced practice in the UK or of the components of the CNS role. Nurses working at advanced levels can be found in primary and secondary care within any setting, and in care homes, the independent sector and charity settings, such as those providing pregnancy terminations.

Advanced practice is a level of practice and not a type of practice. The education required is generally:

1. At Master's level.
2. Assessed as clinically competent in practice using their skills and knowledge.
3. Relevant speciality such as hysteroscopy.

4. Incorporates advanced assessment skills.
5. Incorporates non-medical prescribing.
6. Incorporates evidence-based decision-making and research skills.
7. The freedom to act using autonomy to make decisions in the assessment, diagnosis and treatment of women.

As with any speciality, the evidence base changes all the time and it is part of the practitioner's role to ensure that they stay up to date. This may mean that there are specific re-equipment such as the continuing professional development that is aligned with non-medical prescribing, or there may be employer-specific requirements such as two study days each year and an audit of practice. For hysteroscopy, there is the need to maintain a database of cases, ensuring a certain number and looking at failure rates, and to attend courses recognised by the British Society for Gynaecological Endoscopy. This is again echoed by colposcopy and nurse specialists within the menopause. However, if the role incorporates many of these functions, it can be difficult to obtain all the correct qualifications; therefore, it is necessary to look at certain courses to see if they fulfil all the elements, or whether others may be needed. Many of the updates are multi-professional and it is important from time to time to attend some courses that focus on more generic nursing and advanced practice, as often practitioners can feel isolated and out of the nursing loop.

Advanced practice is moving towards having an advanced practice framework that is multi-professional. This has been developed from the 2014 NHS 5-year forward plan and the 2017 [1] next steps of the 5-year plan. The framework looks at the challenges and demands of advanced practice in the NHS:

• Increased demands
• Increased pressure on the workforce
• Decreased recruitment
• Decreased retention
• Decreased funding

Also included are how to respond to the challenges and ensure that quality and safety are not compromised. It lays out the key skills, which are diagnosis, core skills, capacity and recognises that much has been done to provide national and regional frameworks that brought together so that it is the same specification within each Trust. The key components are operating at a Master's level, practice within one's code of conduct and demonstrating effective practice while working in partnership with others and ensuring ongoing practice evaluation so that the services and role can develop and be responsive to the changes needed. The advanced practitioner should be a role model and be able to assess and develop the team, engage in research and apply this to practice. The employer needs to have a responsibility to show that this is a best-placed post with clear objectives and purpose, and that there is regular assessment of the impact, support and succession planning.

References

1. NHS (2018) Multi-professional framework for advanced clinical practice in England https://hee.nhs.uk/sites/default/files/documents/Multi-professional%20framework%20for%20advanced%20clinical%20practice%20in%20England.pdf
2. O'Connor L, Casey M, Smith R et al (2018) The universal, collaborative and dynamic model of specialist and advanced nursing and midwifery practice: a way forward? J Clin Nurs 27(5–6):e882–e894
3. Anderson C (2018) Exploring the role of advanced nurse practitioners in leadership. Nurs Stand 33(2):29–33
4. http://www.legislation.gov.uk/uksi/2014/1887/contents/made
5. Nursing and Midwifery council. Code of practice. https://www.nmc.org.uk/standards/code/
6. Fulton J (2013) Making outcomes of clinical nurse specialist practice visible. Clin Nurs Spec 27(1):5–6
7. Kendall N (2018) How new nursing roles affect accountability and delegation. Nurs Times [online] 114(4):45–47
8. https://international.aanp.org/Practice/APNRoles
9. Barton TD, Allan D (eds) (2013) Advanced nursing practice: changing healthcare in a changing world. Macmillan, London
10. https://www.rcn.org.uk/womens-health-clinical-topic